HEALTH
AND THE
HUMAN BODY

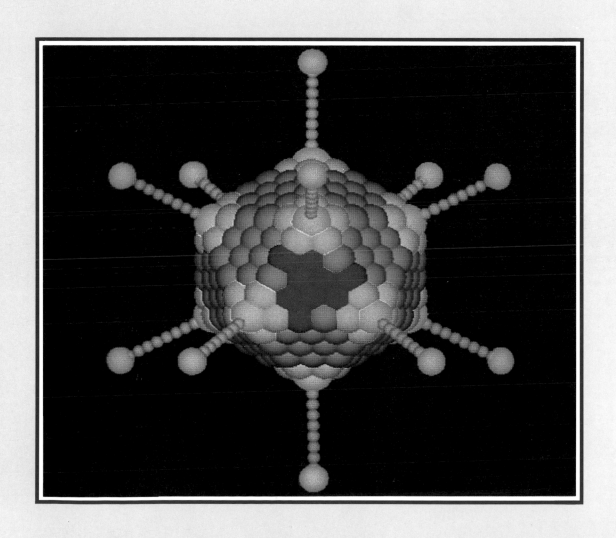

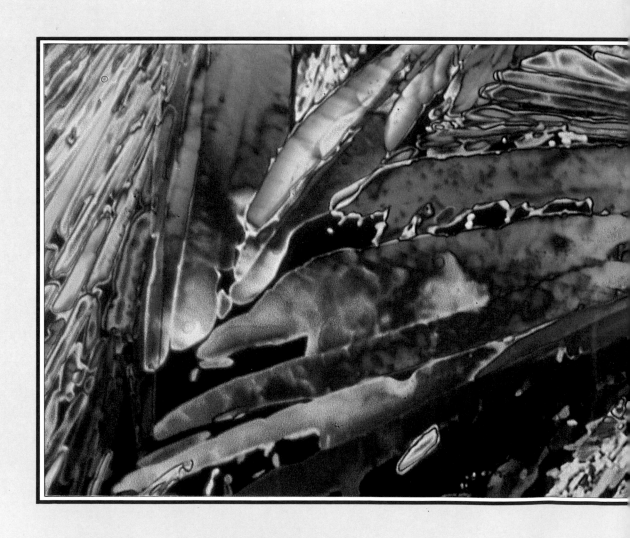

HEALTH
AND THE
HUMAN BODY

An Illustrated Guide to Modern Medical Knowledge

Edited by Dr Bernard Dixon

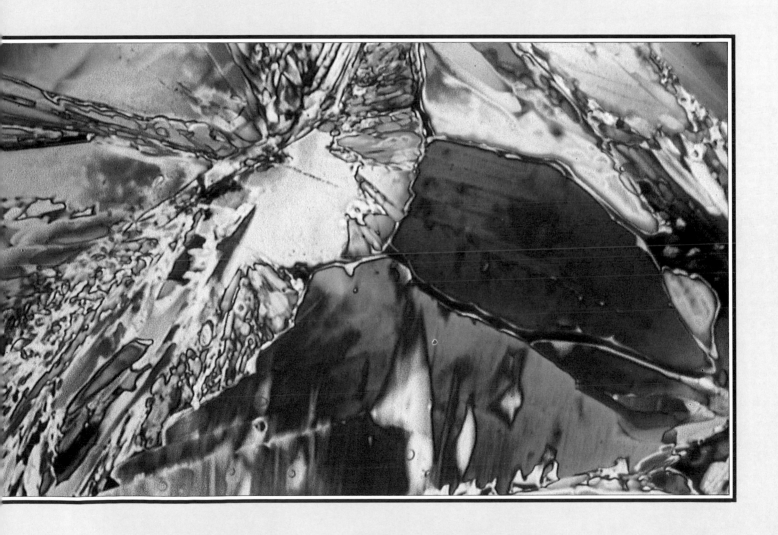

PERSEUS PRESS
An imprint of The Reader's Digest Assn. Ltd.
LONDON · SYDNEY

Editor Peter Furtado
Art Editor John Ridgeway
Designer Ayala Kingsley
Picture Editor Linda Proud

Senior Editor Lawrence Clarke

Advisors
Professor Donald Henderson,
Johns Hopkins University
Sir Peter Medawar, Nobel Laureate
Professor Norman Shumway,
Stanford University
Dr William Brock, University
of Leicester
Professor John Humphrey, Royal
Postgraduate Medical School
Dr Jean Ross, Charing Cross
Hospital Medical School

Contributors
Jenny Bryan (4, 21)
Bernard Dixon (Introduction, 1, 3,
4, 5, 18, 19, 21, 22, 24, 28, 31, 34)
Richard Fifield (15)
Caroline Richmond (1, 6, 7, 8, 9,
11, 12, 13, 14, 16, 17, 22, 25, 29)
Martin Sherwood (20, 23, 26, 27,
30, 32, 33)

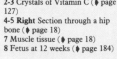

AN EQUINOX BOOK

Planned and produced by:
Equinox (Oxford) Ltd
Littlegate House
St Ebbe's Street
Oxford OX1 1SQ

Published by:
PERSEUS PRESS
An imprint of
The Reader's Digest Assn. Ltd
LONDON · SYDNEY

Copyright © Equinox (Oxford) Ltd
1986

ISBN 0 276 39622 7

Printed in the Netherlands
by Royal Smeets Offset bv, Weert

Introductory pictures (pages 1-8)
1 Computer-image of an influenza
virus (◆ page 171)
2-3 Crystals of Vitamin C (◆ page
127)
4-5 **Right** Section through a hip
bone (◆ page 18)
7 Muscle tissue (◆ page 18)
8 Fetus at 12 weeks (◆ page 184)

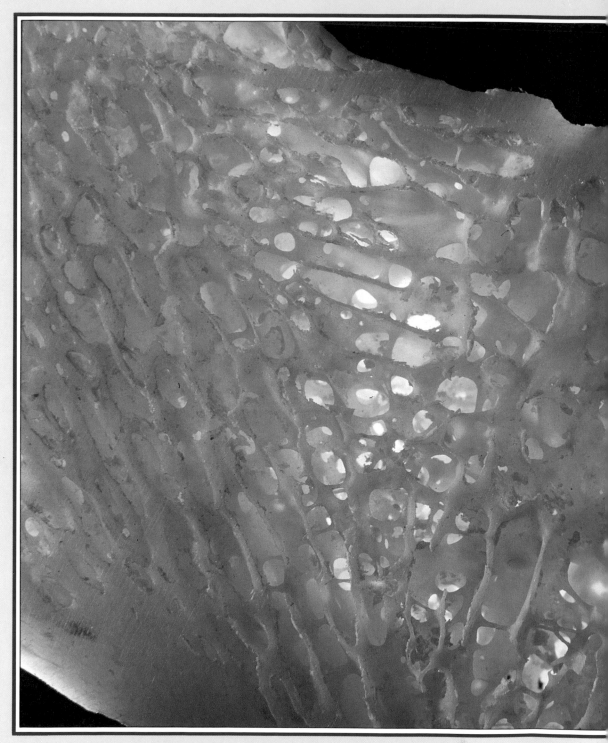

Contents

Introduction

"What a piece of work is Man! How noble in reason! How infinite in faculty! In form and moving how express and admirable! In action how like an angel! In apprehension how like a god! The beauty of the world! The paragon of the animals!"

William Shakespeare found peerless words with which to express a perspective on the human body and spirit that has appealed to poets, philosophers and seers down the ages. This is humanity as a wondrous machine allied with sublime sensibility – the very pinnacle of evolution.

But there is another view of the process that has been responsible for the emergence of life on Earth. "Genetical evolution, if we choose to look at it liverishly instead of with fatuous good humour, is a story of waste, makeshift, compromise and blunder," the distinguished biologist Sir Peter Medawar insisted in 1959. From this standpoint the human body is simply one product, with countless imperfections, of a blind process based upon random, capricious changes in molecules. By this account, the human race seems a cruel caricature of Shakespeare's visionary ideal.

The pediatrician Ronald Glasser highlighted these contrary views with particular force in his book *The Body is the Hero* (1977). Dr Glasser's purpose was to extol the near-miraculous resources of the immune system through which we are able to mount powerful, specific defenses against an infinite variety of different invading microbes. It is the immune system that repels killers such as tubercle bacilli, yellow fever viruses and typhoid fever bacteria – and does so with exquisite precision. Yet Dr Glasser opens his book with an appalling story of uncontrollable infection in a child whose immune system is defective. "Horrified, the parents watch while medicine fails," he writes. "They see the grayish plaques creep down the front of their baby's face, out of his nose. They watch it spill out onto his cheek and neck. The plaques begin to crack and bleed; the round, pudgy face becomes distorted. Hungry, yet unable to eat, the baby struggles and squirms; his mouth begins to rot...."

Not all bodily failures and vulnerabilities are as devastating as this. Yet even the most trivial of them contrast sharply with the physiological excellence which we recognize as health. That contrast is the subject of this book. We shall be considering how the body works in normal health (and how we have reached that understanding) alongside a corresponding picture of the abnormality we call disease. Frailty and robustness will appear in many guises. People are tough enough to swim the English Channel or run a marathon, yet far more sensitive to a few degrees of raised temperature than are primitive tetanus bacilli in the soil. Our tissues, in many ways so delicate, prove to be surprisingly durable in everyday use or under the surgeon's knife. And while we are capable of great strength of mind, we all have areas of profound mental sensitivity too: it is an uncomfortable truth of the modern world that false confessions are as likely to be extracted by subtle psychological torture as by physical ill-treatment.

Health and disease

But robust health and debilitating disease do not give us *alternative* views of the human body. What they do reflect is the concurrent strength and vulnerability of a complex creature. Shakespeare was correct in seeing that our most trivial movements, accomplished without a thought, are "admirable". Even the simple act of getting out of bed or pulling on a shoe, we now know, involves machinery far more sophisticated than that of any modern industrial robot. The same is true of our senses and body chemistry, whose performance out-distances any artificial imitations Man himself has devised.

At the same time, the human animal is susceptible to two types of threat, one external, the other internal. Because *Homo sapiens* is part of a wider, richer pattern of evolution, the body is subject to attack by other evolutionary products, particularly parasites such as viruses and bacteria. Second, an inevitable consequence of the complicated, finely-tuned nature of all bodily processes is that a similarly wide range of things can go wrong with those processes. Even our most mechanical components are founded upon exquisitely delicate interactions and although beautifully adapted for their daily work, these can malfunction in many different ways. The intimate relationship between body and mind throws up further dramatic examples. An 80-year old can emerge triumphant from major abdominal surgery for cancer and live a further 15 years in rude good health. Yet someone a third of that age may be killed by a heart attack as a result of running a few yards for the bus – or receiving a letter carrying bad news.

Such contrasts mean that an increasingly dominant strand of medical thinking is that it is more prudent to maintain health than to rely on treating disease. In the realm of infections, that lesson was learned many decades ago: "magic bullets" such as antibiotics cure the once-incurable, but we owe much of our freedom from communicable diseases to clean water, efficient sanitation and good nutrition. But the importance of preventive measures against non-infectious conditions, particularly cancer and coronary heart disease, is only now being fully recognized and implemented. Although life-saving measures like kidney and heart transplantation epitomize the highest skills of modern medical science, therefore, it is becoming clear that more impressive rewards still may be won by preventing the relevant diseases from becoming established in the first place.

The structure of this book

Because we shall be focusing on modern scientific understanding of the *mechanisms* of health and disease, the book is not organized like a popular health guide with exhaustive lists of diseases associated with particular organs in the body. Our main thrust will be to highlight *causes*, whether internal disorders, or external insults due to infectious microbes or other environmental hazards. Acne, for example, appears as an infection, which it is (◆ page 244), rather than in the section dealing with structural disorders that originate in the skin itself (◆ page 113). Similarly, diarrhea can be found in the module dealing with the infections that are its principal cause (◆ page 141). Our aim is to relate every illness with its root cause – and where relevant to emphasize *multiple* causes of disease, which have been seriously neglected in the past.

What this book does not contain is a section uncritically devoted to the fashionably popular subject of "alternative medicine", because that label covers an infinite variety of different therapies and claims, many of them unsupported by evidence of the sort we rightly expect in other walks of life. It is true that orthodox medicine has sometimes been indefensibly hostile towards ideas from outside its own professional boundaries. We have indicated areas where the validity of such ideas has eventually won the day or looks like doing so – above all in the recognition that the mind has a profound influence on our vulnerability or resistance to bodily disease. It is also true that medicine has always needed the practitioner's art and empathy, as well as the scientist's science. But the science responsible for miraculous feats like the eradication of smallpox from the face of the Earth is based on austere rules of evidence. To accept "alternative" solutions in despair, to pretend hunch and anecdote are as valid as experimental data, or to abandon the simple and elegant protocols which have transformed our health prospects from the cradle to the grave, would be a retrograde step. Only a fool argues that science holds the answer to all things. But only a greater fool disputes the unrivalled explanatory power of science in its proper domain.

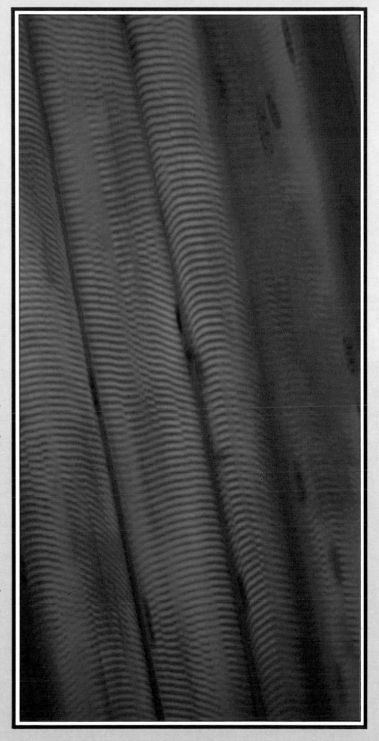

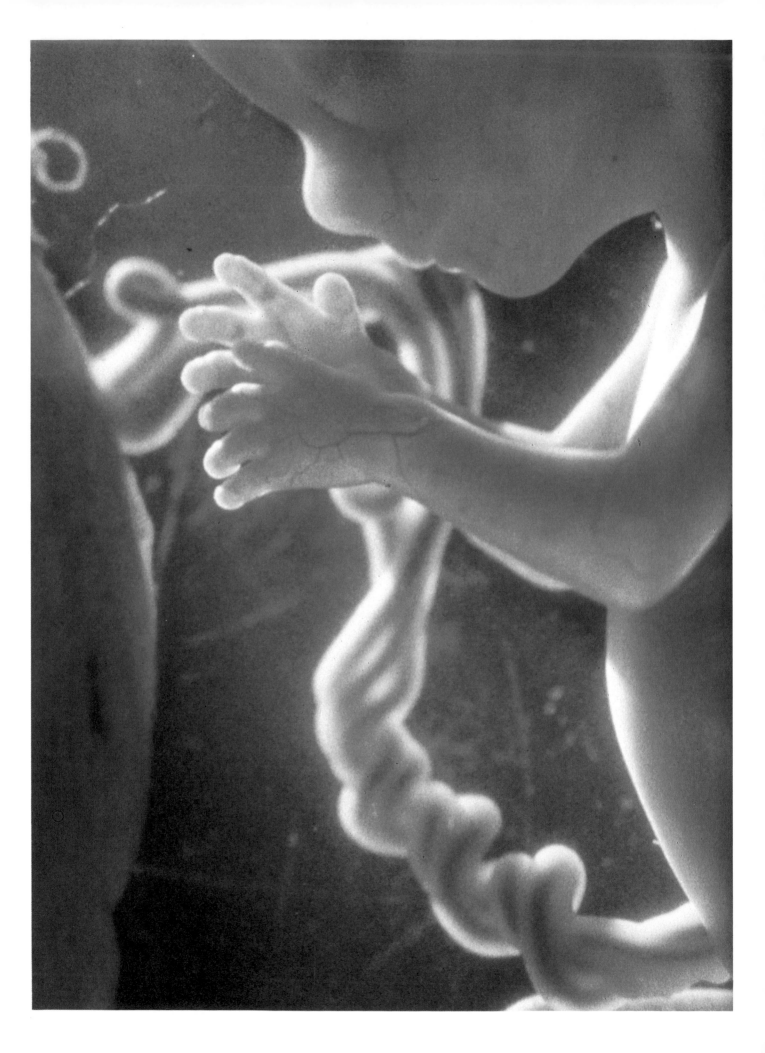

The Human Body

The human species and its variations...Genetic and environmental differences...Population, past, present and future...The organization of the body...The systems of the body...Tissues and cells...Spare parts surgery... Homeostasis, keeping the body in working order... Definitions of health...PERSPECTIVE...Races and racism...Human types...Body rhythms

There is great diversity of size, color and appearance between people, but all are members of a single species, *Homo sapiens*. The diversity is genetic in origin and often reflects the ways in which the body has adapted to the various environments of the Earth, but the fact that members of all the so-called races can breed successfully with each other underlines the similarities rather than the differences.

It is, indeed, debatable whether we can be meaningfully divided into races at all. Most human "racial" characteristics, such as height, pigmentation, texture of hair, are merely adaptations to sunlight, temperature and humidity. People show more affinity with those of a similar climate in another part of the globe than to closer genetic relatives from a different latitude of their own continent. Relationships between human groups are seen better by examining characteristics such as blood groups and genes than external features.

Human groupings are confused by the mixing caused by migrations and by intermarriage across geographical borders. Some groups often thought of as separate races, such as the Jews, are not races at all biologically, but are socio-religious groups. American Negroes are descended mainly from people imported from the Gulf of Guinea, and most have a percentage of European ancestry.

Many differences between peoples that seem to be racial traits are environmental in origin. Japanese raised in the USA are taller than those brought up in Japan, mainly because their childhood diet is higher in meat and dairy products. Adult height is determined by genetics, diet and the incidence of infectious disease in childhood.

Classifying the racial types

Many different schemes have been proposed classifying Homo sapiens into races, and no single system is universally accepted. One widely-used scheme groups us into six main classes:
1. Early Mongoloid (American Indian)
2. Late Mongoloid (East Asians, Eskimos and Japanese). These people tend to have squat bodies, broad cheeks, and a flap of fatty skin over the upper eyelids to adapt them to life in bitterly cold weather.
3. Caucasoid (Europeans, Arabs, Jews, North Africans, Indians, Persians). There is large variation in skin color, but all have prominent noses.
4. Negroid (including Pygmies). These people have flat noses, thick protruding lips, very dark skin and woolly hair – Pygmies have flatter, paler faces and much shorter legs.
5. Khoisan (Bushmen and Hottentots). These people have yellow-brown skin that blends well with the surrounding forest. They are sway-backed.
6. Australoid (Aborigines, Maoris and South Pacific islanders). They are dark people with flat faces and woolly hair.

Politicizing human differences

Racism – the belief in the racial inferiority of other people – dates in its modern form from the 18th and 19th centuries when Negroid slaves were required to work the plantations of America and the Caribbean. Some bizarre theories were formulated to justify their treatment. People deprived of education and torn from their own culture were "proved" to be less intelligent and therefore lower in the evolutionary scale than ex-Europeans.

The American psychologist Arthur Jensen (b. 1923) claims that US Negroids have IQs which average ten points less than those of US Caucasoids (♦ page 65). Other scientists strongly disagree. Even if Jensen's figures were correct, it would be unscientific to use them to predict the IQ or scholastic ability of any individual, because the IQ variation within racial groups is vastly greater than any difference between groups.

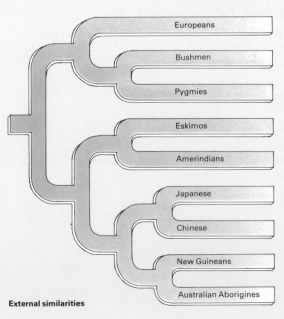

▶ The categorization and grouping of the human races has usually been done by comparing external characteristics; this approach has led to a number of different systems of classification. The study of biochemical features, specifically looking at the variation between the proteins, blood groups, HL antigens (♦ page 32) and enzymes of different populations, suggests that the traditional "family tree" is in need of amendment.

Europeans
Bushmen
Pygmies
Eskimos
Amerindians
Japanese
Chinese
New Guineans
Australian Aborigines

External similarities

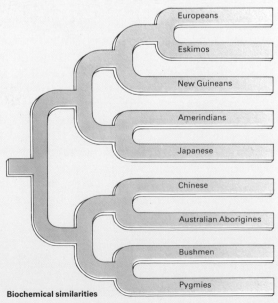

Europeans
Eskimos
New Guineans
Amerindians
Japanese
Chinese
Australian Aborigines
Bushmen
Pygmies

Biochemical similarities

The world's shortest people live alongside the world's tallest

Human variations

Skin color varies individually and with age and gender as well as racially. Women are paler than men, children paler than adults. White people burn, freckle or tan in sunlight; Negroid and Negroid-Caucasoid mixtures tan. Albinos are found in all races, though more commonly in dark-skinned ones. Peoples who have adapted to hot and humid climates have short noses and broad nostrils, and those from arid or mountainous zones have long noses and narrow nostrils. Body hair varies considerably, being scant in Mongoloids and more profuse in Caucasoids and Australoids. Baldness, an inherited trait, occurs in males of all races. People from cold climates are chunkily built to conserve body heat; those from hot climates are more slender. There is wide variation within populations, however, and people can also be crudely classified into endomorphs, who are thickset; mesomorphs, who are athletically built; and ectomorphs, who are willowy. These interpersonal differences are caused by a mixture of heredity, diet and exercise.

Height varies enormously. M'Buti Pygmies of Ituri Forest in the People's Republic of the Congo, are the world's shortest people with a maximum height of 1·38m (4ft 8in), but they live side by side with the Watusi, the world's tallest at up to 2·1m (7ft). The Pygmies, who have lived there longer, are better adapted to their forest environment than the Watusi Negros, who migrated there more recently from the plains. Brain size is greatest in Asiatics, and some 15 percent less in the South Pacific, with Europeans about average. The difference is not related to intelligence (◆ page 53), and Neanderthal Man, now extinct, had a larger brain than anyone living today. Women have a slightly higher ratio of brain to body weight than men, though men's brains are on average slightly larger.

World population

There were about 250 million people on Earth at the time of Christ. Within about 1,600 years the number doubled. It doubled again in the next 250 years, then in 60 years, and again in 30 years. By AD 2000 the present population of 4,000 million will have shot up to at least 6,000 million. A rise of such enormity and speed is placing great strain on the Earth's resources of land, food and materials. The recent rise in population has three main reasons – high fertility, low mortality and the age at which people have children. Since no reasonable person would wish to decrease life expectancy, increasing emphasis has recently been laid on persuading, or in some cases coercing, people to have fewer children and to have them at a later age. An average maternal age of 20 produces five generations per century; one of 33 produces only three.

In the developed world, declining birthrates have stabilized population size, but the average age of the population is rising. In poorer countries, centuries of infant mortality have led to a tradition of large families, to ensure that at least some children survive. Affluence may play a part too – people with assets are reluctant to reduce their wealth by supporting too many children, but people in poverty may regard children as an investment for the future.

Population profiles

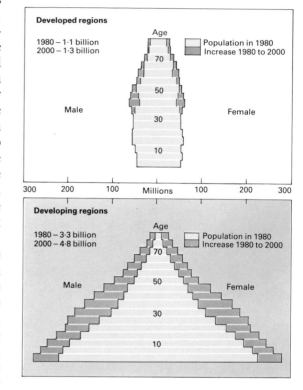

▲ *The very high birth rates in the Third World give a surplus of young people in those countries, whereas the stable populations and low birth rates of the developed countries have led to a possible excess of middle-aged and old people.*

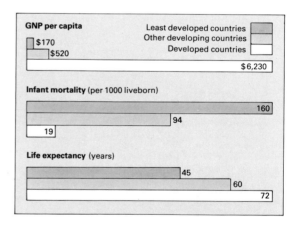

▲ *The difference in wealth between developed and developing nations is directly reflected in the health of their inhabitants. Availability of adequate food, clean water and medical care are the main factors to affect life expectancy.*

▼ *World population grew steadily for many centuries, limited by disease and poverty. Improvements in sanitation and medicine have allowed an exponential curve to develop, with massive ensuing problems of health, food and work.*

4,000

3,000

2,000

1,000

Population (millions)

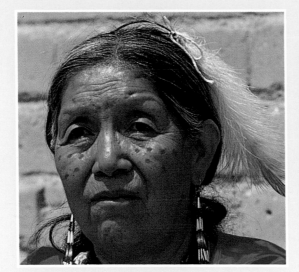

Early Mongoloid

Late Mongoloid

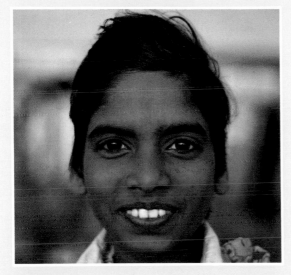

Caucasoid

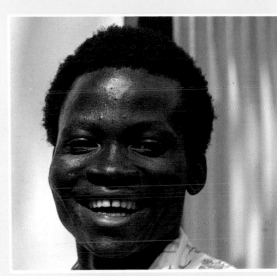

Negroid

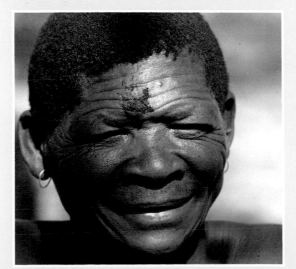

Khoisan

Australoid

The body is a complex of chemical structures and involves many levels of organisation

Internal stability

The body has the capacity to maintain internal stability and equilibrium despite changes in the external environment and internal health. This phenomenon is known as homeostasis, a term coined by the American physiologist Walter Cannon (1871-1945), who noted that strenuous exercise generates sufficient heat to curdle or "cook" body proteins unless rapidly dispersed, and that the lactic acid produced by the muscles during exercise would destroy cells if it were not removed or inactivated.

All the cells in the body need to be bathed in a complex brine of water, salts, dissolved oxygen and other gases, and nutrients. This extracellular fluid is crucial to homeostasis. Without water the cells would dry out; without salts they would become waterlogged (◆ page 235). A constant body pressure is essential or cells would wilt or burst, and high blood pressure would cause damage to the heart and kidneys.

Maintaining an even body temperature

The human body is warm: about 37°C (98·5°F). This temperature is a physiological compromise around the temperature at which enzymes (the proteins that serve as catalysts for the body's innumerable chemical reactions) work best. If we were much cooler, enzymes would work more slowly and we would become lethargic; much hotter and the enzymes would become irreversibly destroyed, just as meat is cooked. Humans become delirious above 40·5°C (105°F).

Temperature differs in different parts of the body; and at waking body temperature is about 0·6°C lower than usual. The heat generated by muscular activity during the day raises the temperature by about 1·1°C, or more in athletes, whose rectal temperature can be 40·5°C, though their skin temperature may be lower than average because heat is lost as sweat evaporates. Women's temperature may rise by 0·6°C after ovulation. The mechanisms that regulate body temperature are not perfect. They are poorly developed at birth – babies drop by 2·2°C in their first three hours of life, and must be kept warm. Babies tend to be warmer than adults, perhaps because of their rapid development; a year-old child has a rectal temperature of 37·6°C, dropping to adult levels by the age of 14 for girls and 18 for boys. In older people the mechanisms controlling temperature work less efficiently, and consequently they may be in danger from hypothermia (◆ page 234). They may not realize their temperature is dropping because they do not always feel cold, and conscious and unconscious mental processes are slowed by the fall in temperature.

The tissues of the body

The body is made up of organs, the organs of specialized tissues and the tissues of specialized cells. The cells themselves are complex units, containing hereditary material and capable of reproduction, which create the proteins necessary to maintain life. Cells are differentiated according to the specialized task they perform within the body, producing or reacting to particular chemicals (◆ page 19). Organs are structures with distinct form and function, such as the heart, lungs, liver, kidneys, stomach or brain. Each is part of a system, such as the digestive or excretory systems. Organs have specialized functions: kidneys to maintain salt and water balance and excrete unwanted and toxic products of metabolism (◆ page 135), lungs to take in oxygen and pour out carbon dioxide (◆ page 156), and the digestive system to absorb food (◆ page 121).

The levels of organisation

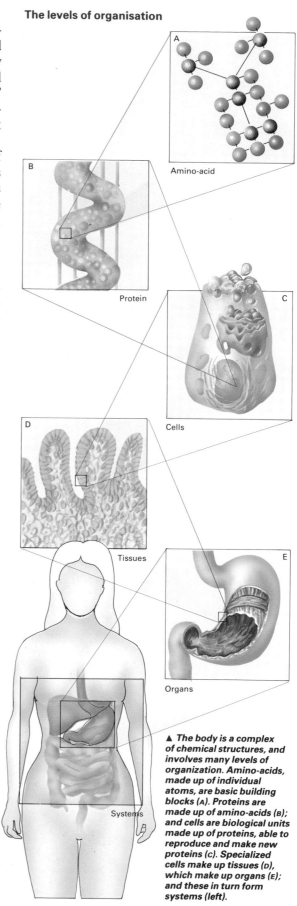

▲ *The body is a complex of chemical structures, and involves many levels of organization. Amino-acids, made up of individual atoms, are basic building blocks (A). Proteins are made up of amino-acids (B); and cells are biological units made up of proteins, able to reproduce and make new proteins (C). Specialized cells make up tissues (D), which make up organs (E); and these in turn form systems (left).*

The systems of the body

The body consists of an organism made up of a number of interlocking systems. In all cases except for the reproductive system, these are identical in male and female. These are:

1 The nervous system, including brain, spinal cord, nerves and sense organs; ◆ pages 41-48, 53-60.
2 The endocrine system, comprising all the glands that produce hormones; ◆ pages 85-92.
3 The skeleton, made up of the bones, the cartilages and joints; ◆ pages 97-101.
4 The muscles, including their associated tendons; ◆ pages 102-3.
5 The skin, or integumentary system, which includes the hair, nails, sweat and oil glands; ◆ pages 113-6.
6 The digestive system, comprising the mouth and esophagus, gut, stomach, and associated organs such as liver, pancreas, gall bladder and salivary glands; ◆ pages 121-6.
7 The urinary system, made up of the kidneys and organs that eliminate urine; ◆ pages 135-6.
8 The cardiovascular system, namely the heart, blood and blood vessels; ◆ pages 149-153.
9 The lymphatic system, comprising lymph, lymph nodes and vessels, and lymph glands; ◆ page 154.
10 The respiratory system, including lungs, and the passages leading to and from them; ◆ pages 155-8.
11 The reproductive systems, including the organs that produce reproductive cells in men and women, and those that store and transport these cells; ◆ pages 177-188.

The nervous system

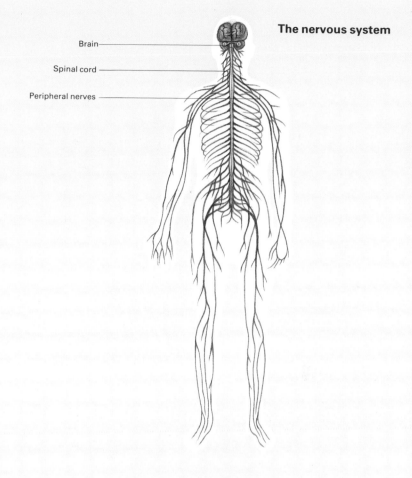

Brain
Spinal cord
Peripheral nerves

The endocrine system

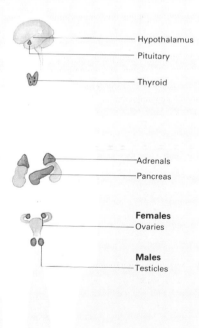

Hypothalamus
Pituitary
Thyroid

Adrenals
Pancreas

Females
Ovaries

Males
Testicles

The skeleton

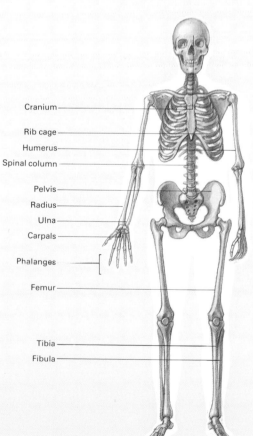

Cranium
Rib cage
Humerus
Spinal column
Pelvis
Radius
Ulna
Carpals
Phalanges
Femur
Tibia
Fibula

The muscles

The skin

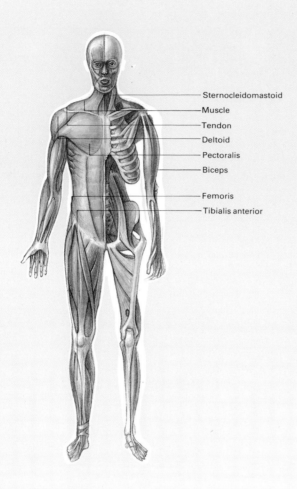

Sternocleidomastoid

Muscle

Tendon

Deltoid

Pectoralis

Biceps

Femoris

Tibialis anterior

Nail

Hair

Skin

The digestive system

The urinary system

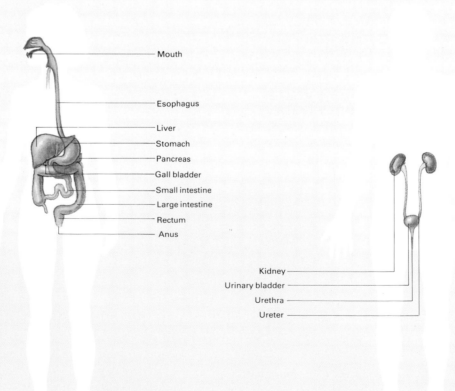

Mouth

Esophagus

Liver

Stomach

Pancreas

Gall bladder

Small intestine

Large intestine

Rectum

Anus

Kidney

Urinary bladder

Urethra

Ureter

The cardiovascular system

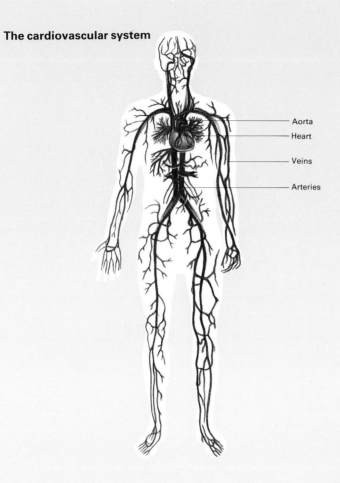

Aorta

Heart

Veins

Arteries

The lymphatic system

Thoracic duct

Lymph vessels

Lymph node

The respiratory system

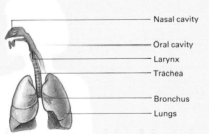

Nasal cavity

Oral cavity

Larynx

Trachea

Bronchus

Lungs

The reproductive systems

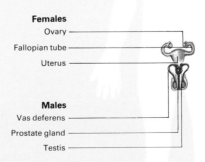

Females

Ovary

Fallopian tube

Uterus

Males

Vas deferens

Prostate gland

Testis

Spare Parts Surgery

Transplants and organ replacements

When just one organ or tissue becomes impaired in an otherwise healthy body, the obvious strategy is to provide a natural or artificial substitute.

The most widespread replacement technique is blood transfusion, using blood from a compatible donor. Particular fractions may be given – concentrated red cells for anemia, for example, and clotting factor VIII for hemophiliacs. Synthetic "plasma extenders" are used to restore blood volume in patients suffering from shock; perfluorocarbons mimic hemoglobin in carrying oxygen to the tissues. Synthetic substances could never replace all the functions of real blood, but they are cheap and effective for specific purposes.

HL antigen typing (◆ page 218) has permitted the grafting of other donor tissues which would normally be rejected by the body's immune system. Bone marrow can be transplanted to overcome conditions such as severe combined immunologic deficiency (SCID; ◆ page 232).

Grotesquely expensive in its early years, and never likely to be appropriate for more than a minority of people with heart disease, cardiac transplantation now gives 35-40 percent of patients five years of extra life (◆ page 163). Victims of certain diseases of the lungs and associated blood vessels may be helped by combined grafting of heart and lungs, though this treatment is still experimental. After several years of poor results, the liver (too complex to be replaced mechanically) is now being transplanted successfully – particularly in children with certain congenital conditions. Other organs grafted with limited success include the pancreas, larynx, trachea, and testicle. Whole knee joints have been accomplished in rabbits, while experiments in rats suggest that brain cells may one day be grafted to treat parkinsonism (◆ page 64). There are also hopes of prompting the body to regenerate organs itself.

No rejection problems attend the use of the body's "self" tissues (◆ page 219). Two examples are arteries taken from the leg to boost blood supply to heart muscle, and skin moved for facial reconstruction or the treatment of burns – an art enhanced by the discovery in 1984 of methods of growing a patient's skin in the laboratory (◆ page 118). Bone grafting is routine in some centers, particularly for replacing bone missing because of injury or tumors. A few muscle grafts have been reported too, including repair of the heart muscle.

Certain synthetic substitutes compete with their natural counterparts. Some surgeons favor plastic heart valves (◆ page 165); others prefer valves taken from pigs. Some plumb the circulation with plastic tubing; others use the patient's own blood vessels. Controversy surrounds the replacement of the entire heart by a plastic pump. Many medical scientists believe that these devices will never prove satisfactory except for temporary support, because of clotting and other problems. Others point to the routine use of devices as large as hip joints (◆ page 110) as evidence that the body will accept major mechanical implants long-term. A few researchers even argue that the brain and nervous system may eventually be repairable with microelectronic implants termed "biochips".

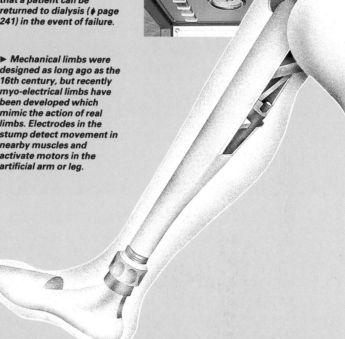

► Transplanting organs such as kidneys may challenge the surgeon's ingenuity, but rejection of the new organ is the most serious difficulty. One solution is to take the organ from a near relative or unrelated person whose tissues match closely those of the recipient. The other is to administer a drug to suppress the immune system. Particularly effective is cyclosporine, which has rendered kidney transplants from cadaver donors so successful that living relatives may soon no longer be asked to donate their organs. Kidney grafting has the great merit that a patient can be returned to dialysis (◆ page 241) in the event of failure.

► Mechanical limbs were designed as long ago as the 16th century, but recently myo-electrical limbs have been developed which mimic the action of real limbs. Electrodes in the stump detect movement in nearby muscles and activate motors in the artificial arm or leg.

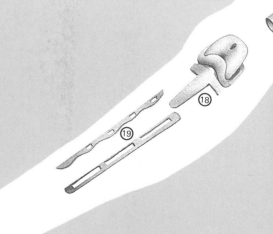

► Accidentally severed limbs can be replanted without rejection problems. Replacement of worn or damaged joints is the most frequent form of spare parts surgery, and offers long-term relief from arthritis. The joints are replaced with plastic, stainless steel or titanium prostheses.

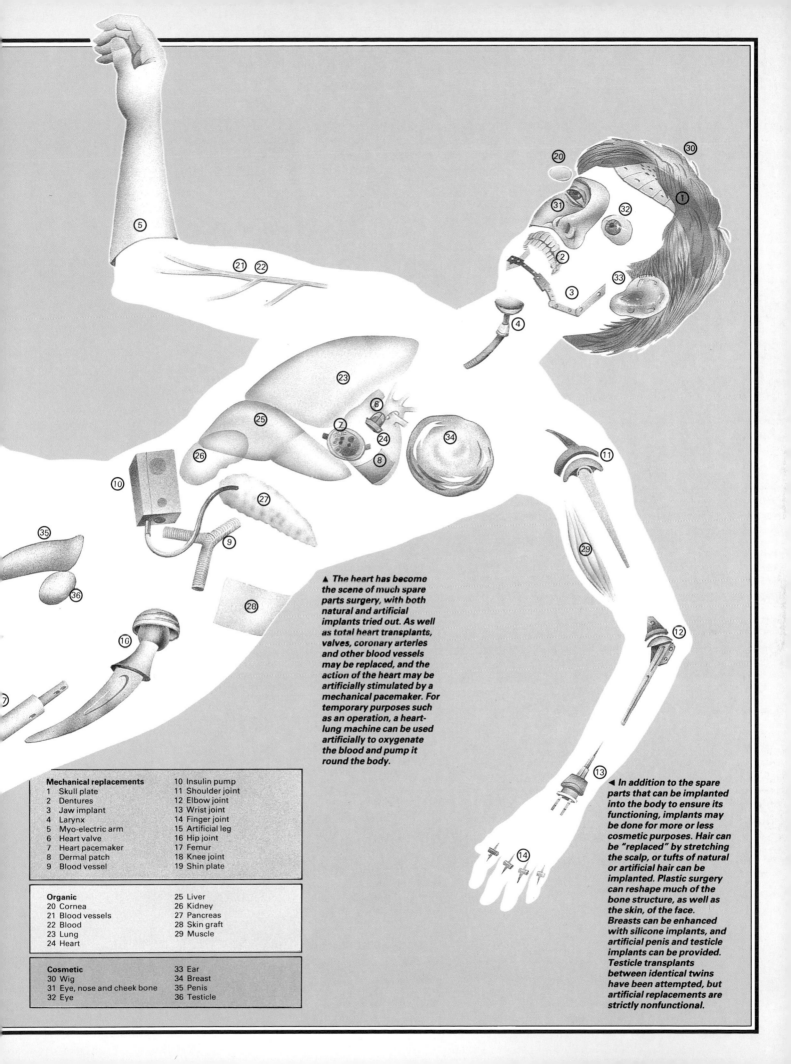

▲ The heart has become the scene of much spare parts surgery, with both natural and artificial implants tried out. As well as total heart transplants, valves, coronary arteries and other blood vessels may be replaced, and the action of the heart may be artificially stimulated by a mechanical pacemaker. For temporary purposes such as an operation, a heart-lung machine can be used artificially to oxygenate the blood and pump it round the body.

◄ In addition to the spare parts that can be implanted into the body to ensure its functioning, implants may be done for more or less cosmetic purposes. Hair can be "replaced" by stretching the scalp, or tufts of natural or artificial hair can be implanted. Plastic surgery can reshape much of the bone structure, as well as the skin, of the face. Breasts can be enhanced with silicone implants, and artificial penis and testicle implants can be provided. Testicle transplants between identical twins have been attempted, but artificial replacements are strictly nonfunctional.

Mechanical replacements
1 Skull plate
2 Dentures
3 Jaw implant
4 Larynx
5 Myo-electric arm
6 Heart valve
7 Heart pacemaker
8 Dermal patch
9 Blood vessel
10 Insulin pump
11 Shoulder joint
12 Elbow joint
13 Wrist joint
14 Finger joint
15 Artificial leg
16 Hip joint
17 Femur
18 Knee joint
19 Shin plate

Organic
20 Cornea
21 Blood vessels
22 Blood
23 Lung
24 Heart
25 Liver
26 Kidney
27 Pancreas
28 Skin graft
29 Muscle

Cosmetic
30 Wig
31 Eye, nose and cheek bone
32 Eye
33 Ear
34 Breast
35 Penis
36 Testicle

The human body consists of 100 million million cells

A tissue is a group of cells and the substances in which they lie. These function together to perform a particular role such as movement, digestion or hormone production. There are four kinds: epithelial, connective, muscular and nervous.

Epithelial tissue lines passages leading into the body, blood vessels and hollow organs. It may be penetrated by nerves but not by blood vessels, and has a base membrane attaching it to connective tissue.

Connective tissue consists of scattered cells in an organic matrix. It includes fat tissue, cartilage and bone (◆ page 97). Connecting other organs to each other, it protects and supports them.

Muscle forms the basis of all movement, maintains posture and generates heat. Muscle is found in three forms, striated or striped, unstriated or smooth, and cardiac, in the heart (◆ page 101).

Nervous tissue forms the brain, nerves and sense organs, including the autonomic nerves (◆ page 58).

Cells are the basic building blocks of the body, and have four parts, the outer membrane, cytoplasm, organelles ("little organs") and nucleus. The cell membrane is made of two layers of fatty compounds called phospholipids, proteins, and small quantities of water, ions and simple fats. Substances cross it by diffusion, osmosis, transport, phagocytosis ("eating") and pinocytosis ("drinking").

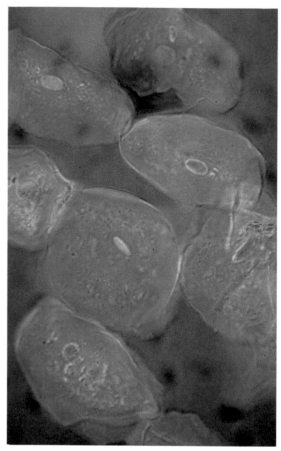

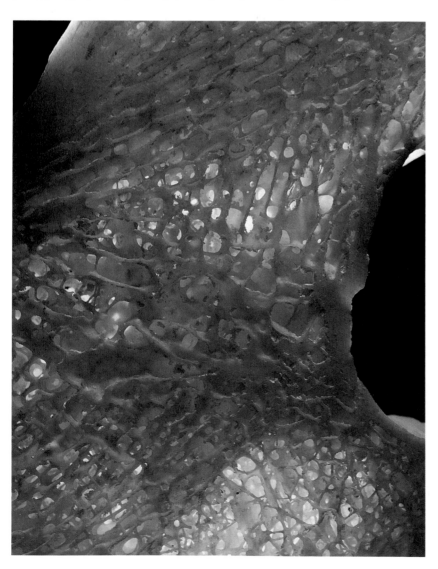

◄ *Connective tissue comprises bone (as in this section through a hip bone), blood tissue, cartilage, elastic and adipose tissue. The cells tend to be loosely packed and contain a rich blood supply.*

▲ *Epithelial tissue, such as this squamous (flattened) tissue from the cheek, makes up sheet-like layers which line body surfaces inside and out, and also make up the hormone-secreting parts of glands.*

▼ *Unlike connective and epithelial tissue, which occur in many forms and perform a number of tasks, muscle tissue is highly specialized to perform the single function of contraction.*

▼ *Nervous tissue, including these neurons from the spinal cord, is designed to receive stimuli from receptors and pass impulses along their length. Like the muscles, nervous tissue is highly specialized.*

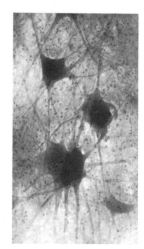

Structure of the cell

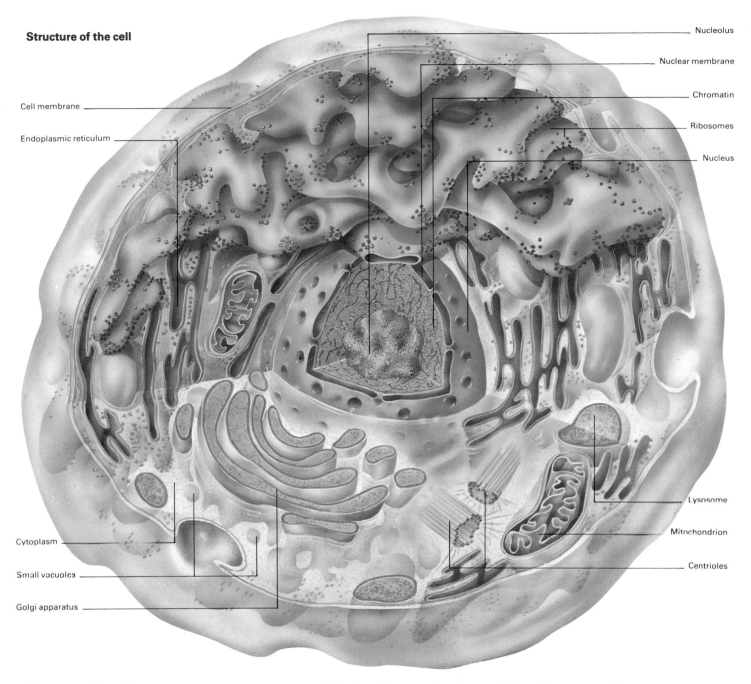

Nucleolus

Nuclear membrane

Chromatin

Ribosomes

Nucleus

Cell membrane

Endoplasmic reticulum

Lysosome

Mitochondrion

Centrioles

Cytoplasm

Small vacuoles

Golgi apparatus

The parts of a cell

The cytoplasm is a fluid in which chemical reactions occur. It contains various organelles.

Endoplasmic reticulum (ER) is a network of channels through the cytoplasm. It conducts materials, provides a surface for chemical reactions and stores molecules made in the cell.

Ribosomes make proteins from amino-acids. Some float freely and synthesize proteins for use within the cell. Others are attached to the endoplasmic reticulum, through which their proteins are transported outside.

Golgi complexes are sets of flat sacks that store proteins made by the ribosomes and lipids made in the ER. At intervals they bud off secretory granules, some of which move to the surface of the cell and discharge. Others, called lysosomes, remain within the cell where they digest unwanted substances.

Mitochondria are small, self-reproducing rods or spheres that make adenosine triphosphate (ATP), the cell's source of energy (◆ page 158).

The nucleus contains the cell's chromosomes. Around the nucleus is a membrane. The chromatin (genetic material) lies in a gelatinous fluid, in which are also two nucleoli made of protein, ribonucleic acid (RNA) and deoxyribonucleic acid (DNA).

The centrosome contains two centrioles, which hold the frame along which the chromosomes separate during cell division (◆ page 205).

Peroxisomes, containing enzymes, are found in most cells, as are microfilaments and microtubules which together form a microskeleton. This is part of the mechanism which allows muscle cells to contract. The microskeleton is often connected with exterior cilia – tiny hairs that move particles along the cell surface.

▲ This generalized cell is a composite of many different cells of the body; actual body cells are designed to perform specific tasks, and may, in the case of neurons, be up to 100cm in length. The human body consists of 100 million million cells.

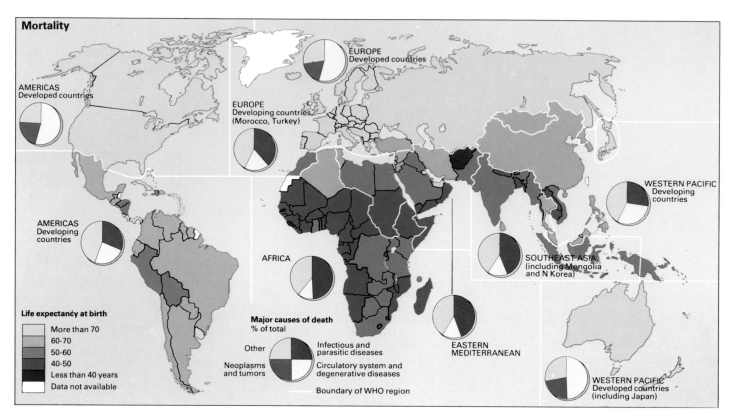

Mortality

AMERICAS
Developed countries

EUROPE
Developed countries

EUROPE
Developing countries
(Morocco, Turkey)

AMERICAS
Developing
countries

AFRICA

WESTERN PACIFIC
Developing
countries

SOUTHEAST ASIA
(including Mongolia
and N Korea)

EASTERN
MEDITERRANEAN

WESTERN PACIFIC
Developed countries
(including Japan)

Life expectancy at birth
- More than 70
- 60-70
- 50-60
- 40-50
- Less than 40 years
- Data not available

Major causes of death
% of total
- Other
- Neoplasms and tumors
- Infectious and parasitic diseases
- Circulatory system and degenerative diseases
- Boundary of WHO region

The body's internal rhythms

*Biorhythms, determined by our "internal clocks",
are cycles that conform to a regular time pattern.
Some last approximately one day, though one – the
menstrual cycle, which has no male equivalent –
takes about a month (page 180). There are also
shorter cycles, such as the "90-minute enigma"
of secretory activity in the stomach and excretion
by the kidney, and the production of several
hormones. These rhythms vary from person to
person by up to ten percent longer or shorter
than average. Individual biorhythms can only be
determined by observation, and are unconnected
with birth dates.*

*The principal cycle is our circadian rhythm, the
sense of day and night and variation throughout
24 hours. We all differ in our preferred bedtime,
need for sleep, time estimates, sensory and
motor responses, drug susceptibility, moods,
performance and alertness. Even the perception of
a "day" varies – people subjected to constant light
and temperature will settle down to a daily cycle of
between 22 and 27 hours, varying with the person.*

*Despite individual differences, there are features
of the circadian rhythm that most people share.
These are important when we do shift work, travel
across time zones, or work for long periods without
sleep. When sleep is reduced or frequently
interrupted, a person's standard of work and
feeling of well-being are related to how long it is
since he or she last slept, rather than to the amount
of sleep actually taken (page 70). Most people
work least efficiently in the early hours of the
morning. Nearly everyone prefers to sleep at
night, and night-workers prefer to sleep in the
morning and early afternoon, rather than the late
afternoon and evening.*

"Health for all"

With the dramatic differences in wealth between the rich and poor countries in the 1980s, variations in the availability of food and hygienic conditions are as important as the number of doctors (page 40) in creating the conditions of health around the world. The charter of the World Health Organization (WHO) describes health as "a state of complete physical, mental and social wellbeing and not merely the absence of disease or infirmity". Such a definition appears more utopian still when coupled with the WHO's current target of providing "health for all" by the year 2000. In reality, it is highly unlikely that modern drugs and vaccines, even with the help of political will and established knowledge about how to thwart infections by sanitation and hygiene, will make it possible even to achieve the more modest objective of conquering disease throughout the planet by AD 2000. But the WHO definition does serve to show that health and disease are relative concepts. Good health means something different for a Kalahari Bushman and a Western office worker, each of whom would become vulnerable to illness if taken abruptly from his usual environment. One tissue of the body can be healthy while another is ailing. Mental health is notoriously difficult to define. Moreover, health is not synonymous with physical condition – as evidenced by a superbly fit athlete who may be suffering from all sorts of diseases. "Health" also implies differing standards of performance from our body in youth and old age – not least in our expectations of its capabilities. Finally, there is a substantial gray area between being well and unwell. For example, while the blood sugar level always rises after a meal, and while the body of a diabetic is unable to cope with this increase, some individuals are intermediate in their capacity to tolerate raised blood sugar. By showing ranges of values, "standard tables" for factors such as blood pressure and heart rate demonstrate how impossible it is to define normality.

*The human species and other animals...
Paleontology, the search for the origins of mankind...
Australopithecus, link between ape and man?...Early
hominids...The growing brain...Adaptation for walking...
Humans and socialization...PERSPECTIVE...An aquatic
origin?... Fossilized footprints... Possible ancestral trees*

If humans were typical mammals, we would run on all fours, be covered with fur, and communicate by noises or gestures. We would be sexually mature within a year or two of birth and be capable of breeding for the rest of our lives, perhaps 20 years at most. Males would be unaware they had offspring and females would lose interest in their young after weaning. We would be adapted to inhabit an environment but not to modify it. We would eat raw food, make only the simplest of artefacts, and die young from disease, starvation or trauma.

In reality, although versatile we are no specialists. We cannot run like gazelles, climb like squirrels, swim like fish, fly like birds, hear like cats, smell like dogs, jump like fleas or even burrow as well as earthworms. Because we live on land we have long limbs for walking, running and jumping, unlike fishes or whales who use their limbs as paddles. Because we live in the warm air rather than cold water, we need and can afford a greater skin area in proportion to bulk than fishes. What hair we have is for decoration and sexual recognition, and does little to keep us warm. Because we are more advanced than other animals, our bodies and brains need longer for development and learning. During this period of childhood we need parental care and sexual maturity is postponed until some ten years after birth.

Our skills lie in forethought, tool-making, language and manual dexterity, which we use to alter the environment. We manage without fur by making clothes, building houses and warming ourselves with fires. Our ability to make fire also means that we can cook food and forge metals. Cooking softens hard food such as grain, and kills bacteria and parasites. With metal and other materials we make tools that extend our bodies' range of acitivites, and machines that run, swim, fly and burrow, store information and "think" for us.

Did humans evolve in water?

The British biologist Sir Alister Hardy (1896-1985) proposed that humans were closely associated with water in their evolutionary past, and that this shows in the design of the human body. Humans differ from other apes in a number of ways which suggest adaptation to water.

They can swim long distances, are unafraid of water even as babies, and can hold their breath under water; swim elegantly, both under water and on the surface; are naked, like whales and dolphins; have hair that follows the direction of water flow when swimming; have streamlined bodies with a layer of blubber under the skin; stand erect, which makes wading easy; and have sensitive hands with fast-growing nails for prising open shellfish.

Opponents of Hardy's theory point out that there is no direct evidence for this aquatic interlude in human evolution, and no need for it. We are not the only hairless land animal – pigs, for example, are nearly as bald and just as well endowed with blubber. Equally, our erect posture and versatile hands are adaptations for many forms of fine manipulative work unrelated to water activity.

The human embryo compared

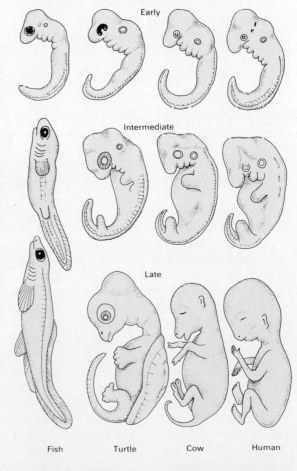

Early

Intermediate

Late

Fish   Turtle   Cow   Human

The human arm compared

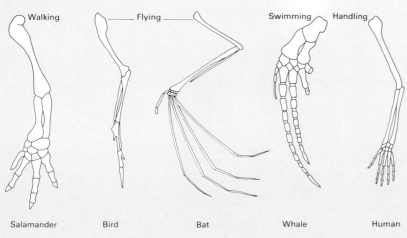

Walking   Flying   Swimming   Handling

Salamander   Bird   Bat   Whale   Human

◄ *The human arm is an adaptation of the basic vertebrate forelimb design, suited for carrying and manipulation of the hand.*

▲ *The gills and tail of the early human embryo, like those of other mammals, reflect the primeval aquatic origins of all life on Earth.*

The Neanderthals, who lived over 35,000 years ago, had a larger brain than modern Man

Human origins

The question of the emergence of *Homo sapiens* is a hotly debated issue; not because of doubt about its occurrence, but because of the difficulty in establishing accurate branching order and timing. These difficulties make this topic more theoretical and notional than much else in the present volume.

Man is a primate closely related to the great apes (the gorilla, chimpanzee and orangutan). The elements that are crucial in the emergence of Man have been variously defined, but include the development of upright walking, and the growth of the overall size and structural complexity of the brain. Using these and other similar criteria, paleontologists attempt to identify fossil remains of early hominids, and to establish lineages that can indicate the moments at which Man diverged from the other apes.

The earliest upright hominids known are 3·75 million years old, found in Ethiopia in the 1970s. These had a brain size less than a third of the modern human brain, and have been designated as *Australopithecus afarensis* (*A. afarensis*). Between three and two million years later are fossils of *A. africanus* and *A. robustus*, which also walked upright. However, their skulls were different from *A. afarensis*. Both had no forehead and a huge, wide and very flat face and large grinding teeth, *A. robustus* being the larger and more solidly built.

Overlapping the younger australopithecines is the first of the fossils called Homo – *Homo habilis* (*H. habilis*). There is not much fossil evidence for this, but it had a distinctly larger brain, and is the first fossil found with manufactured stone tools. *Homo erectus* had a larger brain still, and is the earliest hominid to be found widely outside Africa, from Germany to China.

Finally, between 150,000 and 100,000 years ago there are fossils of fully modern Man, with a higher domed skull, less prominent ridge brows and a flatter face than *H. erectus*. This is *Homo sapiens*. Like *H. erectus*, it is found at several widely separated sites. Several subgroups within *H. sapiens* have been identified, including the Neanderthals. They lived from 70,000 to 35,000 years ago, and had a larger brain than modern Man but a squat build and heavy brows.

Interpreting the fossil story

In the matter of locomotion, opinion is sharply divided as to whether the earliest australopithecines walked upright as efficiently as modern Man, or whether they adopted a bent-kneed, bent-hipped waddle. Although the australopithecines had a small brain, it has been argued that its front portion (the part that is most enlarged in modern Man) was relatively enlarged – even though upright walking may have preceded an increase in brain size, brain organization started very early in our evolution. A complete specimen of *H. habilis* was found in Kenya and designated KNM-ER 1470. About 1·8 million years old, it had a very modern brain. The patterns of its convolutions, seen in a modern brain, would indicate that its owner was capable of speech. By contrast KNM-ER 1805, a slightly younger skull, has an ape-like brain.

Most paleontologists agree that later members of Homo share *H. habilis* as an ancestor, but are divided on exactly how the non-African specimens fit into the pattern. Some believe that the transition to *H. sapiens* took place in Africa and was followed by at least two waves of colonization, the first giving rise to Neanderthal Man, who became extinct or was absorbed by the second wave. Others argue that modern Man emerged independently in Africa, Asia and Europe.

The family tree of humankind

There have been many arguments about the details of the various splits in the lineage of Man. In the 1960s and 1970s, probably the most widely accepted evolutionary tree showed A. africanus as the ancestor of H. habilis, while A. robustus was on a separate branch.

In 1974, the remains of a skeleton about 3.75 million years old were found at Hadar in Ethiopia. Nearly half the skeleton has been preserved. The skeleton, which is probably female, was nicknamed "Lucy". Other finds at Hadar include a large group comprising no fewer than 13 individuals, children and adults. Classification of these remains is critical to determining the family tree of humankind.

Lucy has been named as a new kind of australopithecine, Australopithecus afarensis, after Afar, the region in Ethiopia where she was found. Don Johanson, the discoverer of Lucy, has claimed that A. afarensis is the ancestor of all later hominids, but there are at least three other possibilities, and all are supported to some degree. A. afarensis is lightly built, like A. africanus, and shares many skull features with the lightly-built (gracile) and robust australopithecines. It thus might be the ancestor of the other australopithecines but not of ourselves. But the differences between the two gracile australopithecines and the robust forms could mean that A. robustus is on a limb of its own, with the other two on the branch to modern Man. Finally, it has been argued that the remains currently classified as A. afarensis actually belong to two species – the large specimens (considered by Johanson to be males) are the ancestors of the robust australopithecines while the smaller (Johanson's females) gave rise ultimately to Homo and humankind.

Two versions of Man's family tree

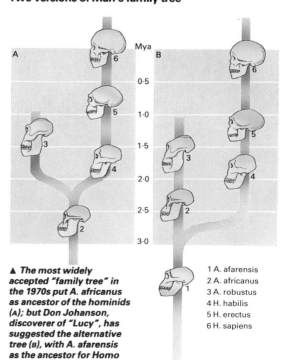

▲ *The most widely accepted "family tree" in the 1970s put A. africanus as ancestor of the hominids (A); but Don Johanson, discoverer of "Lucy", has suggested the alternative tree (B), with A. afarensis as the ancestor for Homo and Australopithecus.*

1 A. afarensis
2 A. africanus
3 A. robustus
4 H. habilis
5 H. erectus
6 H. sapiens

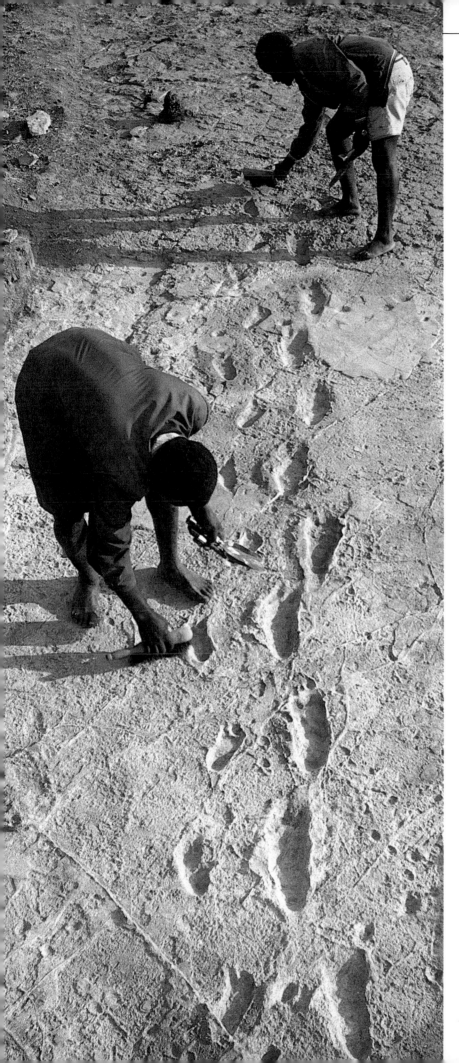

Prehistoric footprints

In 1976 Andrew Hill, a paleontologist now at Harvard University, fell over during a game of catch at the fossil excavations at Laetoli in Tanzania. In front of his nose were animal tracks preserved in the rock. On excavation, signs of spring hares, guinea fowl, rhinoceroses, elephants, pigs, buffaloes, hyenas, antelopes, many baboons and a sabre-toothed tiger were uncovered.

In 1978 unmistakable hominid footprints, described by a trained tracker as incredibly modern, were discovered nearby. Three different individuals walked along for at least 25m. There are two tracks. The smallest footprints are to the left of the double set, made by the largest individual and the medium-sized, who unaccountably placed its feet in the tracks of the larger. At one point the three seemed to pause and half-turn backwards. The prints are roughly 3·75 million years old.

We do not know whether the three individuals walked by as a group, although it is tempting to think that they did. We do know that the footprints were preserved by an astonishing combination of circumstances. Ash from the nearby volcano Sandiman (now extinct) fell on the countryside towards the end of the dry season. Sandiman's ash is known as carbonatite ash, very rare indeed. It contained calcium carbonate and sodium carbonate which, when moistened, form an instant cement. Shortly after the eruption, it rained. The rain that fell was gentle enough to moisten the ash so that it would receive imprints and not blow away, but not so severe as to wash away the prints. When the animals, including the hominids, walked over the ash they left their marks, which were quickly covered by another ash fall, only to emerge 3·75 million years later.

▶ *The remarkably complete skeleton of the australopithecine "Lucy", about 3·75 million years old. She was named from the Beatles' song "Lucy in the Sky with Diamonds".*

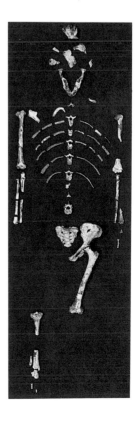

◀ *The 3·75 million-year-old footprints from Laetoli, in Tanzania, which are presumed to be those of a group of australopithecines. Tracks of many kinds of animal were discovered at the same site.*

The making of Man

Between 15 and 10 million years ago Africa's topography changed. The flat central region became uplifted and this altered the climate and vegetation dramatically. The forests shrank and the grasslands expanded. Thus a new habitat was opened, but food in the grasslands was scarcer and of lower quality than in the forests. This necessitated more traveling. For an animal adapted to swing through trees, quadrupedal locomotion is not very efficient. Bipedal locomotion *is*, with the consequent advantage of freeing the hands to carry food.

Brain enlargement and reorganization followed, relative to body size. Humans have brains three times larger than apes of the same body size, and several factors contribute to this. One of the most important, examined by the British scientist Robert Martin, is the mother's food supply. Martin suggests that the upper limit to brain size is determined by the amount of food the mother can supply while the fetus is in the womb (◊ page 185). Once the infant is born, brain growth follows a trajectory set in the womb. In the typical primate this results in a doubling of brain weight, while in humans the brain quadruples. To achieve this growth early humans would have needed a steady and reliable source of energy. This could be found in a forest, but the development of technology and of cooperation, would help ensure a suitable food supply on the savannah too.

Thus tool use, upright walking, brain development and cooperation mutually reinforce each other. There is, for example, a conflict between bipedalism and brain growth, because the larger birth canal necessitated by a big brain makes the female pelvis unsuitable for walking. The conflict is resolved by the development of technology and a social organisation that permits extended childhood and small families.

Parental care is a feature of all primates, but is especially extensive in Man because the human infant is so helpless; most of its brain growth takes places after birth. The modern pelvis, one assumes, permits the largest infant brain compatible with the mother's efficient walking. This is about 350ml. The typical primate doubles in brain size from infant to adult, so if Man were a typical primate the adult brain would occupy 700ml. Any larger and increased parental care would become essential. This theoretical adult brain size of 700ml correlates very well with the observed brain size of *H. habilis*, the first hominid with an enlarged brain and evidence of technology.

The human hand compared

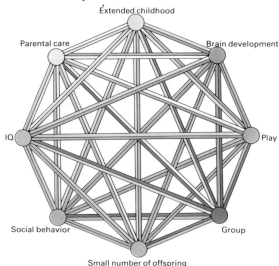

Baboon   Gorilla   Orang-utan   Human

The human skull compared

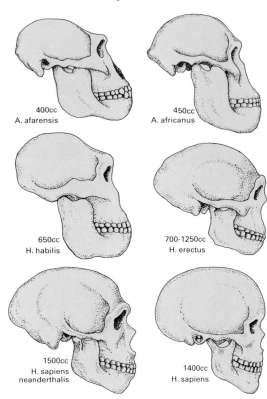

400cc
A. afarensis

450cc
A. africanus

650cc
H. habilis

700-1250cc
H. erectus

1500cc
H. sapiens neanderthalis

1400cc
H. sapiens

▲ The shape of the skull and jaws of hominid fossils offers rich evidence concerning the musculature and posture of the various species. A. afarensis had a brain volume of some 400ml; A. africanus 450ml ; H. habilis 650ml, H. erectus 700-1,250ml; H. neanderthalis 1,500ml, and H. sapiens 1,400ml. By comparison, a modern gorilla has 500ml.

Human development

Extended childhood

Parental care   Brain development

IQ   Play

Social behavior   Group

Small number of offspring

◄ Unlike those of the apes, the human hand allows the thumb to be opposed to every finger, permitting activities needing both power and precision.

▲ Small families, long childhood, intelligence and parental care are all claimed to be interdependent elements in the development of H. sapiens.

Inheritance

Chromosomes and genes...The mechanisms of inheritance... Dominant and recessive traits...Simple and complex inheritance...Blood groups...Inbreeding... Genetics and disease...PERSPECTIVE...Unusual hereditary abilities...Twins and heredity...Gregor Mendel, founder of genetics...The discovery of blood groups...Incest

In 1956, to the embarrassment of colleagues around the world, two biologists in Sweden, Albert Levan and Joe-Hin Tjio, announced that human cells contain 46 chromosomes – the strands of deoxyribonucleic acid (DNA) which carry hereditary characteristics from cell to cell and generation to generation. For decades, scientists had believed there to be 48 – the number found in our evolutionary relatives, the great apes. But improved microscopic techniques had allowed Dr Levan and his Indonesian collaborator to establish that there were no more than 23 pairs. As in other animals, these DNA strands replicate before separating at mitosis (the normal process of cell division; ◆ page 205) so that each new cell will contain its full complement of DNA. On the other hand, they are reduced to only 23 chromosomes during meiosis – the process of creating egg cells and spermatozoa. During meiosis, however, the pairs of chromosomes may twist around each other and exchange sections. By so doing they produce new hereditary combinations to be passed to the offspring.

Males and females have 22 identical pairs of chromosomes. But they differ in the pair which determines sex – a pair of "X" chromosomes is found in females, and one "X" and a smaller "Y" chromosome in males. Thus, after meiosis, egg cells always contain 22 plus X, but there are two sorts of sperm, some with X and some with Y. At fertilization, an egg cell meets either an X-carrying sperm (leading to a female baby) or a Y-carrying sperm (leading to a boy). Just as the stretches of DNA known as genes determine other bodily characteristics, so those peculiar to the Y chromosome ensure maleness.

Inheriting special skills for taste...

The ability to taste phenylthiocarbamide (PTC) is a puzzling hereditary trait. If a child has two parents who can each sense the bitter tang of this chemical, it will be a taster too. Children of non-tasters are all non-tasters. And if one parent is a taster and the other a non-taster, the offspring can be either, but will probably be tasters. Like blue and brown eyes, the bizarre characteristics of tasting and non-tasting are controlled by a single pair of genes, non-tasting being recessive (◆ page 28). PTC tasting is one of those traits for which the prevalence of the genes varies in different parts of the world. About 70 percent of white people in North America and Europe can taste the chemical, compared with only 51 percent of Aboriginal Australians. American Indians (98 percent) and Negros (95 percent) top the league. The biological significance of PTC tasting is not known, although there is apparently a link between non-tasting and a higher-than-average risk of certain forms of thyroid disease.

...and smell

One of the oddest and most recently discovered hereditary traits is the ability to smell the characteristic chemicals that appear in the urine after eating asparagus. Until 1980, it was thought that these substances were produced as a result of a metabolic abnormality found in only a small proportion of people. Then Dr S.H. Blondheim and colleagues at the Hadassah University in Jerusalem realized that excretion of the odorous chemicals is universal. People familiar with the smell can detect it in urine from anyone who has eaten asparagus – whether or not they can smell it themselves. But only a minority of individuals have that sensitivity. Like PTC tasting, the real explanation seems to be genetic, with about 10 percent of the population carrying a gene that gives them the ability to detect the odor and the remaining 90 percent lacking that gene. This is the first example of a specific smell hypersensitivity to have been discovered, and its value is not yet known.

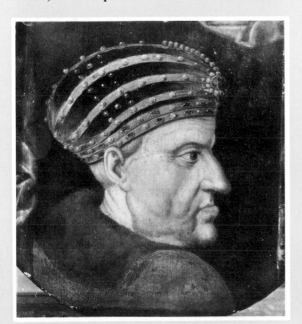

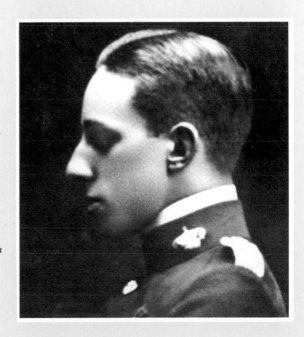

◄ ► *The Hapsburg lip, seen over several centuries in illustrations of the Austrian and Spanish royal families, is a well-known example of a family characteristic produced by a single gene. From the Emperor Maximilian (left) in the 15th century to Alfonso XIII of Spain in the 19th (right), the ugly, protruding lower lip appeared so consistently that geneticists are confident about its origin. When a rare trait turns up frequently in a family and is transmitted only by the affected members, it is almost certainly the result of a dominant gene. The careful genealogical records of the old aristocracy and detailed visual and documentary records of their persons provide invaluable evidence for geneticists.*

Meiosis: mixing genes

1 *Meiosis is the creation of sex cells that may combine to form a new human being. It differs from other forms of cell division in that the sex cells (sperm or eggs) or gametes formed by this process contain only half the normal number of chromosomes and genes. Meiosis takes place in the testes and ovaries.*

2 *The chromosomes form a distinct shape and group into 23 pairs. One from each pair was originally inherited from the person's father, the other from the mother.*

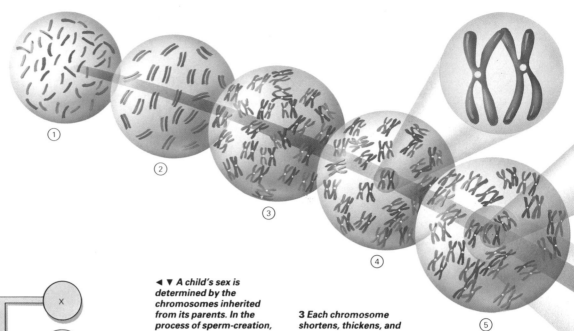

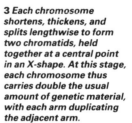

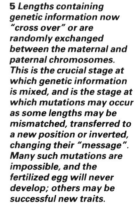

The inheritance of sex

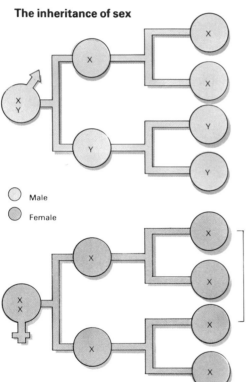

○ Male

● Female

◀ ▼ *A child's sex is determined by the chromosomes inherited from its parents. In the process of sperm-creation, the father's chromosomes are split so that half his sperm carry the X, the other half the Y. Ova creation differs from that of sperm in that only one ovum develops at a time; the remaining three potential ova never reach maturity. If a Y sperm fertilizes an X ovum, the child will be male; if the sperm carries X, the child will be female.*

3 *Each chromosome shortens, thickens, and splits lengthwise to form two chromatids, held together at a central point in an X-shape. At this stage, each chromosome thus carries double the usual amount of genetic material, with each arm duplicating the adjacent arm.*

4 *Paternal and maternal chromosomes line up together closely.*

5 *Lengths containing genetic information now "cross over" or are randomly exchanged between the maternal and paternal chromosomes. This is the crucial stage at which genetic information is mixed, and is the stage at which mutations may occur as some lengths may be mismatched, transferred to a new position or inverted, changing their "message". Many such mutations are impossible, and the fertilized egg will never develop; others may be successful new traits.*

6 *Poles form in the cell and the chromosomes collect in the middle. Chromosomes from each pair are then pulled to opposite sides. (For clarity, stages 6-9 do not show the full number of chromosomes.)*

A fertilized egg-cell divides

▶ *A complete set of human chromosomes seen in a fluorescent micrograph.*

▶ ▶ *The two sets of chromosomes are pulled apart by "spindles" to opposite poles as the division is almost complete.*

▶ ▶ ▶ *A human embryo about 60 hours after fertilization. By a process of cell division known as mitosis (◊ page 205), the original cell has divided into two daughter cells.*

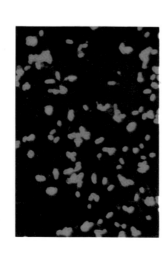

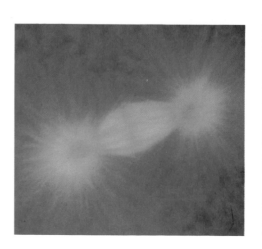

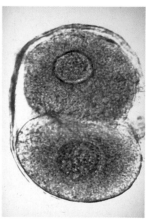

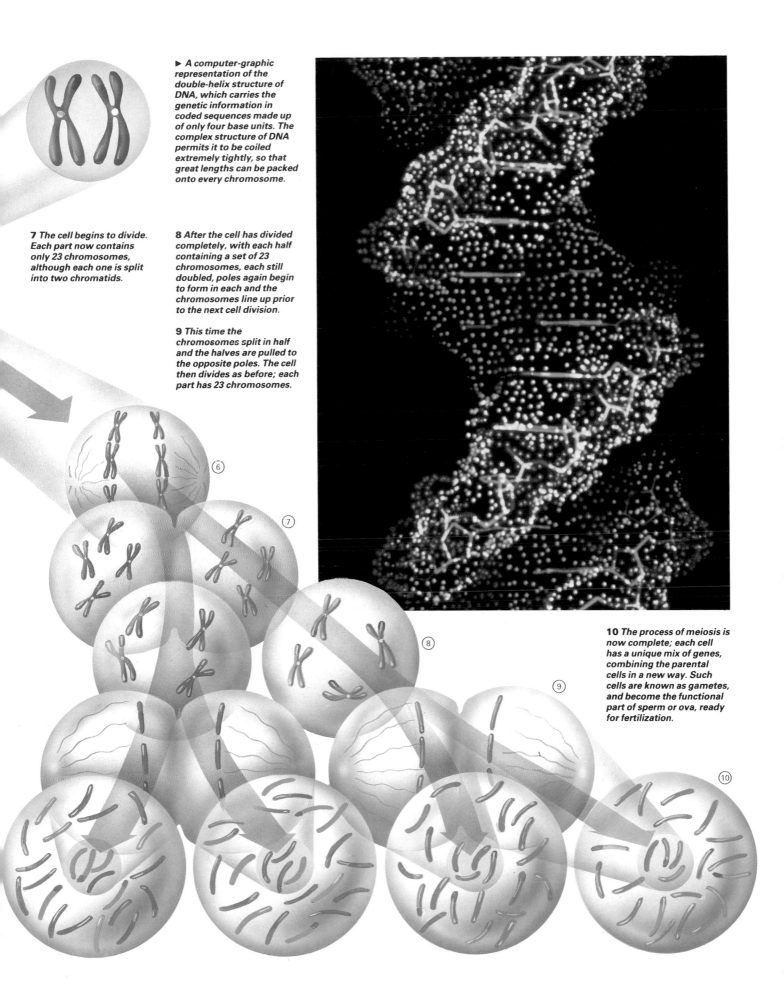

► A computer-graphic representation of the double-helix structure of DNA, which carries the genetic information in coded sequences made up of only four base units. The complex structure of DNA permits it to be coiled extremely tightly, so that great lengths can be packed onto every chromosome.

7 The cell begins to divide. Each part now contains only 23 chromosomes, although each one is split into two chromatids.

8 After the cell has divided completely, with each half containing a set of 23 chromosomes, each still doubled, poles again begin to form in each and the chromosomes line up prior to the next cell division.

9 This time the chromosomes split in half and the halves are pulled to the opposite poles. The cell then divides as before; each part has 23 chromosomes.

10 The process of meiosis is now complete; each cell has a unique mix of genes, combining the parental cells in a new way. Such cells are known as gametes, and become the functional part of sperm or ova, ready for fertilization.

Identical twins are ideal for the study of the relative effects of heredity and environment

The genetic identity of twins

Unless and until cloning becomes a reality, the closest degree of genetic identity possible among humans is between twins. Monozygotic twins come from the same fertilized egg and therefore have identical sets of genes. Dizygotic twins arise from the fertilization of two separate eggs and are no closer genetically than any two siblings born years apart. Studies on both sorts have helped geneticists to explore many questions about the differing influences of genes and environment on behavior.

The usual approach is to compare monozygotic twins who have lived apart – with each other, and perhaps also with pairs who have not been separated. One such survey indicated that the average difference in height between monozygotic twins was less than half that between all other siblings. The strong influence of heredity was confirmed by the very small height difference between the twins who grew up apart and their identical brothers or sisters.

Another study revealed that whereas schizophrenia symptoms occurred in only 15 percent of persons whose dizygotic twin had such symptoms, this "concordance" figure for monozygotic twin pairs was 80 percent. And although tuberculosis is an infection, transmitted between individuals by bacteria, monozygotic twins raised in the same household are much more often concordant for TB than are dizygotic twins.

Identical twins are more likely to be left-handed than other people. Although handedness does not seem to be a genetically determined trait, it could be related to hormone levels in the womb, which may possibly cause an uneven development of the two sides of the brain.

Simple inheritance

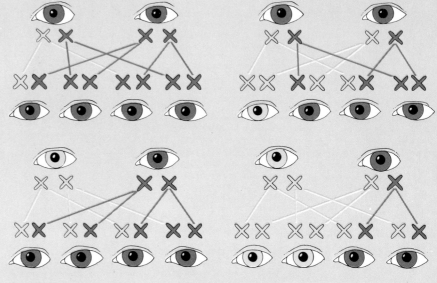

✕✕	Chromosomes carrying blue-eye gene
✕✕	Chromosomes carrying brown-eye gene
👁	Person with blue eyes
👁	Person with brown eyes

▲ *Eye color is a classic example of simple inheritance. The blue-eye gene is recessive, brown dominant, so that a person with blue eyes must inherit that gene from both parents. A brown-eyed person may carry the blue-eye gene, and pass it on to the next generation, but it will not be expressed unless it encounters another similar gene.*

A German zoologist, August Weismann (1834-1914), was the first to suggest that chromosomes contain hereditary substances. We now know that genetic messages, coded by sequences of the four units in the DNA molecule, determine not only characteristics long recognized as carried in families such as brown or blue eyes, but many more subtle ones. Eye color is among the simplest traits to trace. It is determined by a gene found in two alternative versions, known as alleles. That responsible for brown eyes is described as dominant over its blue counterpart. After genes have been randomly assorted at fertilization, a baby may inherit from its parents either two blue genes, two brown genes, or one blue and one brown. But only in the first case will it have blue eyes. With one gene of each type, brown dominates over the "recessive" blue – which expresses itself only when accompanied by another blue. People with brown eyes are therefore commoner; even when carrying blue genes they are likely to produce brown-eyed children if they marry someone with brown eyes. A person with two (dominant or recessive) identical alleles is described as homozygous for that gene. Someone with two different alleles is heterozygous.

Sometimes a dominant trait misses a generation. A study of pedigrees shows that the web-toed condition known as syndactyly behaves as though caused by a dominant gene. Occasionally, however, it is not expressed in individuals known to carry the gene in its double, homozygous dose. DNA coding the relevant (mis)information is in fact present, but the outward effect is so slight as to be undetectable. Such a gene is said to lack penetrance.

Total color-blindness is caused by a recessive gene and is extremely rare. Red-green color-blindness, which affects about one person in 30, provides an example of linkage. Commoner in men than women, the condition is attributable to genes on the X chromosome. When a color-blind man marries a normal woman, their children will probably

Monozygotic twins	Dizygotic twins

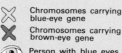

▲ *Identical, or monozygotic, twins are the result of the division of a single egg into two separate embryos; this takes place within two weeks of fertilization. They are both male or both female. They also share a single placenta. Non-identical, or dizygotic, twins originate from separate ova. They have separate placentas, and need not be the same sex.*

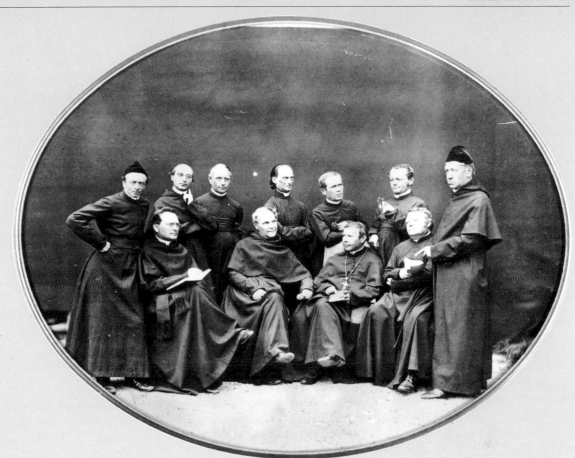

▶ Gregor Mendel (1822-1894), seen here third from the right, was a Bohemian monk who carried out experiments in plant breeding in the 1850s and 1860s. He studied the effects of crossing tall and short pea plants over several generations, and concluded that these characteristics were not merged in the later generations, as should have been expected under the existing theories: the original characteristics of tallness and shortness were fully retained in a proportion of the plants. To explain this he proposed independent factors, some dominant and others recessive. His published results were so theoretically perfect that the British geneticist R.A. Fisher suggested that a zealous assistant may have taken it upon himself to "tidy up" the data. Mendel's work was barely known until the 1900s, when it was seen to solve questions arising from the discovery of chromosomes.

be normal, although all the daughters will be "carriers" (though they will have normal vision themselves). But when a woman carrying the color-blindness gene marries a normal man half their sons will be color-blind and half their daughters will be carriers. Although a girl with a color-blind father inherits his X chromosome and his defective gene, she may also receive its normal allele from her mother. Despite the aberrant gene, the normal X chromosome assures normal vision. In turn, half of her sons will have the defective gene and color-blindness. The other half will have the normal gene and normal sight.

Defects of this sort originate as mutations. These are rare alterations in genes which, though often lethal, also provide the valuable variations upon which natural selection works during the process of evolution. Mutations occur in cells throughout the body, causing differences in the pigmentation of patches of skin, for example. But to be inherited they must take place in the egg cells or spermatozoa. The frequency of mutation in humans is thought to be around one in 100,000 per gene per generation. There are some 500,000 sites for mutation on the human chromosomes, so every individual probably carries at least one such mutated gene. Exposure to X-rays, other forms of high-energy radiation and certain chemicals increases the mutation rate considerably.

Until the rediscovery of Gregor Mendel's work in 1900, people assumed that a father and mother's hereditary traits blended in their offspring. This seemed obvious from the observation that many characteristics in children were indeed intermediate between those of their parents. It was Mendel's demonstration of particulate inheritance in plants which led to the recognition of similar Mendelian patterns of heredity (like that of eye color) in animals, including humans. Further study, however, revealed that some attributes are inherited in a more complex manner than this, their presence depending on the interaction of many genes.

Sex-linked inheritance

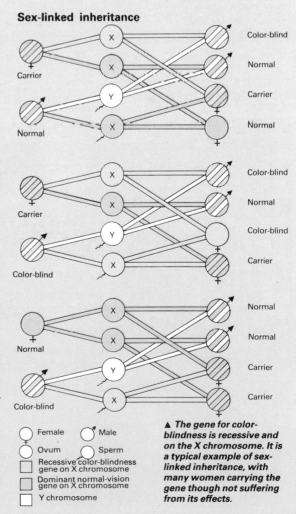

▲ The gene for color-blindness is recessive and on the X chromosome. It is a typical example of sex-linked inheritance, with many women carrying the gene though not suffering from its effects.

Studying the inheritance of blood groups has helped explain why some diseases are more common in certain regions

An early subject of genetic research, and one with great practical significance, was blood groups. The surfaces of red blood cells carry antigens (♦ page 214) which trigger off the production of destructive antibodies if blood is injected into someone with a different genetic makeup. For blood to be transfused successfully, therefore, it has to be "typed", and the donor's blood group matched with that of the recipient. There are 14 different categories of genes controlling the blood group antigens, the most familiar being the ABO system. Instead of two alternative alleles, as with eye color, ABO blood types are controlled by three genes. These multiple alleles are A, B and O. The first two, which are dominant to the third, cause the red cells to produce antigens A and B respectively. If AA or AO blood is transfused into a BB or BO person, it is attacked by anti-A antibodies. The reverse happens if BB or BO blood is given to an AA or AO individual. OO people carry no antigens on their cells, and they do not manufacture antibodies against the other blood types. Such people are known as universal donors.

Enormous numbers of individuals have now been typed throughout the world, and blood group genes are better known than any others in Man. This has led to the recognition that these genes, like many others, have more than one effect. People who develop duodenal ulcers, for example, include more of group O than would be expected by chance, while group A individuals are 20 percent more likely to develop cancer of the stomach than those of the O or B groups. There may be other, as-yet-unknown beneficial effects to balance the risks and benefits and to maintain a "polymorphism" in the population. One example of balanced polymorphism is that of the gene which causes sickle-cell

The discovery of blood groups
Austrian doctor and chemist Karl Landsteiner (1868-1943) was the discoverer of blood groups. He introduced the ABO system in 1909 and received the Nobel Prize in 1930. Working in Vienna, Landsteiner noticed that red blood cells soon disintegrated after being injected into animals of a different species. Later he demonstrated how red cells in blood from one individual sometimes clumped together if blood serum from another person was added. This led him to the idea that blood can be classified into groups. But it was not until the War of 1914-18, with its horrendous toll of injuries, that many clinicians realized the importance of Landsteiner's work. His second major contribution, not fully developed until after he died, was to show how other blood groups (particularly the MN system, which he uncovered in conjunction with Philip Levine) could be used in cases of disputed paternity. MN typing shows, for example, that if a baby is MN and the mother M, its father cannot be M too. Similarly, if a baby is MN and the mother N, the father cannot be N. Such findings are now widely employed in court to settle cases of disputed paternity.

▼ *The incidence of blood groups in the indigenous populations varies widely. The American Indians are the only peoples with a single type (O). The B-group gene is commonest in Asia.*

► *"Lot and his Daughters", by Jan Massys. After his wife turned into a pillar of salt, Lot had children by each of his daughters, in the Genesis incest story. Both families flourished.*

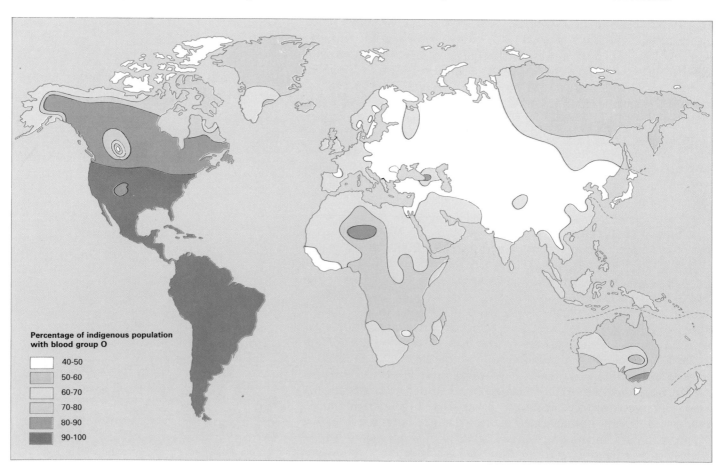

Percentage of indigenous population with blood group O

	40-50
	50-60
	60-70
	70-80
	80-90
	90-100

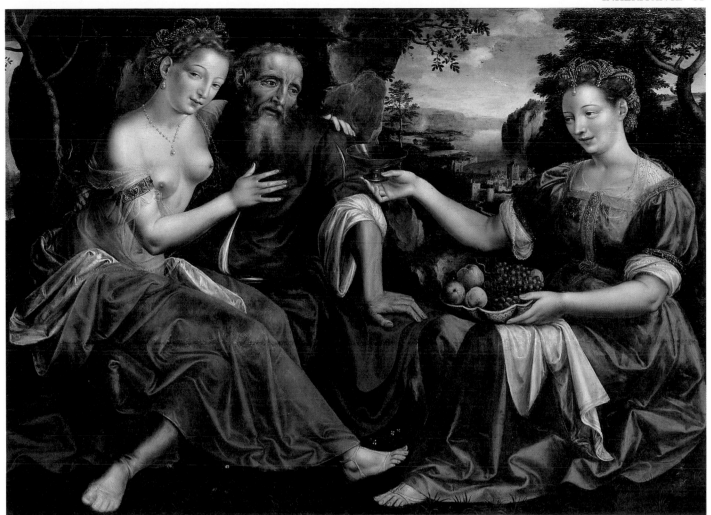

anemia in Africa. Although homozygotes suffer this very serious disease, heterozygotes enjoy some protection against malaria. That is why the gene has not been eliminated during the course of evolution.

More complex again than the simple alternative alleles, like those for eye color, is the interaction of many different genes to produce an end result. Such polygenic inheritance, which mimics the blending inheritance believed in before Mendel, is exemplified by height. Francis Galton (1822-1911), an English mathematician who turned to the measurement of populations, first highlighted the "normal curve" for height, with a few very short and very tall individuals and a bulge of average people in the middle. Here, as with intelligence, weight and other qualities showing continuous variation, innumerable genes are at work. Their influence can be seen from the way in which tallness and shortness run in families. But polygenic inheritance makes it impossible to discern clear patterns or to make firm predictions.

Another factor which complicates efforts to trace patterns of inheritance is the tendency for people to choose partners similar to themselves. Such assortive mating helps explain why correlations are often found between husbands and wives in characteristics such as height, IQ and even skin coloring. Geneticists studying human heredity have to make allowance for this non-genetic factor.

One mating practice proscribed by most societies is inbreeding between close relatives. Although laws to prohibit incest probably arose through the need to maintain social harmony, we now recognize biological objections to inbreeding – particularly in its extreme, incestuous form. Every human being carries dangerous recessive genes, and the chances of two of these coming together are increased greatly when closely-related individuals reproduce.

Skin color

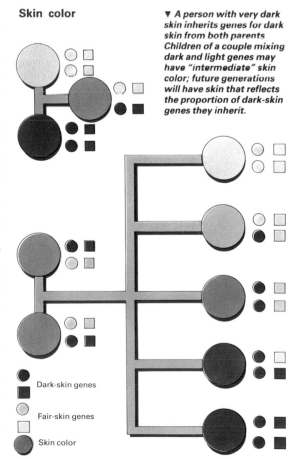

▼ A person with very dark skin inherits genes for dark skin from both parents. Children of a couple mixing dark and light genes may have "intermediate" skin color; future generations will have skin that reflects the proportion of dark-skin genes they inherit.

● Dark-skin genes

○ Fair-skin genes

□ Skin color

See also
The Human Body 9-20
Sex and Reproduction 177-88
Reproductive Defects 189-92
Medicine before Birth 193-200
The Body's Defenses 213-20

The genetic basis of disease

During recent years, our knowledge of the genetic basis of disease has taken two massive steps forward. First, scientists have traced several single-gene disorders much further than just to the defective genes, to the precise DNA regions carrying those defects. Sickle-cell anemia, for example, results from an error in just one of the units in the corresponding stretch of DNA. The new technique of gene-mapping is revealing the molecular basis of many more conditions of this sort. Some types of dwarfism caused by a hereditary shortage of growth hormone, for example, result from deletions of the genes that should regulate production of the hormone. In addition to single-gene diseases such as hemophilia and those (like Down's syndrome; ▶ page 197) which result from chromosomal abnormalities, we now know that many others are related to specific hereditary factors. The starting point for this discovery was the recognition of human leukocyte antigens (HLAs). Like blood groups, these are markers which must be matched if the tissues of a kidney, heart or other transplant are to be accepted rather than rejected by the recipient (▶ page 218). The genes responsible for HLAs are on a short arm of human chromosome six. But certain alleles of those genes, either singly or in combination, occur more frequently in people with particular diseases. Among conditions which are clearly related to HLA genes are rheumatoid arthritis, multiple sclerosis, ankylosing spondylitis, and Hodgkin's disease. A hereditary element has had to be acknowledged, in addition to other more obvious factors such as alcohol in alcoholic cirrhosis of the liver, and *Mycobacterium leprae* in leprosy.

Some HLA genes are more strongly associated than others with their corresponding illnesses. A person with HLA-B27 is over 87 times more likely to develop ankylosing spondylitis than someone without it. The antigen, found in 90 percent of patients, occurs in only 9·4 percent of healthy controls. But HLA-A1, the antigen linked with Hodgkin's disease (▶ page 228), increases the likelihood of developing the disease by only 1·4 times. As molecular biologists build up human gene maps of increasing sophistication, the opportunities will grow for discriminating ever more finely the hereditary determinants of both health and disease.

The incest taboo

Studies of close mating confirm expectations that it increases the risk of harmful recessive genes coming together. In the USA the percentage mortality among offspring during the first ten years is 8·1 percent for first-cousin matings, compared with 2·4 percent for unrelated marriages. Corresponding figures for Japanese children aged one to eight are 4·6 percent and 1·5 percent, while in France those of babies up to one month are 9·3 percent and 3·9 percent. The mortality risk for children from relationships between fathers and daughters, mothers and sons, or brothers and sisters (the relations who have about half their genes in common), is four times higher still. The number of societies in which close unions are usual has declined recently, and greater mobility and other social factors are likely to make such unions less common in future. However, while exogamy or outbreeding will be beneficial in promoting "hybrid vigor" (as is recognized by plant and animal breeders), it will also have adverse consequences. With the death of a malformed child, born to close relatives and carrying a pair of lethal recessives, those genes also disappear. If such matings are avoided, the deleterious genes will be conserved and passed to future generations. A similar problem is posed by the introduction of genetic counselling to discourage unrelated people who carry lethal recessives from choosing each other as mates.

The coming together of two lethal recessives may appear to be an event of Calvinistic determinism; but the fortuitous role of probability should not be overlooked. Like the random mixing which occurs at every fertilization, there is also an element of chance in the assortment of two portfolios of genes containing potentially harmful combinations. As exemplified in the past by the Rothschilds, described by Miriam Rothschild in her book "Dear Lord Rothschild" (1983) as a "truly incestuous family", consanguineous matings can and do occur without disastrous consequences.

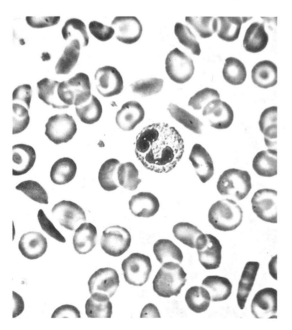

◀ ▶ **Sickle-cell anemia is a disease in which the red blood cells contain abnormal hemoglobin, which tends to form stiff, rodlike structures and distort the blood cells into the elongated, flat and pointed form characteristic of the disease. They lose their oxygen-carrying abilities and may tend to clog up the blood vessels, thus causing damage to body tissues. The incidence of sickle-cell anemia (which is caused by a recessive gene and must be inherited from both parents) tends to be related geographically to the incidence of malaria, since the sickle-cell gene seems to confer a degree of immunity from malaria. Thus it has flourished in malarial regions of Africa and the Middle East.**

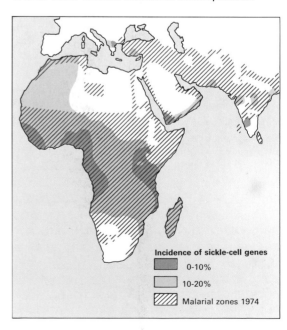

Incidence of sickle-cell genes

▨ 0-10%

☐ 10-20%

▨ Malarial zones 1974

The multiple causes of illness...The challenge to medicine...Health for rich and poor...The development of modern medicine...PERSPECTIVE...Ancient medicine... Medieval and Renaissance medicine...Medicine and science...Identifying microbes...Medicine in the 17th century...Seeing into the body...Paying for medicine

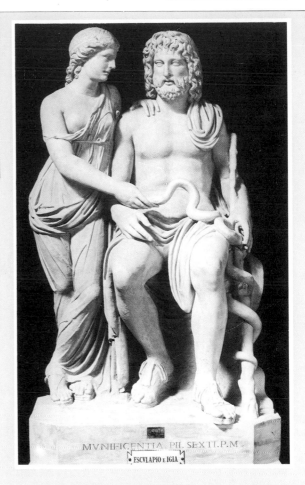

From earliest times, efforts to understand how the body is constructed and how it works have gone hand-in-hand with attempts to comprehend and treat ill health. Whether by probing human anatomy or by charting physiological processes, investigators have provided insights not only into normality but also into the abnormality that we call disease. Erratically at first, and with many false trails, this rational approach led to modern medical science, whose spectacular triumphs range from the global eradication of smallpox to the transplantation of ailing organs and the exquisite intricacies of brain surgery. Today, recognition of these achievements is tempered by two cautions. First the benefits of science-based medicine have been applied inequitably, leaving appalling imbalances in the burden of disease between countries of the North and the South. Second, mechanistic methods have been so successful that they may have obscured the subtle interplay between mind and body, and eclipsed healing as an art.

Health and illness

The achievements of medical science in this century, and the possible limitations of those achievements, both derive from the idea that particular diseases have particular causes (♦ page 37). In recent years scientists have found that, for a number of reasons (♦ page 40), people vary considerably in their innate susceptibility to many illnesses, including infections. A prime example is coronary heart disease. While arguments continue about their relative weight, many different factors influence the condition's onset and course (♦ page 161). For this reason, and because personality and mental attitude are also relevant, coronary heart disease is one of those which critics of wholly materialistic medicine have highlighted as needing a holistic approach. While not repudiating medical science, holistic practitioners advocate a return to the Hippocratic approach of treating the whole person rather than tinkering with specific malfunctioning parts.

The multifactorial nature of disease is the principal explanation for the contrasts in health between and within different societies. Thus many of the conditions responsible for mass mortality in the Third World are not exotic tropical diseases confined to those regions by accidents of geography. They are infections like measles, made more virulent by poverty and malnutrition. "Diseases of civilization", on the other hand, are those (like coronary heart disease) which are associated with overeating and other aspects of the affluent lifestyle. Even within developed countries, different socio-economic groups show persistent disparities in measures such as perinatal mortality rate (stillbirths and deaths in the first four weeks). There are, in turn, several causes of these contrasts, including differences in nutrition, living conditions, and access to and use of medical services.

▲ *Asclepius, the Greek god of medicine, mentioned by Homer in the "Iliad" as a physician, but later deified as the god of medicine and son of Apollo, was killed by Zeus in case he passed his knowledge on to humankind. His cult was celebrated at temples at Epidavros and Kos, where a ritualistic form of treatment was offered for many diseases, involving interpretation of dreams and purification.*

The origins of scientific medicine
Knowledge of anatomy, physiology and pathology as we now understand them began to emerge with the Greeks. They were also the first to recognize the distinction between internal and external causes of illness, which became a vital strand in the emergence of scientific medicine.

Hippocrates (c.460-c.377 BC) was a blend of scientist and artist, who examined his patients at the temple-hospital on the island of Kos with both empathy and rationality. He believed that disease occurred when four humors – blood from the heart, yellow bile from the liver, black bile from the spleen and phlegm from the brain – became out of balance. Although long discredited, this theory was important in combining a picture of the body as a machine, subject to adjustment when it malfunctioned, with an awareness that the whole person was much more than the sum of the individual parts, and should be given treatment accordingly. In this, Hippocratic medicine paralleled the even older Chinese tradition, founded on the complementary principles of yin (female principle) and yang (male), whose correct proportions were essential for health.

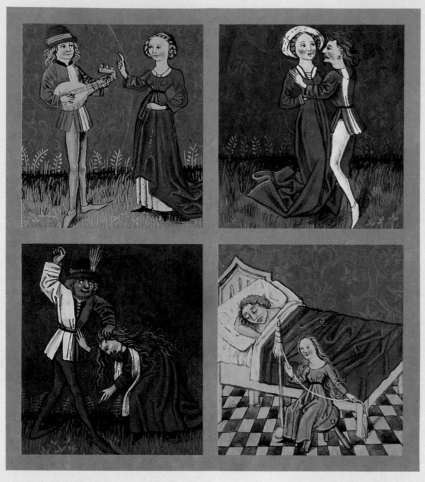

Egyptian medicine

The ancient Egyptians seem to have been the first to realize the possibility of rational therapy, albeit through attempts to placate evil spirits. Many of their drugs were foul substances, given in the belief that they would be unwelcome to the demons possessing patients' bodies. Gradually, however, cause and effect became apparent as practitioners noted the difference between poisonous, ineffective and genuinely potent preparations. The Egyptians also anticipated the scientific stance in another sense, with doctors specializing in eyes, bellies, heads and other parts of the body.

The authorities of medieval medicine

Although more often remembered for his erroneous ideas about the physical world, Aristotle (384-322 BC) was a prime figure in the history of Greek medicine. By dissecting small animals and describing their internal anatomy, he laid the foundations for the later scrutiny of the human body. The person who took the next major step was Galen of Pergamon (AD 129-199), who dissected rhesus monkeys and possibly also human bodies. He described the arteries and veins, itemized tendons and muscles, classified bones, and even revealed the working of the nervous system by severing a pig's spinal cord at different points and demonstrating that corresponding parts of the body became paralyzed. After Galen's death, however, anatomical research ceased and his work was considered infallible for 1200 years.

Challenging Galen

It was only with the work of Andreas Vesalius (1514-1564) that Galen's ideas were challenged. Vesalius became professor of anatomy and surgery at Padua immediatey after graduating in 1537, and began a lifetime of scrupulous dissection of the human body. In his "De Humani Corporis Fabrica" he illustrated not just what bodily parts looked like, but how they worked.

▲ **Temperaments associated with the four humors – phlegmatic, sanguine, choleric and melancholic. The humors were said to govern character as well as health.**

▼ **A medieval illustration of collecting and preparing herbs. In the 16th and 17th centuries this skill formed the essence of pharmacy and was based on empirical knowledge and on folklore.**

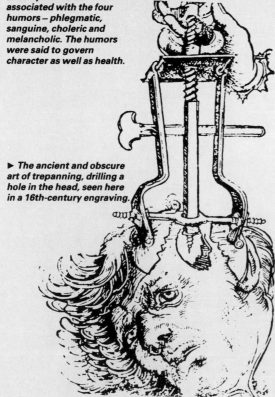

► **The ancient and obscure art of trepanning, drilling a hole in the head, seen here in a 16th-century engraving.**

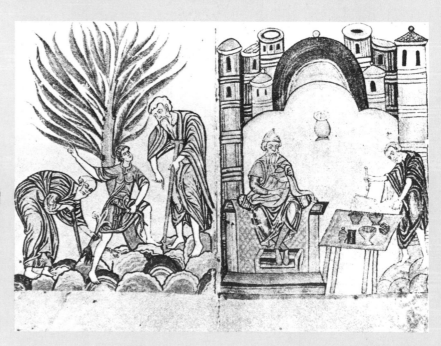

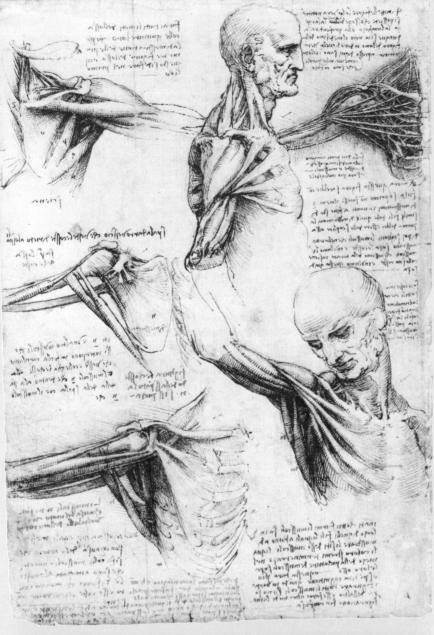

Renaissance medicine

The tradition established by Vesalius was continued by a succession of researchers at Padua including Gabriello Fallopio (1523-1562), discoverer of the Fallopian tubes, and Sanctorio Sanctorius (1561-1636) who initiated the serious study of body chemistry. A remarkable phase of conquest was completed when William Harvey demonstrated the circulation of the blood in the early 17th century and Marcello Malpighi revealed the blood capillaries as the link between arteries and veins.

Such efforts were greeted with skepticism by vitalists, who believed that the body's workings could never be fully understood in material terms. Similar opposition confronted the physicians and biologists who were increasingly successful in understanding living creatures as machines. It was Thomas Sydenham (1624-1689), an English physician with little interest in anatomy, who took the next rational step, by trying to specify and classify different illnesses. Distinguishing diseases from their victims, hc also suggcstcd that at least some were due to particular agents fighting against the healing powers of the body. This led to a spate of accurate descriptions of diseases – notably by Bernardino Ramazzini (1633-1714), an Italian physician who founded occupational medicine by listing the conditions associated with 40 trades.

The increasingly close liaison between medicine and science was furthered in the 18th century by such figures as Stephen Hales, the first person to measure blood pressure; Albert von Haller, pioneer in the study of nerves and muscles; and Claude Bernard, who began to delineate the process of digestion and founded experimental medicine.

◄ **The muscles of the shoulder, by Leonardo da Vlncl (1452-1519). Leonardo's very detailed anatomical studies were in advance of any in his time, but they were never published and his knowledge was lost or ignored at the time. Only very occasionally, as in a drawing of the circulation of the blood through the heart, did his work show any reliance on Galenic ideas rather than on individual observation.**

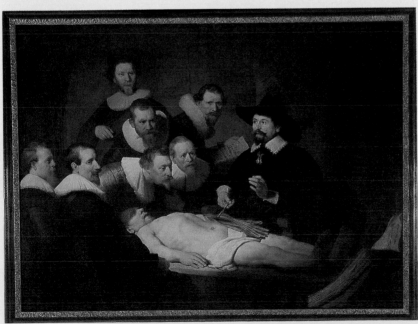

◄ **"The Anatomy Lesson", (1632) by Rembrandt in which the students intently observe dissection.**

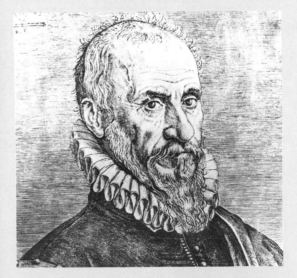

▲ **Ambroise Paré (c. 1510-1590), the French military surgeon who introduced more humane surgery.**

Bacteria were discovered a century before they were known to cause illnesses

► *Louis Pasteur (1822-1895), seen here testing a vaccine on himself; his observations of the exact relationships between microbes and diseases revolutionized medical science.*

▼ *Florence Nightingale (1820-1910), the English woman who established the first professional nursing service, for British soldiers in the Crimean War (1853-1856). On her return she helped to lay the foundations for a new style of health care, with well-run and hygienic wards in airy hospitals.*

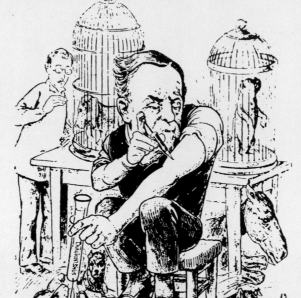

Discovering microbes

The marriage between medicine and science was consummated in the late 19th century by a group of scientists who finally showed that unseen micro-organisms caused epidemics and other diseases now known as infections. This idea was a venerable one, supported by the efficacy of measures such as the quarantine which kept bubonic plague out of Venice between 1370 and 1374. Yet there was no proof – not even when Anton van Leeuwenhoek (1632-1723) used his finely-ground lenses to discover "animalcules" (which we would now recognize as microbes such as bacteria) in the late 17th century. The Dutch linen draper was well ahead of his time – further investigations of the microbial world, and of its relationship to health had to await technical improvements in the microscope, which did not come for over 100 years.

Even when micro-organisms were more widely recognized, proof that they are transmitted from person to person, causing particular diseases, was not possible until the idea of spontaneous generation had been discredited. In 1688 the Italian physician Francesco Redi (1626-1697) had demonstrated that maggots did not develop in decaying meat when it was protected from contamination by flies. But it was not until the mid-19th century that the French chemist Louis Pasteur (1822-1895) confirmed that "animalcules" too did not appear, unless introduced from the outside, in food materials that had been sterilized by boiling.

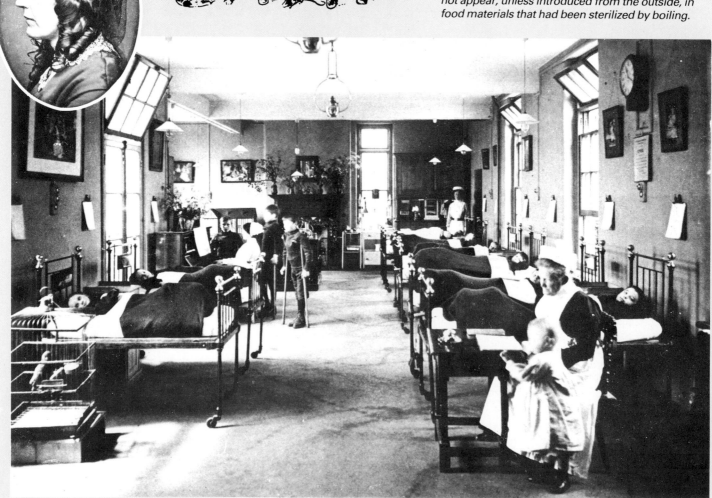

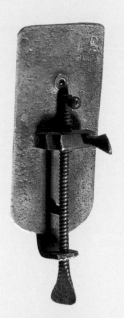

▲ The first microscope, made by Anton van Leeuwenhoek (1632-1723), with a single, powerful lens set within a brass plate.

▶ The introduction of ether and chloroform as anesthetics revolutionized surgery for surgeons as well as patients.

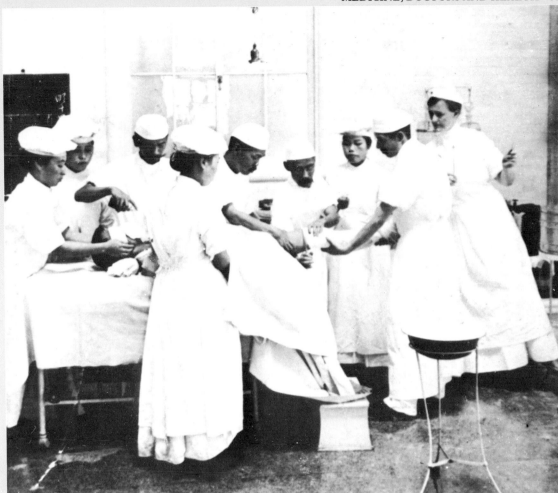

Medicine in the 19th century

Pasteur made a second discovery that was to transform the practise of medicine. Asked to investigate occasional irregularities in wine and vinegar making, he found that each was promoted by a particular sort of microbe and that when the processes went awry a different organism was present. Undrinkable "ropey" or "oily" wine, for example, always resulted from contamination with specific, atypical types of microbe. It was a short but brilliant step from these "diseases" of wine to the idea that human and other animal maladies might also be produced by specific, characteristic sorts of micro-organism. But so it proved. Beginning with chicken cholera, and anthrax in sheep, Pasteur found that they too were caused by corresponding bacterial species. This led him to highly successful efforts to weaken the organisms by aging them so that when injected into healthy animals they no longer triggered the disease but did elicit specific immunity. Although Edward Jenner had pioneered vaccination against smallpox nearly a century before, Pasteur's was the demonstration that established the feasibility of immunization in general and led to the conquest of conditions such as diphtheria and poliomyelitis.

Another result of Pasteur's earliest experiments was that the English surgeon Joseph Lister (1827-1912) devised a method of overcoming a severe problem created by the very success of another branch of medicine. In the mid-19th century, the American dentist Thomas Morton (1819-1868) and the Scottish physician James Simpson (1811-1870) pioneered the use of ether as an anesthetic. Chloroform was introduced shortly afterwards.

These developments were a great boon to practitioners of surgery – transforming amputation, for example, from a maneuver that was agonizing for patients and required unrealistically speedy dexterity from surgeons. They had also made it possible to contemplate sophisticated and time-consuming operations deep inside the body. By facilitating surgery, however, the availability of anesthesia had focused more attention on one of its complications: vile, suppurating wounds. It was Lister, shortly after Pasteur had shown that suppuration too was caused by micro-organisms, who began using a carbolic spray to play over the operation site. By reducing postoperative infection dramatically, antiseptic surgery (soon superseded by aseptic methods in which all materials and dressings were sterilized) transformed the work of surgeons. Together with the later introduction of blood transfusion, it also encouraged further innovation in operations.

The German bacteriologist Robert Koch (1843-1910) took Pasteur's work further and established the supreme importance of specific etiology – the idea that particular diseases have particular causes. Between 1879 and 1900, the causative agents of at least 22 infections were confirmed using Koch's approach. In turn this prompted the idea of a specific therapy, the use of drugs targeted like magic bullets to seek out and kill "pathogens" without harming the tissues of the body. The founder of the science of chemotherapy, based on this hope, was the German bacteriologist Paul Ehrlich (1854-1915). Ehrlich's greatest triumph came in treating human syphilis with an arsenic compound, Salvarsan, in 1911.

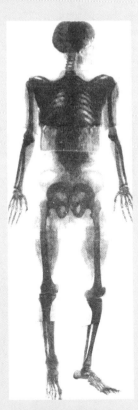

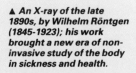

▲ An X-ray of the late 1890s, by Wilhelm Röntgen (1845-1923); his work brought a new era of non-invasive study of the body in sickness and health.

Imaging the Body

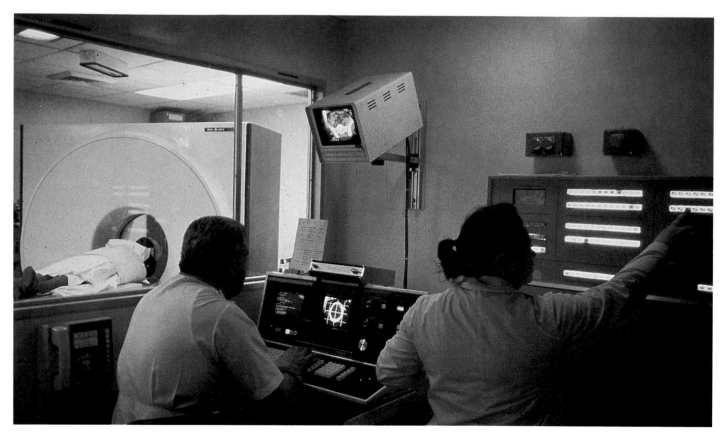

Seeing into the body

Ever since X-rays were first used in 1895 to capture a likeness of the bones of the human hand, scientists have been looking for better and safer ways of monitoring the internal workings of the body. The X-ray remains the most frequently used diagnostic imaging test. For routine screening for lung disease and detection of simple fractures, it is quick, cheap and effective. But it does have limitations in detecting abnormalities deep inside the body, and its risk of damaging the fetus makes it unsuitable for monitoring pregnant women.

Three developments in imaging which have occurred since the 1950s – two of them since 1970 – have enabled doctors to get a better view of the body than ever before. In the first of these, ultrasonography, sound waves inaudible to the human ear are bounced off the internal structures of the body. The "echoes" which are picked up as the sounds leave the body vary according to the density of the tissues through which they have passed. Ultrasound is especially useful in detecting objects lying in a watery environment, a fact that makes it perfect for monitoring the growth of the fetus. Recent developments with the technique give moving pictures of the baby.

Ultrasound is frequently used to detect fetal abnormalities such as spina bifida, as well as to check for normal growth; and some of the most skilled technicians can recognize abnormalities inside the heart of the fetus.

Ultrasound is also useful in imaging some other organs such as the gall bladder which are difficult to pick up with other techniques because of their position in the body.

In computerized axial tomography (CAT, or CT) scanning, X-rays are passed through the body and a computer converts data on the amount of X-ray absorbed by each tissue into a picture of the internal structures. Each picture is made up of thousands of tiny dots, and can differentiate between bone, fat, muscle and water because of the variations in the amount of X-rays absorbed by these tissues. "Slices" of tissues are examined to detect tumors, blood clots and other abnormalities which would be invisible to normal X-ray machines.

CT scanning is increasingly used in hospitals, but it too has limitations; and the risks which accompany exposure to X-rays from regular CT scans cannot be ignored. These problems may be avoided if the newest technique, nuclear magnetic resonance (NMR), fulfills its initial promise.

NMR does not use X-rays. Instead, radio waves of a known frequency are passed through the body in a huge magnetic field. When the magnet is switched on, the atoms in the body are excited by the radio waves and move into a high-energy state. As they lose this energy they give off weak radio signals which can be picked up and converted into a picture of tissues. The frequency of the radio waves can be tailored according to elements most common in the particular tissues to be investigated. So if doctors wish to check the pattern of hydrogen (most common in watery tissues), carbon (bone), phosphorus (muscle) or other elements in a tissue, they can choose the appropriate frequency.

Although NMR is safer and more effective it is too expensive and experimental to take over from CT scanning and ultrasound in the near future.

▲ A CT scan computer detects differences between radiation emitted and the rays detected after passing through the body.

▼ Thermography detects variations in the heat given off by parts of the body; it is particularly useful in detecting cancers.

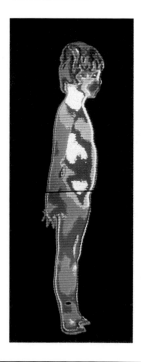

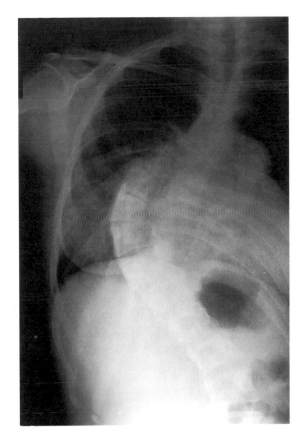

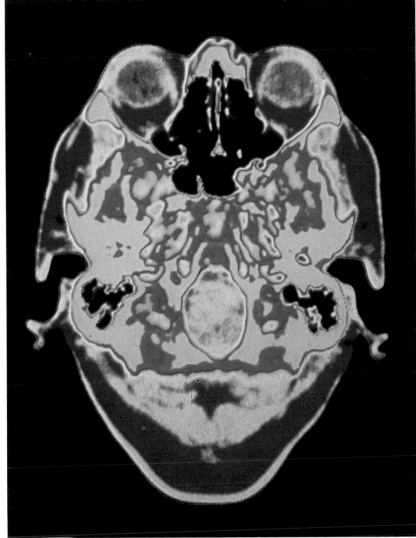

▲ *X-ray of a malformed vertebral column. X-rays remain the most common diagnostic aid used for skeletal and lung disorders.*

▶ *CT scans allow doctors to investigate the relative position of the organs. This is a slice through the base of the skull and eyeballs*

▼ *Ultrasound offers an opportunity to study pregnancy, without the dangers of X-rays. Here the head of the fetus is visible.*

▶ *NMR scans, as of this slice through a chest, can detect subtle changes in tissue composition, and are completely non-invasive.*

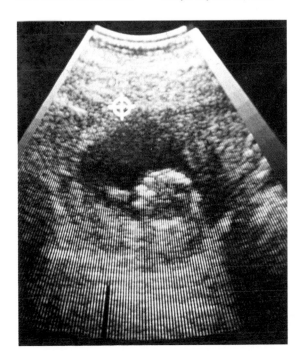

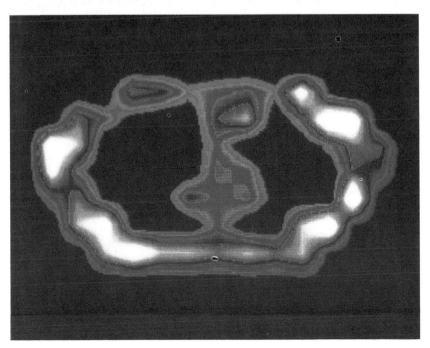

Towards the modern age

During the early 20th century, many drugs were discovered to destroy infections without harming the patient. In 1932, German physician Gerhard Domagk (1895-1964) introduced the first of the sulfa drugs, which produced near-miraculous cures for scarlet fever, meningitis, gonorrhea and several other infections. During the Second World War, the Australian pathologist Howard Florey (1898-1968) and the German biochemist Ernst Chain (1906-1979) developed penicillin on the basis of observations made ten years earlier by the Scots bacteriologist Alexander Fleming (1881-1955), thereby launching the golden age of antibiotics – substances produced by one organism which destroy or inhibit the growth of others. Penicillin was even more effective than the sulfa drugs, had virtually no side-effects and acted against a wide range of bacteria. Together with the wide-spectrum tetracyclines and streptomycin, the anti-tuberculosis antibiotic isolated in the USA during 1944 by emigré Ukrainian Selman Waksman (1888-1973), later semi-synthetic versions of penicillin have transformed the treatment of infectious disease.

The idea that diseases have particular causes did not just apply to infections; it was underlined by the discovery early this century of vitamins – specific chemicals whose absence created characteristic patterns of symptoms. Around the same time an English physician, Archibald Garrod (1857-1936), described several hereditary defects such as phenylketonuria, the end-results of particular defective genes. Specific etiology gained further support when a lack of insulin was found to be the cause of diabetes, and when certain forms of anemia proved to be attributable to irregularities in the hemoglobin molecule. During very recent years the theory has been strengthened further with the detection of oncogenes – particular fragments of the DNA double-helix which are thought to be the basic causes of certain types of cancer. There are also suggestions that some forms of mental illness are caused by certain associated aberrations in the chemistry of the brain.

The complex causes of disease

Despite this succession of triumphs in accounting for disease, specific etiology has had its critics. At the outset, two skeptics (◆ page 141) demonstrated their disbelief over the alleged discovery of the cholera bacillus by consuming large amounts of it with impunity. This led to a recognition that an encounter with a pathogenic microbe is rarely sufficient for it to produce its relevant illness. Although the tubercle bacillus, for example, is necessary for tuberculosis to develop, and is in one sense therefore the cause of the disease, other factors such as malnutrition and fatigue play an important part in determining the outcome of infection. A healthy, well-nourished body may respond vigorously by repelling the invaders and becoming immune, without the individual concerned even being aware of the fact. But someone whose diet has been inadequate to sustain those defenses may succumb to what used to be called consumption and die an early death. Such discoveries, plus those of the HL antigens which are genetically determined markers on our tissues but are apparently related to the likelihood of contracting particular diseases (◆ page 32), and the knowledge that the state of mind can influence one's susceptibility to diseases (including cancer) and chances of recovering from them, have made the medical profession increasingly aware in recent years that understanding the causes of disease is not simplistic.

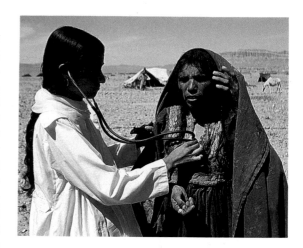

▲ ▼ *A "barefoot doctor" in Pakistan, trained in simple techniques of recognizing and treating diseases. The number of patients to each doctor in different countries underlines the problem of aiming at "health for all" by AD 2000.*

Population per physician

East Africa
Central Africa
West Africa
South-East Asia
South Central Asia
North Africa
Southern Africa
East Asia
South West Asia
Caribbean
Central America
South America
Oceania
Europe and North America

0   2,500   5,000   7,500   10,000   12,500   15,000   17,500

Paying for health

Modern medicine is too expensive for most individuals, even in wealthy areas, and many countries run health insurance schemes. Germany was the first nation to institute health insurance when, in 1883, the government launched a plan by which employers and workers in certain industries contributed payments towards a fund covering medical care in the event of illness. Since then, many other public and private schemes have come into being, providing full or partial settlement of physicians' and hospital fees, drug bills, and ancillary expenses. Britain's National Health Service, inaugurated by the post-war Labour administration in 1946, was designed to ensure that medical attention was free at the time of need, all working persons and employers making compulsory contributions. At the other extreme, American schemes such as Blue Cross are entirely private and optional, with gradations of dues and benefits. Some governments subsidize private insurance plans of this sort. Cover for hospital charges is the commonest form of private medical insurance, particularly in countries like the USA where medical expenses can be cripplingly severe.

The Senses

The major senses...The varieties of touch...How the eye works...Color vision...The structure of the ear... The sense of balance...Taste and smell, mysterious senses...Pain...PERSPECTIVE...Blind sight...Magnetic sense?...Sensing your own body...Pheromones, sexual attraction?

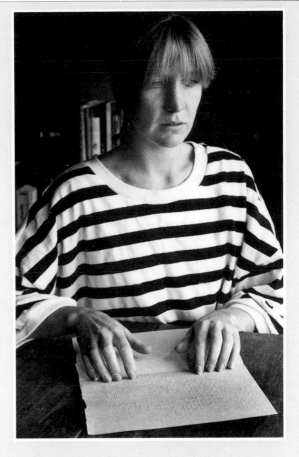

Touch, sight, hearing, taste and smell – the five senses classified by the Greek philosopher and biologist Aristotle (384-322 BC) – were supposed to be the windows of the soul. We still tend to think of them as the primary senses, but we now recognize additional "modalities" such as balance, and the sensitivity of the skin to temperature, pressure and pain. Although the sensations they perceive differ widely, the cells responsible for the various senses resemble each other in occurring on body surfaces and in reacting only to particular stimuli.

We are also more conscious than Aristotle of the fact that information provided by one of the senses may interact with that from another, although the information is of a quite different quality. It is possible for one set of sense impressions to conflict with and even begin to override those coming from another category of sensory organ. The peculiar sensation experienced when stepping off an out-of-action escalator, for example, occurs because the image of the escalator – which is normally moving – is contradicted by messages from cells which monitor balance and orientation. These tell us that the escalator is stationary.

▲ Fingertips are sufficiently sensitive to localization and discrimination between points to enable the sense of touch to be used for reading, as in the Braille system, invented in the 19th century by Louis Braille, for the blind. Each letter is represented by up to six raised dots. An experienced reader can read at up to 50 words a minute.

Touch, the mysterious sense

The sense listed by Aristotle which has proved less clear-cut than any of the others is touch. Towards the end of the last century, physiologists began to map the human skin with fine bristles and with probes at different temperatures, showing that areas differed in maximum sensitivity to pressure, warmth and cold. More recently, studies of patients with certain diseases have extended this knowledge. Individuals suffering from the spinal cord degeneration associated with syringomelia, for example, lose their awareness of pain and temperature, but remain sensitive to pressure.

Physiologists now believe that there are distinct senses for light pressure, heavy pressure, warmth, cold and pain. The skin contains several sorts of nerve endings, including Meissner's corpuscles and Pacinian corpuscles, which are thought to respond to particular stimuli. But efforts to relate them to the five categories of sensitivity have not been completely resolved.

The skin's sense receptors

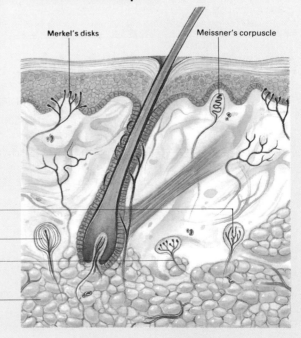

Merkel's disks

Meissner's corpuscle

Bulb of Krause

Pacinian corpuscle

Organ of Ruffini

Sebaceous fat

▶ The skin contains a number of different sense receptors (♦ page 114).Pain receptors have free ends which can be in the epidermis. Other sensory receptors have encapsulated ends of some kind. Meissner's corpuscles are small oval masses of connective tissue, each with one or more nerve fibers; they are most common in hairless regions, and are most sensitive to motion and light touch. Pacinian corpuscles are large elliptical structures in the subcutaneous layers, especially of hands, feet, sexual organs, tendons and joints. Organs of Ruffini are elongated, embedded in the dermis, and detect heavy touch sensations. Merkel's disks are dendrite formations in the epidermis. Bulbs of Krause, in the dermis, may be one of the organs involved in the detection of cold.

The brain detects motion, depth and color separately and constructs its own total image

Focusing

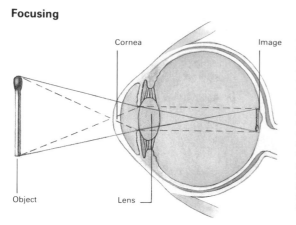

◄ ► The eye consists of a lens (which can be focused by being squeezed or extended); an aperture to control (the iris) and an area in which the image is resolved (the retina), from which light-sensitive cells pass information to the brain. Part of the focusing is done by the transparent, bulging cornea. The fovea, surrounded by the macula, is the part of the retina with most receptor cells, and so the part that forms the best image. The blind spot is where the optic nerve leaves the retina.

Anatomy of the eye

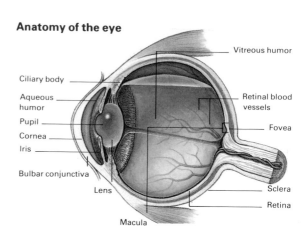

The optic pathways

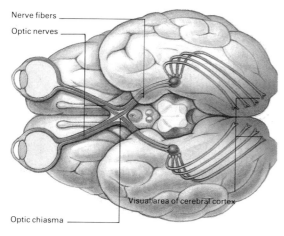

▲ *The optic nerves from each eye meet in the optic chiasma, then divide as the fibers pass impulses to the visual cortex at the back of the brain. Some nerve fibers (those from the medial part of the eye) cross over in the optic chiasma, while the lateral fibers do not. The left side of the brain receives impulses from the left side of each retina, and vice-versa.*

▼ *The visual receptor cells of the retina consist of millions of rods and cones. Rods have long thin projections; cones are shorter and blunter. Each cell is fired by light striking it; the brain assembles their information into a coherent image.*

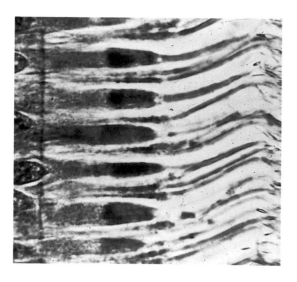

Sight, the obvious sense

Apparently the simplest sense to fathom, eyesight has proved to be more complex than was once supposed. For many years, the science of optics and an understanding of the eye ran in parallel, yielding a simple analysis of vision. Light waves enter the eye via the protective cornea, which, together with the lens focuses the image on the retina. The lens differs from that in an optical instrument only by its surrounding ring of muscle, which can alter the shape and thus the focus of the lens. The pupil – a circular opening in the iris, which gives the eye its external color – is comparable to the iris diaphragm in a camera, serving the same function of regulating the amount of light admitted. At the back of the eye, the retina contains some 125,000,000 rods and 7,000,000 cones – light-sensitive cells which pass their information to the brain via the optic nerve. Rods, capable of detecting only shades of gray, are for night vision, while cones sort out the colors. As in a camera, the lens in the eye produces a tiny inverted image of whatever its owner looks at. According to the old view, this image is broken down by the retinal cells (just as a photograph is processed into dots for printing in a newspaper) and the sense impressions conveyed to the brain, where they stimulate corresponding cells and give a continuous picture of the outside world.

Recent research has not invalidated this sketch, but has certainly modified it. The image on the retina is not as sharp or clear as that on a film in a camera. Nor do the rods and cones break it down to precise units, like a newspaper photograph. The brain has to do some complex computations to make sense of the image – as when we instantly recognize different versions of a letter of the alphabet, a task well beyond the scope of the most advanced electronic scanning devices.

Clues as to how the brain works in processing visual data have come from studies of animals. A toad, for example, will try to eat a line moving across a screen (because it "sees" the line as a worm) but not if the line travels vertically (because worms do not crawl on their ends). The human brain has prior expectations too, as shown by optical illusions and its brain cells are not hooked up to a corresponding mosaic of cells in the retina. Instead, different regions of the visual cortex look after different aspects of what we see. Thus in a human brain there are cortex cells concerned with lines, others concerned with depth, others responding to color and others dealing with motion. Their efforts are combined to sort out the image on the retina and make sense of it. Instead of the brain putting together a facsimile of the vertical and horizontal lines of, say, a goalpost, different banks of brain cells respond to lines at different angles.

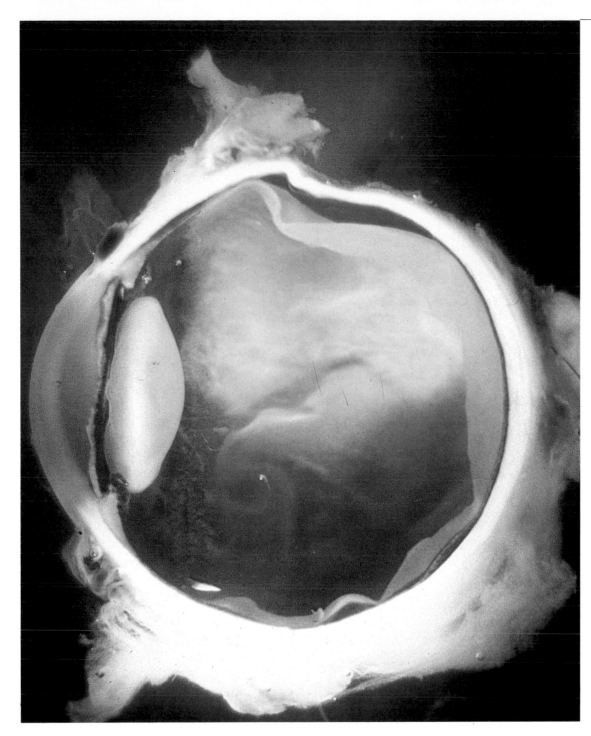

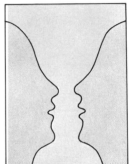

◄ *The eye-ball contains internal muscles that control the iris and lens, and external muscles that move the eye within its socket.*

▼ *The image is interpreted by the brain, which may introduce elements not objectively present on the retina. This forms the basis of many optical illusions, such as these in which the brain's assumptions about what is image and what is background, or about perspective, influence the way the image is seen.*

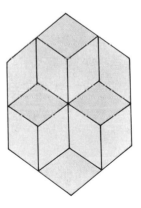

We do not perceive color in a straightforward way either. The theory first advanced by the English physician and scientist Thomas Young (1773-1829) that the retina contains three types of sensitive cells reacting to three primary colors, is now thought to be only approximately true. There are three groups of retinal cells, but their color responses are not as distinct as the theory requires. The American Thomas Land (b. 1914), inventor of Polaroid when a student, and later of the Land camera, has discovered that we can see a much greater wealth of colors when Young's red, green and violet are arranged in complex patterns. Thus a color slide, although based on the primary trio, gives us brown and other colors which Young was unable to produce by overlapping red, green and violet in a simple pattern. It seems that cortex cells operate not by reacting to specific, unambiguous messages but by comparing the color of an object with that of its surroundings. That is why a red area reflecting more green and blue than red light can sometimes still be seen as red.

The sense of "blind sight"
A chameleon has only three positive choices to make about something in its line of sight: whether to eat the object, mate with it or run away. So its brain has a relatively simple visual department. Man, in addition to the sophisticated visual cortex, retains this elementary machinery. The midbrain contains colliculi, corresponding to structures in the chameleon, fish and toad, which direct our gaze towards an object, before the cortex analyzes the image in detail. A basketball player uses his midbrain colliculi to sense the position of the ball, though he needs his visual cortex to analyze the changing image on the retina. Remarkable evidence about the colliculi comes from people whose visual cortex has been damaged. They are, strictly speaking, blind. Yet when asked to guess at the position of flashing lights, they can do so very accurately. This is "blind sight".

There are 30,000 nerve fibers in each ear, detecting different frequencies of a sound

Hearing, the delicate sense

Although Aristotle recognized the ear as the organ of his second sense, we now know that it is responsible for two senses, hearing and balance, of which the latter is arguably the more important for survival. Both are located in the inner ear set deep inside the bone of the skull. Sound waves are first collected by the outer ear and then transmitted by the ear drum (tympanic membrane) to the middle ear. To ensure the ear drum is free to vibrate when sound reaches it, the air pressure has to be equal on both sides. This is achieved by the eustachian tube, connecting the middle ear to the nasopharynx, which opens every time we yawn or swallow. The vibrations from the eardrum finally transfer to the inner ear by an exquisitely sensitive sequence of three bones – the hammer, anvil and stirrup. At the inner ear the vibrations pass through a membrane in an oval window. Because the membrane is far smaller than the ear drum it also amplifies the sound.

Within the inner ear is a complex of tiny membranous tubes called the labyrinth – the working machinery. Fitted inside a similarly shaped bony structure, the labyrinth contains no air but is filled with fluid and has fluid between it and the bone. From front to back, the bony labyrinth is divided into a bony cochlea (concerned with hearing), and a vestibule and semicircular canals (concerned with balance and orientation). The cochlea (from the Latin word for a snail), consists of a gradually tapering spiral tube. Inside are channels, each filled with fluid and containing the organ of Corti, first described by the Italian microscopist Alfonso Corti (1822-1888). Vibrations from the oval window, transmitted through the fluid, press on this organ, stimulating sensitive hairs attached to hair cells, which then pass impulses to the brain. Some 30,000 nerve fibers leading from the 16,000-20,000 hair cells in each ear, combine to become the auditory nerve which conveys all signals to the brain. Sounds of different frequencies seem to activate different regions of the organ of Corti, with a gradual progression from one end to the other. The brain recognizes which cells are being stimulated, and interprets the pitch accordingly. The organ of Corti can measure both the intensity and frequency of sound waves from 20 to 20,000 cycles per second.

The vital sense of babance

We owe our sense of orientation, acceleration and rotation to the remaining parts of the inner ear. Inside the bony vestibule are two membranous sacs – the utricle and the saccule – both of which have a thickened area of specialized cells called the macula. In turn, each macula contains sensory cells with tiny hairs attached. These project into jelly-like material, within which float innumerable crystals of chalk. When we are stationary, the sensory cells indicate the weight of crystals resting upon them. When we move, they tell the brain that the crystals have changed position. Because the maculae of the utricle and saccule lie at right-angles to each other, they are affected differently by gravity, and also make us sensitive to direction. Continuous stimulation of the sensory cells by movement (particularly when the messages reaching the brain conflict with visual information such as a newspaper held with a fixed gaze) can cause motion sickness.

The three bony semicircular canals, set in planes mutually at right-angles to each other, indicate balance and rotation in a similar way. When we move our head, up, down, right or left, fluid in the canals also moves – but it lags behind, and the relative movement stimulates hair cells like those in the maculae, sending messages to the brain.

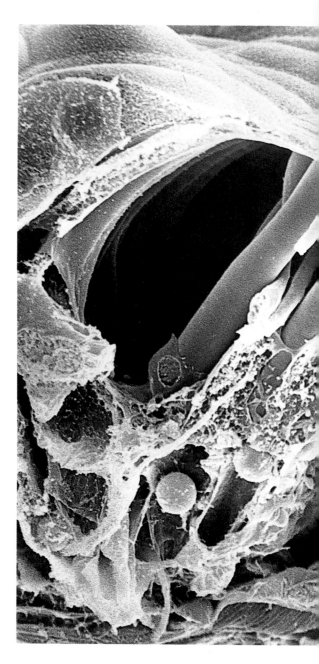

Magnetic sense?
In 1980 Robin Baker, a psychologist at the University of Manchester, reported evidence suggesting that humans have a magnetic sense. He had taken some children, blindfolded and wearing apparently identical helmets, on a winding route into the countryside. At their (unknown) destination, some were able to point roughly in the direction of their school. Others pointed about 90° to the right of that direction, and others to the left. What the children did not know was that two-thirds of the helmets contained magnets. Those worn by the youngsters erring to the right had magnets in the right-hand side, and vice-versa. The individuals with an unimpaired sense of direction had worn helmets without magnets. Robin Baker believes that these results show that humans can discern the direction of the earth's magnetic field and use it to navigate.

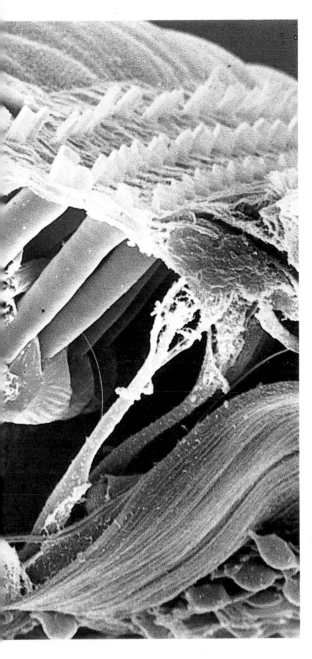

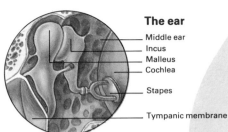

The ear

- Middle ear
- Incus
- Malleus
- Cochlea
- Stapes
- Tympanic membrane

▲ ▶ *The outer ear collects sound waves and directs them to the middle ear. Here they are transmitted and amplified by three bones, the auditory ossicles, and passed to the inner ear where sensory receptors pick them up.*

◀ ▼ *The hair cells of the organ of Corti in the cochlea. These detect movements in the cochlear fluid and generate nerve impulses that the brain hears as sounds. Different parts of the cochlea pick up different frequencies.*

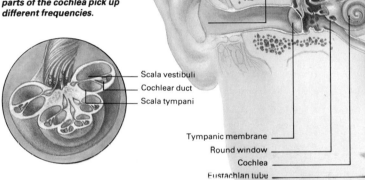

- Scala vestibuli
- Cochlear duct
- Scala tympani

- Middle ear
- External auditory canal

- Tympanic membrane
- Round window
- Cochlea
- Eustachian tube

Kinesthesis — sensing your own body

In addition to senses of balance and equilibrium provided by the vestibule and semicircular canals, we also have "kinesthesis" or proprioception – the awareness, even with closed eyes, of the position of our limbs and of their movement and direction. This sense enables us to judge the effort needed for a task, and to carry out actions without using our eyes continuously. The information for kinesthesis comes from sense organs in the muscles, tendons and joints. They give the cerebellum region of the brain (◊ page 54) information about active contraction of muscle fibers; passive stretching; tension, whether caused actively or passively; and the degree of angulation within the joints. Unlike the other senses, which tend to adapt to regular stimuli (so that we lose our awareness of, say, a regular noise of medium loudness), the kinesthesis sense organs adapt only slightly.

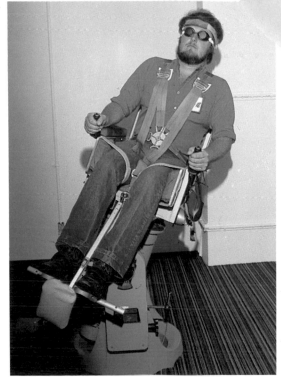

◀ *The balance mechanism consists of three semicircular canals in the inner ear, at right angles to one another. As the head moves, fluid in each canal disturbs receptors. The brain combines information from each plane to produce a sense of threedimensional movement. Here the balance mechanism of a trainee astronaut is tested on a chair that moves through many planes.*

Taste and smell, the chemical senses

Unlike balance, hearing and vision, which are based on physical inter-actions, taste and smell are known as the chemical senses because they depend on responses to chemicals in food and the environment. They also differ in being far less completely fathomed by science. Greek philosophers speculated about both taste and smell, but it was not until the 19th century that rigorous investigation began, when experimental psychology established itself in Germany as an independent discipline. That was the beginning of efforts, still unresolved, to break down tastes and smells into their individual components.

The anatomy of taste is well understood. Taste buds on the tongue, palate, pharynx, tonsils, epiglottis and (in some people) the surface of the lips and cheeks, contain the two types of cells responsible. These are groups of "gustatory receptor cells" – ends of specialized nerve fibers – and of supporting cells. Most taste buds cluster near papillae, visible protuberances on the tongue's surface. Each papilla is surrounded by a trench, forming a container for solutions to be tasted.

Before we can taste anything, it must be dissolved in saliva. The tasty substance then contacts the tips of the gustatory cells, which protrude through the surface of the tongue and other areas, and stimulates them. Different nerves – including the facial nerve for the front of the tongue and the glossopharyngeal nerve for the rear – then transmit the sensation to the brain (◆ page 57). How dissolved chemicals elicit particular tastes is uncertain. Most physiologists now believe that there are four basic qualities – sweet, sour, salty and bitter – which combine to form specific tastes just as different wavelengths of light blend to produce colors. The idea that individual gustatory cells correspond with particular tastes has been dismissed, though researchers still do not agree on whether single nerve fibers correspond in this way.

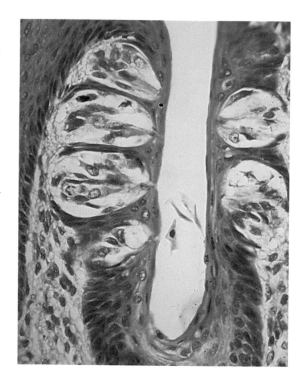

▲ *A taste-bud consists of taste cells within a small opening on the tongue known as a taste pore. Projections or taste hairs are the sensitive part of the cells. Taste buds mostly occur in groups surrounded by a trench in which solutions collect for tasting.*

▼ *The tongue is covered with taste buds, with the large nipple-like papillae at the rear. These mainly detect bitter tastes. Sweet taste buds are mainly on the tip of the tongue; sour receptors on the sides, and salt along the upper front portion.*

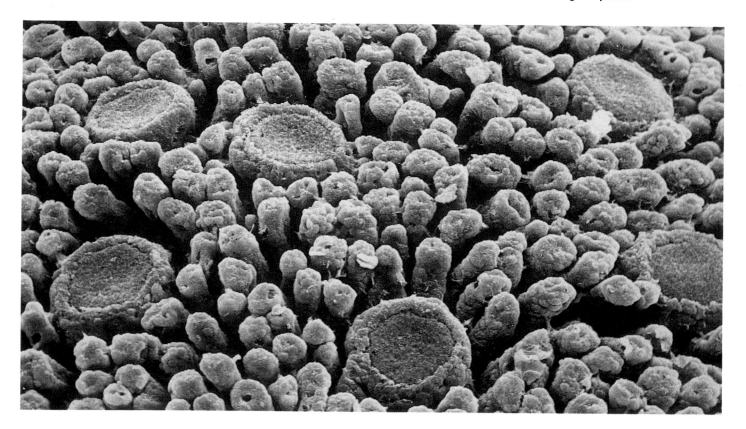

Olfactory nerves

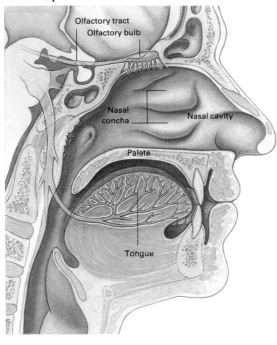

Olfactory tract
Olfactory bulb
Nasal concha
Nasal cavity
Palate
Tongue

▲ The sense of smell depends on the olfactory organs; the receptor cells have cilia which project down into the nasal cavity. The receptors respond to a smell very quickly, but also adapt so that half the intensity is lost within a second.

▼ A wine-taster uses a combination of taste, smell and sight to evaluate the quality of the wine. Though taste and smell receptors die off in large numbers during life, his overall judgement is able to make good any deficiency in perception.

Contrary to general belief (especially the beliefs of chefs and gastronomes) taste and smell are completely separate systems. Although they both operate in the oral cavity and react to chemical stimuli, the cells responsible are quite distinct. The confusion probably arises via the term flavor, which actually has three components – taste, smell and "texture-temperature". When food enters the mouth, these three senses are stimulated independently, the net result being the experience of a particular flavor.

When we breathe, odorous particles escape from the main airstream and reach specialized sensitive tissue at the top of the nasal cavity. This contains millions of tiny olfactory nerve endings, plus supporting cells, which are somehow stimulated by the particles. The nerve fibers converge into larger and larger bundles as they leave the area, and send their messages, perhaps amplified en route, to the brain. As with taste, investigators have tried to resolve smells into their component parts. Suggested schemes range from Plato's elementary division ("pleasant" and "unpleasant") to the sevenfold system introduced by Carl von Linné (1707-1778) – aromatic, fragrant, ambrosial (musky), alliaceous (garlicky), hircine (goaty), repulsive and nauseous. A Dutch physiologist, Hendrick Zwaardemaker, enlarged the Linnean scheme earlier this century to include ethereal (fruits and wines) and empyreumatic (roasted coffee and creosote).

While perfumers and others find such classifications of practical value, today's odor researchers are seeking to understand how molecules elicit particular smells. There are three main theories. Odorous substances may react chemically with olfactory nerve endings; they may stimulate the nerves by radiation; or they may interact with them by vibration. Interest in solving this problem has been heightened by the need to help people with defects of taste or smell, but there is as yet no agreement.

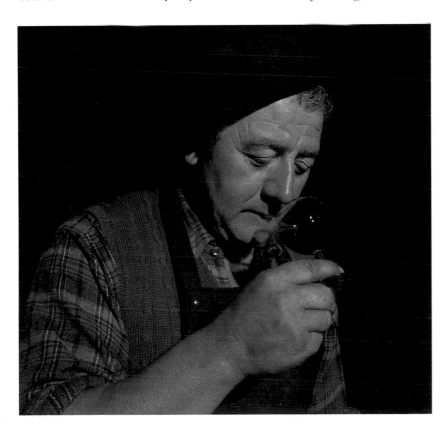

A sense of sexual attraction?

Pheromones (odor substances that operate below the threshold of conscious sensitivity) are used by ants as alarm signals. Wolves employ them as territorial markers; dogs produce them as sexual attractants. Most scientists believe that humans too respond to these chemical agents of silent communication. The search for a human smell that is not consciously detectable began in 1970 when psychiatrist Richard Michael and others at the Georgia Mental Health Institute in Georgia discovered substances such as acetic acid in the vaginal secretions of female rhesus monkeys. Because they stimulated male sexual interest when daubed on the genitals of spayed and otherwise sexually undesirable females, they were termed copulins. The meaning of this work has been questioned (on the grounds that sexually bored males were simply responding to a novelty), but the possibility of pheromones functioning in humans remains. The synchronization of menstrual cycles, which has been noted among friends and room-mates, may depend upon pheromones. This was confirmed in 1977 when Michael Russell of Sonoma State Hospital in Eldrige, California, synchronized university students' cycles by giving them perspiration three times weekly from cotton wool pads worn under the arm by another woman. Efforts are now under way to isolate the substances responsible for this subconscious communication.

48

See also
Disorders of the Senses 49-52
The Nervous System 53-60
Consciousness and Intelligence 65-72
The Skin 113-6
Growth, Aging and Renewal 205-12

Pain – a state of the body or mind?

Though universal, pain is far from completely understood. Philosophers debate whether it should be described as a sense at all, rather than the result of genuine senses overstimulated. It can be painful to have a strong light in the eyes, for example, though the sensation is quite different from that of a cut finger. Some parts of the body, particularly deep tissues, are relatively insensitive to pain or respond to only certain types of trauma. The organs in the abdomen produce pain if stretched but not if cut or burned. Damage to other tissues causes acute pain. Patterns of stimulation, and the psychological context, are all important. A single electrical shock to the skin may hardly be noticed, whereas repeated shocks can produce severe pain. Some pains vary from one moment to the next although their causes seem to remain unchanged. To account for such variations, and the occasional total absence of pain with severe injury, the British physiologist Patrick Wall has evolved his "gate theory". In contrast to the simplistic view that the intensity of pain depends on the number of nerve endings sending pain messages to the brain, Wall believes that a "gate" operates to regulate the forward passage of those signals. He argues that messages from the brain instruct the nerve receptors in the spine not to send the pain signals. Because about 40 percent of injuries are not immediately painful, such a gate may close off the flow of pain signals at first. Conversely, a wide-open gate could account for the heightened sense of pain which anticipation can create. There is much support for Wall's ideas, but as yet no physiological proof.

Referred pain

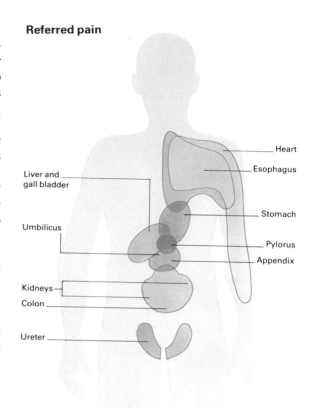

Liver and gall bladder
Umbilicus
Kidneys
Colon
Ureter

Heart
Esophagus
Stomach
Pylorus
Appendix

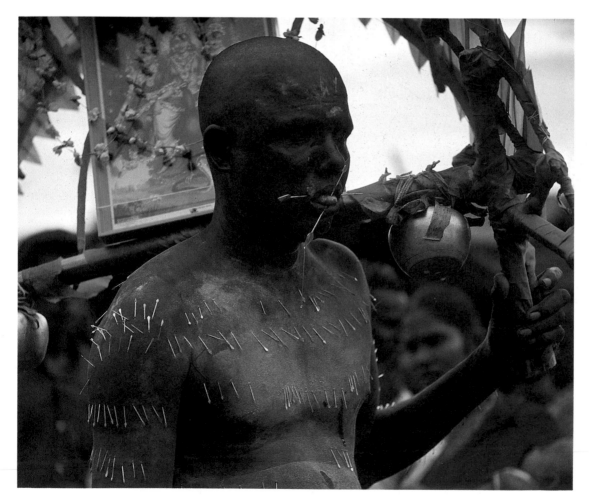

▲ Pain from disorders to many organs may be experienced in quite other parts of the body. This referred pain results from the fact that the affected organ and the region to which the pain is referred usually receive nerves from the same segment of the spinal cord. Thus pain from the heart may be felt down the left arm.

◄ A man covered in needles for ritual purposes may be able to suppress all sensations of pain. The mind seems to be capable of preventing pain impulses from reaching it under certain circumstances, while the brain also contains substances known as endorphins (♦ page 59) which relieve pain.

Short-, long- and farsightedness...Blindness and partial blindness...Color blindness...Astigmatism... Cataracts... Conduction and nerve deafness... PERSPECTIVE...Contact lenses...Lazy eye and squints... Failures of balance

Anatomy of the eye

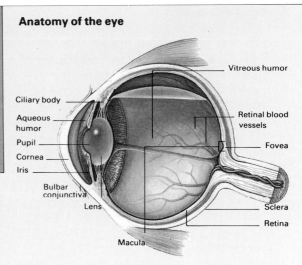

When the sense organs are damaged or destroyed, either through disease, injury or the normal processes of aging, their functions are impaired. We lose some of our sense of smell and taste when we get older, but the most noticeable changes are in our sight and hearing.

Correcting poor vision

Normal vision, once called 20/20 but now 6/6 vision, is the ability to see a standard chart from a distance of 6m (20ft) with either eye. A 6/5 eye can see at 6m what a normal eye must be within 5m to see, and is therefore better; a 6/9 eye is worse. Near-sightedness (myopia) is the inability to focus on distant things. The eye's lens bends the light rays too far inwards, so they meet before they get to the retina, and diverge again. Longsightedness (hyperopia) is the inability to focus on close things. The eye's lens does not bend light rays sufficiently to converge them on the retina. Farsightedness (presbyopia) is decline of the near-focusing muscles. Astigmatism is imperfect vision in particular planes caused by uneven curvature of the cornea or lens.

The need for glasses indicates faulty focus; it cannot be improved by exercises. Wearing glasses of the wrong strength is harmless, as is reading. Shortsighted people need concave lenses; longsighted and farsighted people need convex lenses. In spectacles both types of lense distort vision – concave lenses make objects (and the wearer's eyes) look smaller; convex lenses make them look larger. Lenses for astigmatism differ in thickness vertically and horizontally.

Contact lenses fit directly over the cornea and give better correction than spectacles, as they do not enlarge or reduce the size of objects. Hard contact lenses present an optically even surface, correcting astigmatism. In the USSR nearsightedness is cured by making tiny radial scars in the cornea to change its shape.

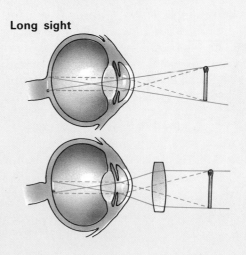

▲ *The earliest recorded use of spectacles was by a Dominican friar in Italy in the mid-14th century; by the 16th century, when this engraving was done, various forms were available, including a pinhole design to assist with myopia.*

▶ *In myopia, or short sightedness, the image forms in front of the retina, usually because the eyeball is lengthened; presbyopia, the weakening of the lens-focusing muscles, has a similar effect. A concave lens is used to correct this, by making the light rays diverge before entering the eye. In hyperopia, or long sightedness, the opposite is true, and a convex lens is used to converge the light rays so that they can focus exactly on the retina. Some conditions require bifocal or trifocal lenses, offering the wearer a variety of focusing options through various parts of the lens.*

Short sight　　　　　　**Long sight**

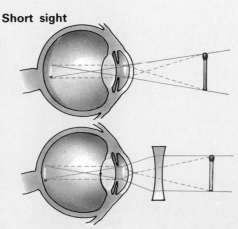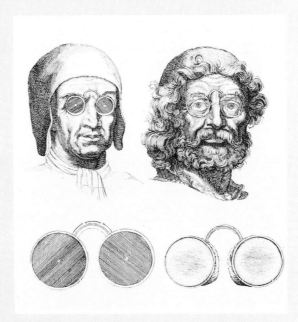

General visual defects

Vision is impaired if the retina becomes detached from the choroid behind it or the vitreous matter in front, and is worst when the detachment is near the center or over the macula. Though painless, this produces spots and flashes before the eyes and loss of part of the visual field. Causes include a general tendency to poor adhesion, blows to the eye, cysts, tumors, scar tissue, bleeding or retinal tearing. Detached retinal tissue tends to tear, and torn retinal tissue to detach. Treatment is by sealing around the tear and re-attaching it to the choroid, using an ice probe or laser beam.

Spots before the eyes are usually caused by floaters, small cell clusters released from the eyeball's lining. They are untreatable but disappear spontaneously. Bloodshot eyes, from burst blood vessels on the eye's surface, occur spontaneously or after injury. They are harmless and disappear within 10 to 14 days.

Color blindness is an untreatable, retinal condition commoner in men but inherited through both parents (◀ page 29). Usually the sufferer cannot distinguish between red and green; occasionally the confusion is between blue and yellow.

Night-blindness is the inability, usually inherited, to see in dim light. It is occasionally caused by deficiency of Vitamin A or can be an early sign of retinitis pigmentosa, an inherited disease in which the retinal pigment degenerates, causing eventual blindness.

Cataract – clouding of the lens – occurs with aging but may also be congenital, or caused by injury, infection, metabolic disorders or some drugs. It cannot be made better or worse by reading or lighting levels. Treatment is by removing the lens under local or general anesthetic. Healing and permanent adjustment takes three months. Lack of a lens to focus light entering the eye is overcome by using glasses or contact lenses.

Blindness

Total blindness occurs only when eyes or their nerves are lost through injury. Ordinary blindness – absence of useful sight – is caused by degeneration in old age, diabetes, trachoma (◆ page 241), glaucoma, detached retina or corneal scarring. In degeneration or diabetes, the blood vessels in the retina or macula burst and then heal to form an overgrowth of new vessels which interferes with vision. Lasers or xenon arcs can be used to arrest their growth and partly remove them; these potent light rays can be focused onto an area of one micrometer.

Glaucoma, high pressure within the eyeball, damages and gradually kills nerve fibers and blood vessels. Treatment is by eyedrops that widen the pupil's drainage channel, tablets that reduce the eye's fluid production, or an operation to widen or make new drainage channels. Early stages of glaucoma, and damage from diabetes and high blood pressure, can be detected by inspecting the retina for bleeding or fluid exudates, descriptively called "cotton wool patches".

Corneal scars can be caused by diseases including ulcers and glaucoma, and may lead to blindness because they are opaque. Removing the damaged cornea and replacing it by a graft is successful in 85 percent of cases. The grafted cornea is removed from the donor within ten hours of death and can be stored for up to 20 days before use. Grafted corneas are not rejected by the body's immune system because they require no blood supply and do not provoke the body to produce antibodies (◆ page 221). Corneal ulcers heal slowly and with difficulty because there is no blood supply.

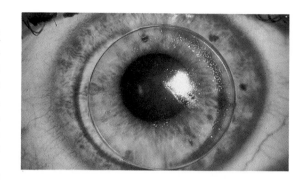

▲ *Hard contact lenses automatically correct astigmatism, as do some soft lenses. These are made thicker and heavier at the bottom, and thus orient themselves correctly in the eye. Bifocal contact lenses similarly orient themselves by gravity.*

Contact lenses

The first glass contact lens was made in 1887 by A.E. Fick, a Swiss physician. Today, of the two types of lens, hard lenses are made of perspex or oxygen-permeable plastic. Because they are rigid they present an optically even surface to the world, correcting astigmatism. They remain in the eye because of the capillary action of tears, which provide a form of suction. They may fall out if the eyes become dry and they become uncomfortable if tiny particles of dust slip underneath them.

Soft lenses are made of thin plastic, and contain water. They have the texture, thinness and appearance of cellophane and cover a larger area of the eye than hard lenses. Without this extra size they would be difficult to insert and remove. Their flexibility means that they cannot correct astigmatism, but they do allow a more intimate fit over the cornea, so dust does not get under them. Because they are permeable to water and tears they can hold bacteria, which breed in them if they are not kept very clean. Contact lenses cannot slip behind the eye because the junction of the conjunctiva and eyelid prevents them.

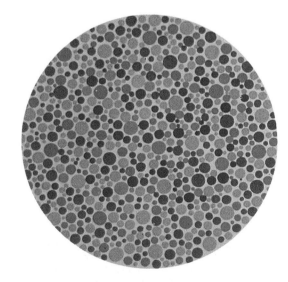

▲ *Color blindness, tested with charts in which images are concealed in a random network of dots, is usually caused by a defect in one of the three groups of primary-color-sensitive cone cells of the retina. It cannot be corrected.*

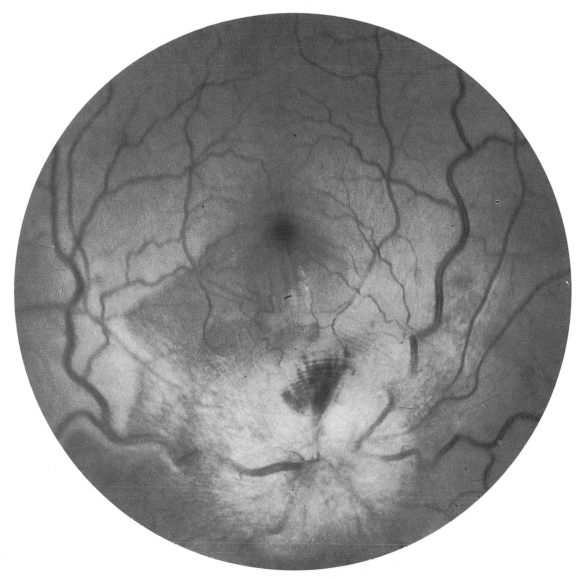

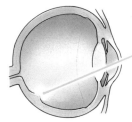

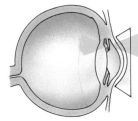

▲ ◄ *A diseased retina, often found in diabetes, can result in the profuse growth of new blood vessels. These may grow over the macula and cause the retina to detach. A recent treatment uses an argon laser to fuse the blood vessels, thus preventing further growth. Lasers are also used to correct defects to the iris.*

▼ *When a cataract develops, the lens grows steadily more opaque; the operation to remove the lens with the cataract is relatively simple. Since some of the focusing work of the eye is done by the cornea, the patient is able to see with the help of spectacles.*

"Lazy eye", cross-eyes and squints

Better known as amblyopia, "lazy eye" is not lazy at all. It is caused by focusing defects that prevent the brain from combining information from both eyes. In an adult this causes double vision but in children the brain simply ignores information from one eye. It must be corrected by the age of six; after that age, the brain cannot learn to interpret information from the "lazy" eye.

Strabismus – squint or cross-eyes – results from faulty alignment of the six muscles that surround the eye. One or both eyes may be affected. It has a number of causes including attempts to overcome focusing defects. Children do not spontaneously "grow out" of strabismus, which is usually cured by glasses. If not, an operation to reduce the length of some external eye muscles produces improvement if done before the age 5-6. Corrective therapy such as eye exercise rarely helps.

Half-closing the eyes, which is sometimes also called squint, is an attempt to improve short sight. Like reducing the aperture of a camera, it increases depth of field. It can be corrected by either glasses or contact lenses.

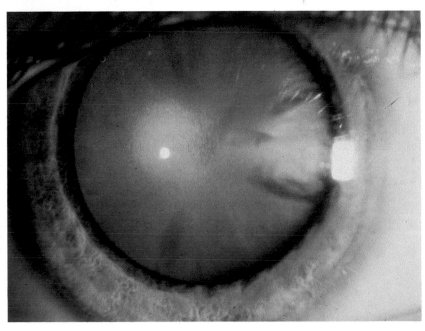

Hearing failure

Deafness is caused by a selective lack of perception or by loss of conduction. Conduction deafness is due to ear or nose infections, which can inflict long-term damage, or otosclerosis, where new bone growth fixes the stirrup (one of the three bones of the middle ear ◀ page 45), so it cannot vibrate and transmit sound. The stirrup can be freed, or replaced with a plastic substitute, by an operation. People with conduction deafness speak quietly because they hear their own voices amplified through their skull bones (a similar effect is produced by talking with hands over the ears). One way of detecting this type of deafness is to place a ticking watch near the ear; the watch sounds louder when touching the head.

People with perceptual (nerve) deafness speak loudly as they hear their own voices faintly. They cannot hear high-pitched noises or sounds like s, f, p, k, t and hard g. Nerve deafness may be congenital or caused by noise pollution, degeneration in old age (presbyacusis), head injuries, and some drugs and poisons. It is often compounded by tinnitus, an intermittent ringing or buzzing in the ears, and by an inability to select certain sounds while disregarding others.

Hearing aids consist of a miniature microphone, amplifier and loudspeaker. They are a great help in conduction deafness but less so in nerve deafness, as it is difficult to amplify some sounds selectively without others. Each person with nerve deafness has a different loss of perception for pitch, loudness and selectivity, so hearing aids must be tailored to individual needs.

The eardrum can rupture when subjected to pressure from within (pus from infections) or outside (poking with hard objects, head injuries, diving or a slap on the ear with a hollowed palm). It is accompanied by great pain, deafness and nausea. Small perforations heal spontaneously if kept free from infection, but larger ones may need surgical repair or a graft, usually from the wall of a vein.

Failure of balance

Menière's disease consists of giddy attacks, often during sleep, with nausea and vomiting. It can be preceded by tinnitus and usually begins with mild fluctuating deafness on one or both sides. It is caused by excess fluid in the inner ear, brought on by hereditary factors, stress, disease or high doses of quinine or aspirin. Treatment includes restricting fluid intake, diuretics, seasickness remedies, antihistamines or blood-vessel dilator drugs. Motion sickness is provoked by fluid movement in the semicircular canals (◀ page 45), which have nerve receptors. Drugs prevent or relieve it.

Hearing in old age

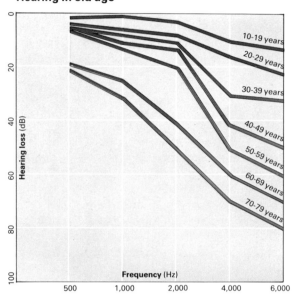

▲ The ability to hear declines steadily with age, starting from the late teens. The highest pitch disappears most quickly.

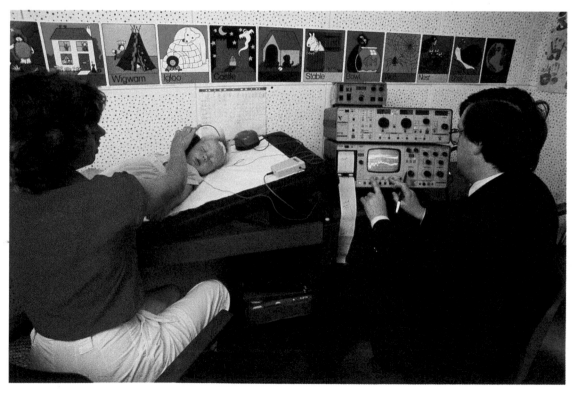

◀ Testing the auditory evoked response in a child.

The Nervous System

*Anatomy of the brain...Fore-, mid- and hindbrain...
The spinal cord...The peripheral nerves...Reflexes...
Structure of the nerve cells...Neurotransmitters...
PERSPECTIVE...The size of the brain...The hole in
the head of Phineas Gage...The cranial nerves...
The autonomic nervous system...Endorphins*

The nervous system is the body's major control and communications system, detecting changes in the environment, determining how to react and instructing the organs to respond. It is divided into the central nervous system, which deals with sensation, movement (motor functions) and conscious thought; the peripheral nervous system which relays messages to and from the organs and muscles; and the autonomic nervous system which controls many of the body's organs.

The central nervous system consists of the brain and spinal cord. The brain is one of the body's largest organs. Its functions include thought, movement, the senses, emotion, behavior, learning and memory. It controls the endocrine system (♦ page 85). The brain's three divisions are forebrain, midbrain and hindbrain. The cerebrum – the large cerebral hemispheres – constitutes 95 percent of the forebrain and over 90 percent of the brain as a whole. The remaining 10 percent – the mid- and hindbrain – together make up the brainstem.

The brain and spinal cord are covered by three membranes. The two cerebral hemispheres have hollow cavities – ventricles – connected to a single central ventricle. This in turn is connected through a rear fourth ventricle to the hollow center of the spinal cord. The ventricles and the membranes enclosing the brain contain the watery cerebrospinal fluid. This acts as a shock-absorber and circulates nutrients filtered from the blood. The brain also has a rich supply of blood, but its capillaries have thick linings that prevent diffusion of most larger molecules, thus protecting the brain from harmful substances.

The cerebral cortex – the seat of learning

The cerebral cortex is the outer layer of the cerebral hemispheres. It is the seat of higher mental processes, including movement, the senses, emotion and intellect. More convoluted than a walnut, it covers 2,600 sq cm. It consists of columns of gray matter (nerve cells) covering white matter (nerve fibers). The gray matter is a 3mm-thick layer of sensory and motor nerve cells, and an inner layer of nerve cells whose fibers – white matter – cross-connect with other parts of the same or opposite hemisphere. Those fibers going to the opposite hemisphere form the corpus callosum, a band of 100 million fibers linking the hemispheres. Major grooves in each hemisphere separate the five lobes – prefrontal, frontal, parietal (top), temporal (side) and occipital (rear). Prefrontal lobes determine intensity of reactions rather than intellect, and damage to them makes a person passive. Frontal lobes contain the areas for movement, including the eyes and the mechanics of speaking. Parietal lobes contain skin sensory areas, receiving touch, pressure, temperature and pain sensations from specific parts of the body. They also include hearing, taste and smell, and association areas. Temporal lobes deal with coordination of space and movement. Occipital lobes deal with vision and visual association.

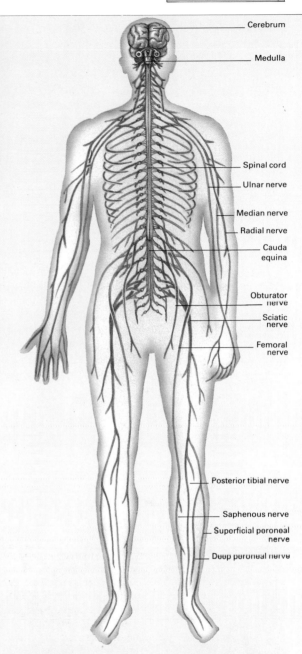

Cerebrum
Medulla
Spinal cord
Ulnar nerve
Median nerve
Radial nerve
Cauda equina
Obturator nerve
Sciatic nerve
Femoral nerve
Posterior tibial nerve
Saphenous nerve
Superficial peroneal nerve
Deep peroneal nerve

▲ The nervous system consists of the brain, spinal cord and peripheral nerves. There are 31 pairs of spinal nerves: 8 in the neck go to the throat, shoulders and arms; 12 thoracic nerves supply the trunk; 5 lumbar go to the front of the legs and upper feet; 5 in the coccyx and 1 in the sacrum go to the back of the legs and soles.

Brain size
The average male brain weighs 1,350g, that of females 1,200g; but females have a slightly higher proportion of brain to body. The brain is often weighed at autopsy – the writers Jonathan Swift and Ivan Turgenev both had brains weighing over 2,000g, the French anatomist Baron Cuvier 1,830g.

In fact the overall weight of the brain is not significant, but its surface area is, since the cerebral cortex is convoluted to increase the area of grey matter. Brains are roughly in proportion to body size. Brains shrink at the rate of 20-30g per decade until the age of 60, and 30-40g thereafter.

The bridge linking the two sides of the brain contains 100 million nerve fibers

The brain

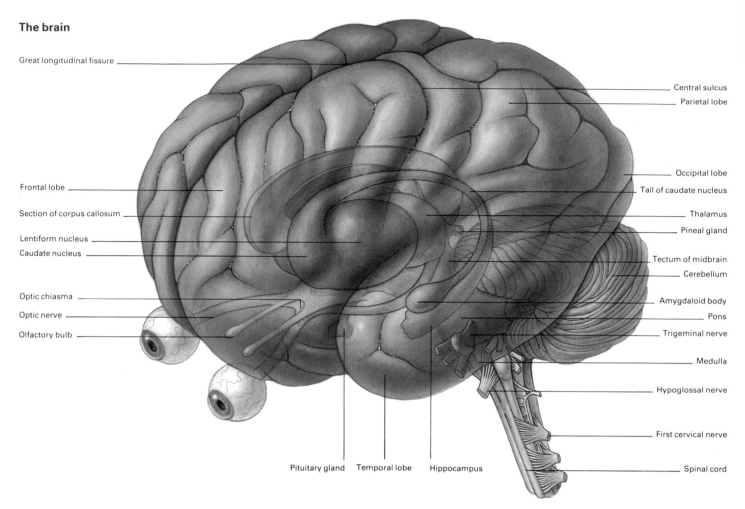

Great longitudinal fissure

Central sulcus

Parietal lobe

Occipital lobe

Frontal lobe

Tail of caudate nucleus

Section of corpus callosum

Thalamus

Lentiform nucleus

Pineal gland

Caudate nucleus

Tectum of midbrain

Cerebellum

Optic chiasma

Amygdaloid body

Optic nerve

Pons

Olfactory bulb

Trigeminal nerve

Medulla

Hypoglossal nerve

First cervical nerve

Pituitary gland   Temporal lobe   Hippocampus

Spinal cord

The visual cortex

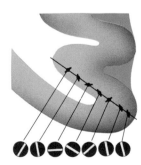

▲ A section through the primary visual cortex, in the occipital lobe; the individual cells of the region are stimulated by specific inputs. Thus if a vertical bar of light is shown, one particular cell will fire; if the bar is turned through 45 degrees, another cell in the visual cortex is stimulated. From the vast number of individual pieces of such information, the brain then assembles a coherent image.

The parts of the brain

The main forebrain structures are the cerebral cortex, thalamus and hypothalamus. The thalamus channels to the hemisphere all the senses except smell, voluntary actions, arousal and sensory impulses from other forebrain areas, brainstem and spinal cord. It is an interpretation center for sensory impulses such as pain, temperature, touch and pressure, emotions and memory. The hypothalamus, which lies under the thalamus, has many functions, mainly to do with homeostasis (♦ page 12). Its different areas control the autonomic nervous system and most of the endocrine system. It receives sensory impulses from the guts, and is the center for temperature control, mind-and-body phenomena such as panic reactions, psychosomatic illness (♦ page 73), rage, aggression, hunger and thirst. It is the center for the biorhythms (♦ page 20).

The limbic system is sometimes called the emotional brain. Shaped like a wishbone, it consists of some inner areas of cortex, hypothalamus and basal ganglia. It is concerned with pleasure, punishment, rage, docility, fear, sorrow and sexual feelings. Altogether it regulates behavior relating to social survival.

Between forebrain and midbrain (and belonging to both) lie the basal ganglia, paired masses of gray matter within each hemisphere, interconnecting with cortex, cerebellum, thalamus and hypothalamus. They are concerned with unconscious movement (such as swinging the arms when walking), and muscle tone. They include the substantia nigra ("dark substance"), which ensures smooth movement of limbs, and the red nucleus, part of the reticular formation (see below). It transmits fibers from cerebellum and cortex to spinal cord, and connects with the cranial nerves that control the muscles of the eye.

The midbrain contains relay stations passing motor fibers down (from cortex to pons and spinal cord) and sensory fibers up (from spinal cord to thalamus). It also contains the tectum, consisting of four colliculi, with reflex centers for head and eyeball movement in response to sights, and for head and trunk movement in response to sounds.

Between midbrain and hindbrain (and belonging to both) is the centrally-placed lemniscus, which conveys impulses for fine touch, vibration and body position from medulla to thalamus.

The hindbrain consists of medulla oblongata (often known simply as the medulla) and above it, the pons, meaning bridge. The pons has crossways fibers connecting with the cerebellum, and longitudinal motor and sensory fibers connecting the medulla with higher parts of the brain. The medulla contains all the ascending and descending tracts between the brain and spinal cord. Most of them cross sides in the medulla, so the brain's left side receives most of its information from the

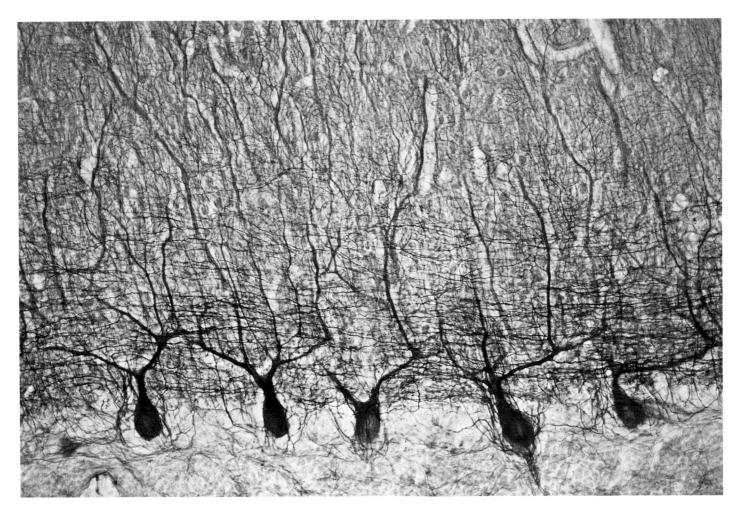

▲ *Nerve cells in the cortex of the cerebellum, each with a large number of dendrites, axons and fibrils, provide connections with other brain cells.*

body's right, and vice-versa. Centered in the medulla is the reticular formation, which extends into the spinal cord and higher parts of the brain. This is concerned with consciousness and arousal and has several centers, three of which are considered vital. The cardiac center regulates the heartbeat; the rhythmicity center adjusts breathing, and the vasomotor center regulates blood vessel diameter. The "non-vital" centers coordinate swallowing, vomiting, coughing, sneezing and hiccuping. Also in the medulla is the vestibular complex, essential for maintaining balance.

Many functions are not shared by both cerebral hemispheres, but allocated to one side, often to a temporal lobe. Most people are right-handed and, for them, the left side of the brain is important for right-hand skills, language (spoken and written), numerical and scientific ability and reasoning. The right side is more important for left-hand control, musical, literary and artistic awareness, space and patterns, insight, imagination, and remembrance of sounds, sights and sensations recalled for everyday comparison. However, the centers for these attributes and skills are probably arranged slightly differently in everyone; left-handed people frequently have their language areas on the right. They may compete for space, which would account for peoples' different skills, and for defects in "lateralized" skills such as dyslexia, tone-deafness or lack of arithmetical ability.

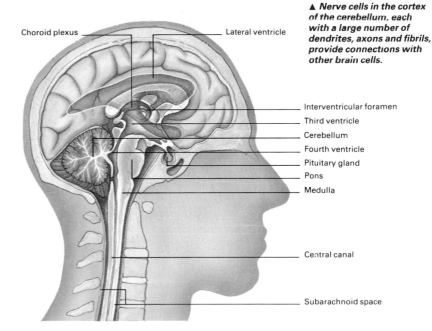

Choroid plexus

Lateral ventricle

Interventricular foramen

Third ventricle

Cerebellum

Fourth ventricle

Pituitary gland

Pons

Medulla

Central canal

Subarachnoid space

▲ *The brain and spinal cord are surrounded by two layers of meninges, which contain the cerebro-spinal fluid. This filters, protects and cleans the brain cells, passing through a series of ventricles in the brain, then down the central canal of the spinal cord before recirculating up to the head. It also adds an effective watery cushion against jarring.*

Most of the brain's sensory and motor nerves are devoted to the head, hands and feet

The spinal cord and reflexes

The spinal cord passes down the center of the vertebrae. It consists of white matter – myelin-coated nerve fibers (axons) – and gray matter, comprising nerves cells and naked axons. The tracts of white matter transmit impulses between body and brain. Columns of gray matter on the inside have sensory tissue at the back and motor tissue at the front. They are joined in the center by a band with a tiny canal containing cerebrospinal fluid. All spinal nerves entering the cord divide into two roots – sensory at the back and motor at the front. Sensory roots have a swelling or ganglion containing cell bodies of its nerves. These extend from the receptors (usually in the skin) to the gray matter of the spinal cord. Here they connect with sensory nerves to the brain or motor nerves to muscles, or both. The front motor roots have their cell bodies in the gray matter of the spinal cord, and receive axons from the brain. They extend directly to muscles, where they branch into a cluster of "fingers" – motor end plates – at their termini.

A reflex is the conduction of impulses from a receptor (such as a Pacinian corpuscle in the skin ◀ page 41) to an effector (such as a motor end plate). Transmission between the two may take place in the brain, or in the spinal cord. Reflexes are fast responses to internal or external changes, and help to maintain homeostasis (◀ page 12). The British physiologist Sir Charles Sherrington (1857-1952) shared a Nobel prize in 1932 for showing that integration in the nervous system takes place at different levels and that reflex pathways are inborn. Somatic reflexes such as the knee-jerk involve skeletal muscle; autonomic reflexes such as salivation or increased heartbeat involve smooth muscle (◀ page 103). The knee-jerk is the simplest kind of reflex, involving only one junction, between a sensory and a motor neuron in the spinal cord. Most reflexes are more complicated, and involve interneurons, "go-between" cells in the spinal cord that have many connections. These can instruct several muscles to contract, for example when a person stumbles but regains balance. Autonomic reflexes can sometimes be made controllable by biofeedback or by yoga. A conditioned reflex is one that has been installed by training or habit.

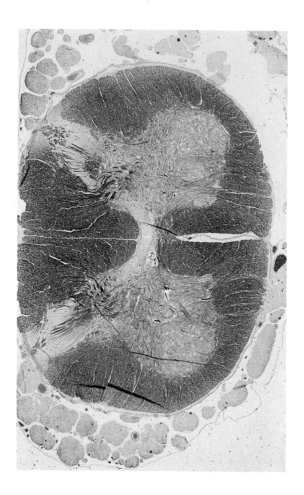

▲ **The spinal cord, seen here with the back to the right, consists of gray matter comprising unmyelinated axons and nerve cells surrounded by white matter. The spinal cord has a dual function of conveying information to and from the brain, and providing reflexes to certain responses. These can be simple, as in the case of the knee jerk or can involve more complex pathways, involving more than one nerve synapse.**

The hole in the head of Phineas Gage

In 1848 a road-gang foreman in the USA, Phineas Gage, poured gunpowder into a rock for blasting. His assistant forgot to cover the powder with sand, and Gage failed to check. He dropped in a tamping iron which struck rock and blew the 1,300cm-long, 4cm-wide iron rod into his left cheek, through his brain and out of the top of his head. Gage was stunned for an hour and then, helped by his mates, set off on foot to find a surgeon, talking about the hole in his head as he went. The wound became infected and took a long time to heal, but eventually Gage was pronounced fit for work. But he never did work again; he suffered no loss of intellect or memory, but his personality changed. Once considerate and well-balanced, he became fitful, irreverent, foul-mouthed, inconsiderate, obstinate and capricious. He had little inclination for work, but traveled around the USA, exhibiting himself and his tamping iron. In 1860 he died in San Francisco in circumstances that warranted an autopsy, which showed destruction of his left lobe and damage that had spread to his right lobe.

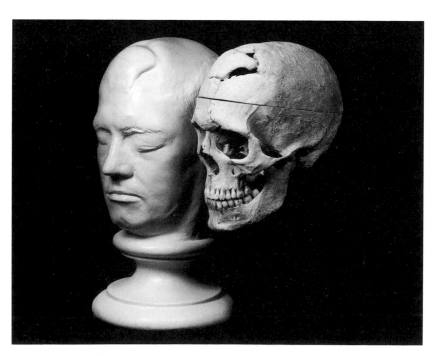

◀ **The damaged skull of Phineas Gage.**

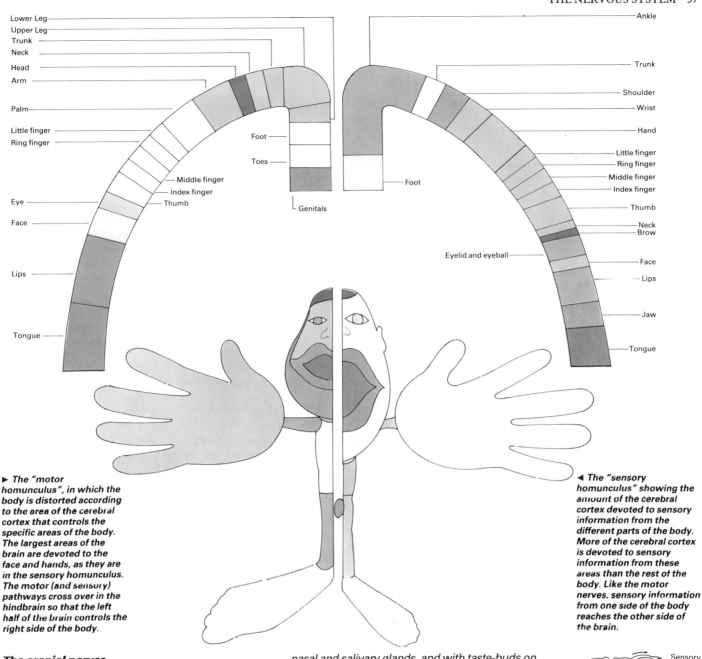

Lower Leg
Upper Leg
Trunk
Neck
Head
Arm
Palm
Little finger
Ring finger
Middle finger
Index finger
Thumb
Eye
Face
Lips
Tongue

Foot
Toes
Genitals

Foot

Ankle
Trunk
Shoulder
Wrist
Hand
Little finger
Ring finger
Middle finger
Index finger
Thumb
Neck
Brow
Eyelid and eyeball
Face
Lips
Jaw
Tongue

► The "motor homunculus", in which the body is distorted according to the area of the cerebral cortex that controls the specific areas of the body. The largest areas of the brain are devoted to the face and hands, as they are in the sensory homunculus. The motor (and sensory) pathways cross over in the hindbrain so that the left half of the brain controls the right side of the body.

◄ The "sensory homunculus" showing the amount of the cerebral cortex devoted to sensory information from the different parts of the body. More of the cerebral cortex is devoted to sensory information from these areas than the rest of the body. Like the motor nerves, sensory information from one side of the body reaches the other side of the brain.

The cranial nerves

Twelve pairs of nerves leave the brain through openings in the skull. Some of these cranial nerves are purely sensory, some mixed and some motor (all the motor nerves going to skeletal muscle bring back sensory information about position).

Information about smell is conveyed from the nose to the cortex by cranial nerve I. The eyes, which are outgrowths of the brain, are linked to it by sensory fibers forming cranial nerve II. Most are relayed from the thalamus to the cortex, but some fibers go to the tectum, where they connect with cranial nerves III, IV, and VI, which moves the eyeballs. Cranial nerve III also focuses the lens and dilates the pupils.

The trigeminal nerves (V) branch in three. The upper branches carry sensory fibers from the upper half of the face, eyeball, tear glands and nasal cavity. The lower two branches transmit motor fibers for chewing, and sensory fibers from the rest of the face, teeth, insides of nostrils, palate, front of throat and tongue (excluding taste). Facial expression is controlled by motor fibers in cranial nerve VII, connected with face, scalp and neck muscles; the same nerve also connects with tear,

nasal and salivary glands, and with taste-buds on the back of the tongue.

Information from the inner ear is conveyed via the medulla to the thalamus and cortex on the acoustic (vestibulocochlear) nerve (VIII). This also carries balance sensations from the semicircular canals via medulla and pons to thalamus and cerebellum.

Motor impulses to the chewing muscles and salivary glands are conveyed on the glosso-pharyngeal nerves (IX). These also bring sensory information from the rear of the throat, back-of-the-tongue taste-buds and from blood-pressure receptors from the carotid artery near the heart. Motor fibers from the medulla to the respiratory system, muscles for swallowing, voicebox, heart, gall bladder, and all the gut except the rectum and anus are carried on the vagus nerves (X), which also bring back sensory information from the larynx, gut and ears. Accessory nerves (XI) arising from medulla and spinal cord, transmit motor impulses for swallowing and moving the head, and motor fibers for moving the tongue in speech and swallowing are carried on the hypoglossal nerves (XII).

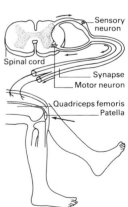

Sensory neuron
Spinal cord
Synapse
Motor neuron
Quadriceps femoris
Patella

▲ The knee jerk reflexes in which a tap on the knee stimulates stretch receptors in the quadriceps femoris muscle. This impulse is passed to the spinal cord, where a single synapse passes the impulse to the motor nerve to flex the muscle.

The autonomic nervous system controls the unconscious activities of many of the body's organs

The autonomic nervous system

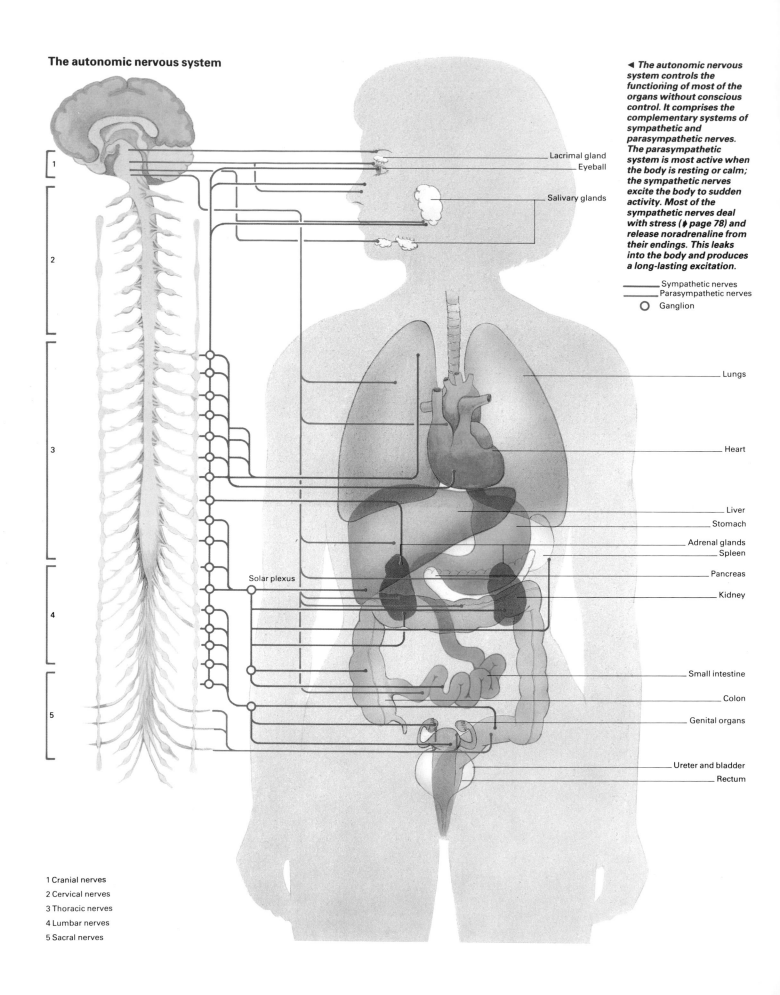

◀ The autonomic nervous system controls the functioning of most of the organs without conscious control. It comprises the complementary systems of sympathetic and parasympathetic nerves. The parasympathetic system is most active when the body is resting or calm; the sympathetic nerves excite the body to sudden activity. Most of the sympathetic nerves deal with stress (♦ page 78) and release noradrenaline from their endings. This leaks into the body and produces a long-lasting excitation.

——— Sympathetic nerves
——— Parasympathetic nerves
○ Ganglion

Lacrimal gland
Eyeball
Salivary glands

Lungs

Heart

Liver
Stomach
Adrenal glands
Spleen
Pancreas
Kidney

Solar plexus

Small intestine
Colon
Genital organs

Ureter and bladder
Rectum

1 Cranial nerves
2 Cervical nerves
3 Thoracic nerves
4 Lumbar nerves
5 Sacral nerves

Nerves to the viscera

The autonomic nervous system regulates the activities of smooth muscle, cardiac muscle and glands. It is regulated by the brain, particularly the hypothalamus and medulla, but is normally outside conscious control. Entirely motor, it is run by fibers that exit with the main nerves but soon branch off and terminate in autonomic ganglia that lie on the vertebral column. Nerves entering the ganglia are covered in myelin, but those leaving them are naked. The system has two effects, which are produced by separate subsystems – the parasympathetic nerves dealing with everyday administration, and the sympathetics reacting to excitement and emergency.

The cranial part of the parasympathetic system arises from nerve cells in the brainstem. They leave the brain in cranial nerves III, VII, IX and X, and pass to separate ganglia. Here each fiber forms connections with many nerve cells, which send nerve axons to iris and lens muscles, tear-producing glands, those producing nasal secretions and saliva, lungs, heart (which receives 80 percent of all upper parasympathetic fibers) and rectum. The lower "paras" have their cell bodies near their exits from sacral nerves 2, 3, and 4.

The sympathetic system arises from the twelve thoracic nerves and the first two lumbar nerves. These have two rows of plexuses. The first is interconnected from top to bottom, and extends upward and downward to additional plexuses – there are four pairs of neck ganglia above the thorax and seven more pairs below the second lumbar nerves. They ascend to a second row – the solar plexus and five smaller ones. Like the parasympathetics, they send fibers to the eyes (but not the tear glands), nasal and salivary glands, lungs, genital organs, kidneys, ureters, bladder and the gut. Unlike the "paras", they also innervate the colon, spleen and adrenal glands.

▶ *A nerve's end-plates in muscle fibers.*

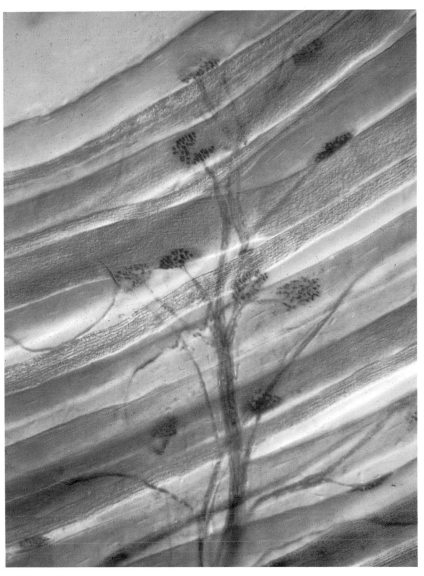

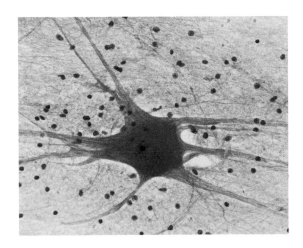

▲ *A motor neuron in the spinal cord, showing the cell body and associated dendrites. The cell body may be at one end of a long nerve cell, or have arms reaching out equally in several directions. It contains the nucleus and is essential to maintaining the activity of the neuron and manufacturing substances that are to be passed along the axons to the synaptic knobs.*

Nerve cells – neurons – consist of a cell body, dendrites (short feathery fibers that conduct impulses towards the cell body) and an axon (a long thin projection carrying each impulse to another neuron or tissue). Each axon may give off colateral branches, which may be wrapped in myelin. They end with feathery branches, finer than dendrites, and terminate in tiny knobs that release transmitters onto a muscle or the dendrites of the next cell. Most neurons in the brain and spinal cord have several dendrites and one axon; some (as in the retina, inner ear and smell receptors of the nose) have one dendrite and one axon.

Transmitters are produced by nerve cells to enable them to communicate with each other at synapses. Many different chemicals are used as transmitters in the brain and elsewhere, but the most common is acetylcholine. The endings of the transmitting nerve contain sacs of acetylcholine, and this is released when an impulse is received. It crosses the synaptic space, combines with receptors on the receiving nerve and makes them permeable to electrically charged particles of sodium and potassium. This enables the nerve message to pass through into the receiving nerve. Acetylcholine is destroyed within 0·002 of a second, and the receiving nerve becomes quiescent again. The next most common transmitter is noradrenaline.

More than 40 other chemicals act as neuro-transmitters in the brain. Eight are so-called "classical" transmitters, acting in a similar way to acetylcholine and noradrenaline but these may be present at fewer than half the brain synapses. The rest are peptides (sequences of amino-acids), which are involved in many other tasks; some are similar or identical to hormones found in other parts of the body, such as insulin. Unlike classical transmitters, peptides are not made at the nerve endings but are produced near the cell nucleus and then transported to the nerve endings, which can store several days' supply. It has been suggested that each nerve cell secretes many different peptides, the effects of which depend on what receptors are present on the receiving cell. In addition to endorphins, which suppress pain, other neuropeptides are linked with satiety after meals and learning and memory.

Excitatory transmitters work by reversing the electrical charges in the membrane of the receiving neuron, and inhibitory transmitters by strengthening it. This was discovered in the early 1950s by the British physiologists Alan Hodgkin (b. 1914) and Andrew Huxley (b. 1917). A resting neuron has 30 times more potassium ions than its surrounding medium, and one one-fifteenth of the sodium ions. Though both ions tend to leak through the nerve membrane, the difference is maintained by a pump than transports potassium in and sodium out. The effect is to make the cell electrically negative – by 70 millivolts – compared with its surroundings. When the nerve receives a strong stimulus – for instance when a skin receptor is fired or a transmitter is released onto it – the sodium channels of the pump open. The electrical charge goes down to zero and then to 30 millivolts. This charge is immediately transferred along the membrane (it can only travel in one direction). After firing, a part of a nerve needs a few milliseconds rest before it can conduct another impulse. Each nerve cell works on an all-or-nothing principle – a weak impulse will not fire it; we feel some impulses stronger than others because they fire more nerve fibers. Large fibers recover faster after firing, 2·5 milliseconds compared with 25 for smaller fibers.

Speeding nerve conduction

The speed of an impulse also depends on the size of the fiber through which it is traveling. The smallest (leading from gut receptors, or going to smooth muscle) are slowest; the thickest fibers (from skin receptors or going to skeletal muscle) are fastest. These are the nerves of split-second reactions, and unlike the smaller fibers they are all covered by a sheath of myelin. Myelin consists of the protoplasm of Schwann cells, found near peripheral nerves. Each Schwann cell gives out three or four flat protoplasmic extensions, each wrapping around three of four axons. Each axon has a succession of myelin cell wrappings; the gap where two meet is called a node of Ranvier. The myelin sheath acts to insulate the nerve, and so the electrical impulse jumps rapidly from one node to the next. Thus myelin speeds up nerve conduction. Unmyelinated nerves are also enclosed by Schwann cells, but they do not have the multiple binding.

In the brain and spinal cord, myelination is performed by four kinds of accessory brain cells called glial cells. These have several functions – they attach neurons to blood vessels; form strong, flexible connections between neurons and form a supporting network; destroy microbes and cellular debris; and provide a ciliated lining for the central cavity containing the cerebrospinal fluid.

Structure of a neuron

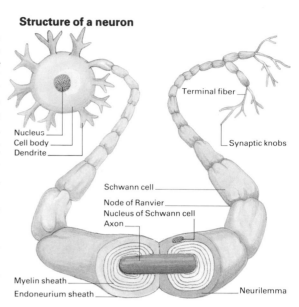

▲ *The neuron consists of a cell body, axon and synapse. The axon is surrounded by a myelin sheath created by Schwann cells wrapped around the axon. The impulse is transmitted along the nerve by the differential between the axon and surrounding tissue. The Schwann cells act as insulation in a myelinated cell so the impulse jumps from node to node and is therefore passed more quickly along the nerve.*

Transmitters of pain and relief

Among the many substances found in the brain that act as transmitters, there are more than 15 connected with the transmission of pain. One of these is known as Substance P, which is also found in the retina and in blood vessels behind the forehead (areas associated with migraine). Endorphins (short for "endogenous morphines") are a group of peptides that resemble morphine and suppress pain; they may act by suppressing the release of Substance P. They also enhance learning and memory, regulation of hormones that affect the onset of puberty, sexual drive, depression and schizophrenia (♦ page 82).

Enkephalins (peptides similar to endorphins) were discovered in 1975 by John Hughes (b. 1924) and Hans Kosterlitz (b. 1903) at Aberdeen University, Scotland. Mammal brains have receptors that react exclusively to opium, extracted from poppies, a fact that seems extremely odd since very few mammals are ever likely to encounter an opium poppy. To investigate this phenomenon, morphine, an extract of opium, was measured for strength on various tissues, including the vas deferens of a mouse. The vas deferens was dissected out and placed in a solution resembling normal body fluid. When a small electrical charge was passed through, the tissue contracted; but this contraction could be prevented by the application of a certain concentration of morphine. Hughes discovered the existence of enkephalins by looking for morphine-like activity in extracts of pig brain. His choice of mouse vas deferens was fortunate, since most other tissues destroy enkephalins.

Both of the two endorphins so far isolated are three times as potent as morphine, yet we do not become addicted to them.

Epilepsy...Motor neuron disease...Parkinsonism, multiple sclerosis and other disorders of the brain... Headaches and migraine...Fainting and stupor... Neuritis, neuralgia and diseases of the nerves... PERSPECTIVE...Famous neurologists...Boxing and brain damage...Brain cell transplants?

The two parts of the nervous system vary greatly in their reaction to damage and disease. The cells of the peripheral nervous system can regenerate; those of the central nervous system – the brain and spinal cord – are susceptible to damage, and once lost are irreplaceable.

Epileptic fits

Violent electrical activity in the brain produces epilepsy (fits). Fits can also be induced by brain infections, strokes, heatstroke, drugs, poisons and drug withdrawal. Only 25 percent of chronic sufferers have an obvious cause such as brain tumors (♦ page 62). Most sufferers are mentally and physically normal between fits, and their EEG may show no abnormalities. There are three kinds of epileptic fit. In *grand mal*, which is preceded by a premonition ("aura"), the sufferer shouts and falls down unconscious with muscles tensed, and then twitches and writhes, salivating, incontinent, and with eyeballs rolling. After two to five minutes movements cease and the patient regains consciousness, feeling tired, dazed, with aching head and sore muscles. *Petit mal* begins and ends abruptly. The patient becomes pale and normal activitites are suspended for 5 to 30 seconds as the eyes stare or blink rapidly. In focal epilepsy, the patient undergoes muscle spasms for several minutes, starting at the mouth, thumb, or big toe and moving over the body. There is a temporary loss of awareness, sometimes followed by hallucinations. Nothing can cut short any kind of epileptic fit but recurrences may be controlled by drugs.

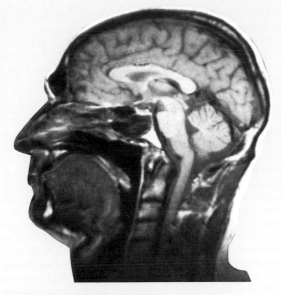

▲ *NMR section through the brain.*

EEGs – recording the brain's activity

The electrical activity of the brain's surface can be recorded from the scalp. The technique, electroencephalography and the recording made, an electroencephalogram, are both called EEGs.

Electrodes, usually 16, are placed in standard positions on or just under the scalp, and the electrical differences between them are chaneled through the encephalograph, which converts the impulses into the vertical movement of a pen over a sheet of paper. The resultant encephalogram takes about 30 minutes to record.

Most normal adults have an alpha rhythm, which is abolished by thinking or opening the eyes. Beta rhythms, which are fast, are found in anxious people and can be induced by drugs. Theta waves, slower than alpha, are found in many normal adults, probably arising from the temporal lobes. Delta waves, which are very slow, are often found between epileptic fits.

Normal EEGs vary between individuals, and with age, emotions, metabolic changes, drugs and state of consciousness, including sleep. Despite these variables, EEGs reveal a lot about many brain and metabolic diseases, from epilepsy and dementia to myxedema (♦ page 93) and liver disorders. EEGs alone are not a good measure of brain death – patients have recovered from barbiturate coma and hypothermia although their EEGs recorded no brain activity.

Other methods of comparable, non-invasive brain investigations include ultrasound and scanning (♦ page 38), which can show cerebral blood flow and the site of blood vessel and brain tissue damage and tumors. The brain is also investigated by injecting into arteries dye that shows on X-ray, and radioactive chemicals, including some that penetrate the blood-brain barrier only where there is disease.

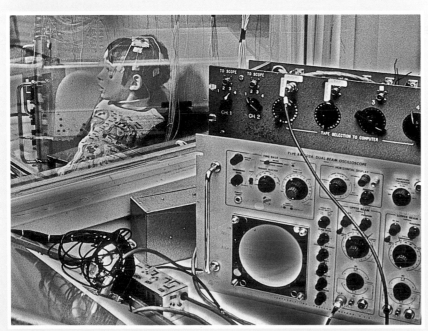

◀ *Taking the EEG of a child. The electrical activity of the brain was first demonstrated by the German psychiatrist Hans Berger in 1929, when he identified alpha waves. It was many years before the value of his work was generally appreciated.*

Wasting diseases, tumors, concussion, migraines...

Motor neuron disease, which often runs in families, is a wasting disease starting in tongue, hand and arm, with intermittent cramp. The disease gradually spreads over the body and death, usually from pneumonia (◆ page 172), takes place within three years. Its cause is unknown and there is no treatment. It was first described in 1865 by French neurologist Jean-Martin Charcot (1825-1893), Freud's teacher; Charcot also made the first distinction between Parkinson's disease (parkinsonism) and multiple sclerosis.

Senile dementia and Alzheimer's disease, severe insanity caused by brain degeneration, are related conditions starting in mid- or later life. A few cases are caused by poisoning, liver disease, tumors or alcoholism. Early symptoms are mental deterioration and apathy. Death takes place within five to ten years, but some sufferers benefit from an operation to drain the cerebrospinal fluid.

Multiple sclerosis results from progressive loss of the myelin sheath covering nerves in the brain and those leading around the body, resulting in visual disturbances, abnormal movement, and loss of coordination, strength and stamina. The sufferer may also experience emotional upsets, apathy and an inability to concentrate. Onset is usually in early adult life, and the disease goes through cycles of improving and relapsing. Patients survive for an average of 20 years.

Parkinsonism, caused by cell death in the substantia nigra, starts in late middle age. It may be caused by drugs, follow encephalitis or arise spontaneously. Patients suffer tremor and apathy, and have difficulty starting to move and stopping once they are moving. Unlike multiple sclerosis, for which there is no treatment (◆ page 248), parkinsonism can be treated with the drug L-dopa and physiotherapy.

Brain tumors vary in effect depending on their site and which brain structures they compress. There may be loss of senses, movement or speech; or sustained headache, nausea and mental deterioration.

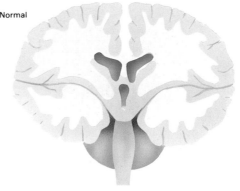

Boxing and brain damage

"It started two years ago and it's been getting more acute. I'm always tired. I go to bed and sleep eight, ten hours, but two hours after I get up I'm tired and drowsy again...for 33 years I've been taking punches." These were the words of Muhammad Ali (b. 1942), former world heavyweight boxing champion, when brain damage was diagnosed in September 1984. Ali has been slurring his speech and repeating himself – symptoms of damage to the brain – since 1980.

Boxers occasionally get brain hemorrhages in the ring, and often suffer the accumulated effects of thousands of blows. Frequently these lead to "punch-drunkenness" – slurred speech, unsteady gait, poor memory and clumsiness. Ex-boxers may be impotent, insomniac and have deteriorating vision. Most of the damage is in the substantia nigra, a key part of the brain's motor system; other damage is to the cortex and cerebellum. There is often retinal detachment and dementia.

Shortly before Ali's condition was known, both the American and British Medical Associations published reports on boxing and brain damage and adopted policies in favor of banning professional boxing. Those who support professional boxing point out that the number of known injuries, serious or otherwise, is small in proportion to the number of contests.

Normal

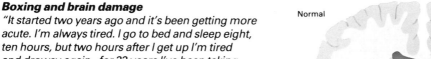

Damaged

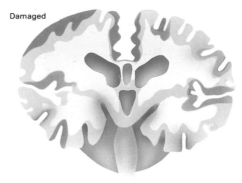

▲ ◄ Muhammad Ali and Leon Spinks in the ring, fighting for the heavyweight championship of the world. When a boxer is hit on the head his brain is slammed against his skull. This may result in internal bleeding. In the long run this can cause brain damage and even death; a boxer's brain in section may appear shrunken, with enlarged spaces and separated tissues.

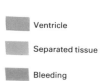

Ventricle

Separated tissue

Bleeding

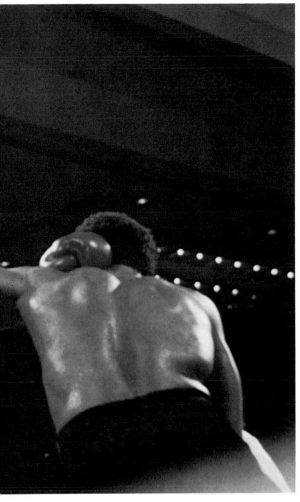

Patients are frequently cured, and usually improved, by surgery. Stroke, loss of blood supply to part of the brain (♦ page 168) and brain damage can cause paralysis, or loss of speech or vision, depending on their location.

Fainting is loss of consciousness because insufficient blood is reaching the brain. Sufferers must be allowed to remain with their heads low until they recover. Narcolepsy, abnormal desire for sleep and repeated daytime sleeping attacks and paralysis, is a rare disease running in families; it is treated by stimulation drugs. Concussion is temporary loss of consciousness, lasting a few minutes, after head injuries. Stupor is partial loss of consciousness and has a variety of causes. Concussion and stupor often indicate brain damage or bleeding, and medical help should be sought promptly, even though there are usually no lasting effects. Coma, prolonged unconsciousness, is a sign of serious damage or disease.

Frequent ordinary headaches are usually a sign of tension or worry. They occasionally indicate eye strain but are almost never a sign of a brain tumor. Migraine (sick headache) is found in children and adults, and usually fades after 60. It is often preceded about 20 minutes earlier by a premonition ("aura") including numbness, nausea, dizziness or speechlessness. An attack consists of throbbing head pain, often with vomiting, chill, tremor, dizziness and an aversion to lights and sounds. It affects five women to every two men, and is commoner in people who live stressful lives. It is often precipitated by allergies to food such as red wine, cheese, chocolate and onions. It can be reduced in frequency by avoiding foods to which the sufferers know they are allergic, and by regular meals, rest and relaxation. Attacks can be cut short if medicines (including ergotamine) are taken when the aura first appears. People suffering frequent attacks can prevent many recurrences by taking beta-blocker drugs (♦ page 144).

Stroke

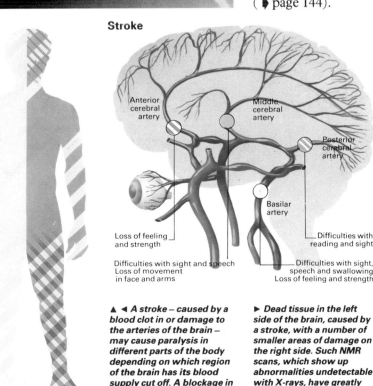

Anterior cerebral artery

Middle cerebral artery

Posterior cerebral artery

Basilar artery

Loss of feeling and strength

Difficulties with sight and speech
Loss of movement in face and arms

Difficulties with reading and sight

Difficulties with sight, speech and swallowing
Loss of feeling and strength

▲ ◄ A stroke – caused by a blood clot in or damage to the arteries of the brain – may cause paralysis in different parts of the body depending on which region of the brain has its blood supply cut off. A blockage in the anterior artery is the most common (♦ page 162).

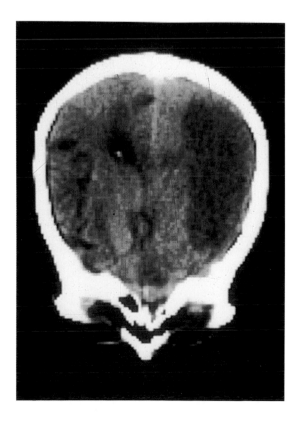

► Dead tissue in the left side of the brain, caused by a stroke, with a number of smaller areas of damage on the right side. Such NMR scans, which show up abnormalities undetectable with X-rays, have greatly improved diagnosis of brain diseases and tumors.

Neuralgia, sciatica, tics, tremors...

Inflammation of the nerves is called neuritis. Degeneration and other diseases in the nerves is neuropathy. Their effects are similiar and each can be caused by pressure, oxygen shortage, infection, poisons, diabetes, gout or vitamin B1 deficiency. There is prolonged numbness, tingling or paralysis as the nerve loses its sensory or motor function, and the area it innervates becomes acutely painful for some days. Bell's palsy is a neuropathy of the nerve controlling facial expression and eyelid closure on one side of the face. Paralysis is complete after two days, but 85 percent of cases recover over a few weeks; other cases recover slowly and incompletely regenerate. Neuralgia – nerve pain, found in older people – can occur anywhere in the body but is commonest in the trigeminal nerve (◀ page 57). Carpal tunnel syndrome, compression of the nerve at the wrist, is commonest in people who work with their hands. Minor surgery can relieve the compression. Sciatica is inflammation and pain in the sciatic nerve (◀ page 53). Commoner in men, it can start around 40.

Tics are involuntary nervous twitches such as blinking, grimacing or shaking the head. Commonest in teenagers, they are a sign of stress and neurosis. Choreas are diseases with involuntary tremors, tics and jerks. Some cause only mild disability; others, like Huntington's chorea, are fatal. Torticollis, muscle spasm turning the head to one side, is a lifelong disease. The cause is unknown. Restless legs syndrome consists of tingling or pain in the legs when they are still, so that the sufferer feels obliged to walk or move. It can be associated with iron deficiency, and is often relieved by iron or sedatives.

Brain transplants

In recent years, scientists have been able to make a brain graft "take" in animals. Pieces of implanted fetal brain, or brain cells separated and injected as a suspension, will grow fibers into the host brain. The host brain is less good at growing fibers into the graft. British biologist Steve Dunnett has used grafts to restore lost agility and memory to aged rats. Scientists in New York and Oxford have used grafts to cure rats with inherited absence of brain-secreted hormones. Swedish biologist Anders Bjorklund has cured rats with experimentally-produced parkinsonism, by grafting fetal substantia nigra neurons into their brains. He achieved the same result by transplanting adrenal medulla cells. These are derived from the spinal cord and have the same transmitter chemical, dopamine, as the substantia nigra. Swedish neurologist Erik-Olof Backlund has transplanted adrenal medulla cells into two severely ill parkinsonism patients, in 1982 and 1983. The first showed marginal improvement; the second was unchanged. In the future, despite such disappointing results, transplants are likely to help patients with diseased or damaged brains.

▼ *Paraplegic athletics. Paraplegia, paralysis of the legs, and tetraplegia, paralysis of all four limbs, occur when the spinal cord is partially or wholly severed. The limbs affected lose all sensation and voluntary movement. Despite recent experimentation on regenerating severed spinal cords in animals, human paraplegia and tetraplegia remain incurable, but rehabilitation may improve the quality of life.*

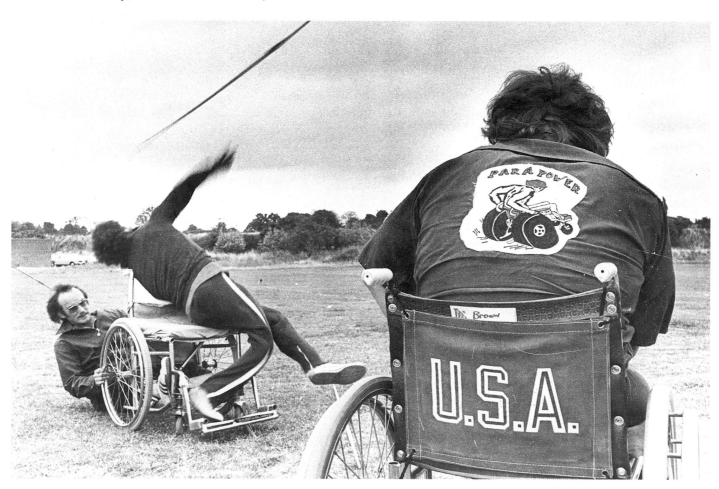

*Defining intelligence...Emotions...Personality traits...
Speech, a unique ability...Language and grammar...
What is learning?...Memory...PERSPECTIVE...IQ testing...
The two hemispheres of the brain...Can chimpanzees
be taught to speak?...Hypnosis...Phrenology...
Parapsychology*

Intelligence, said the British computer scientist Christopher Evans (1931-1979), is "one of the most important concepts in psychology and one of the least understood". It is even harder to define. Evans saw it as "a quickness of response to changes in the environment, the ability to scan a variety of solutions to any problem, and in particular to perceive new relationships between any aspects of a problem".

Adult intelligence quotient (IQ) is commonly measured on a scale, devised by psychologist David Wechsler (b. 1896), which tests knowledge and use of words, numerical skills, and ability to recognize patterns. The average score for a population is 100; more than two-thirds of the population fall within the range 85-115. Those scoring below 70 are ranked subnormal; only one percent score above 150.

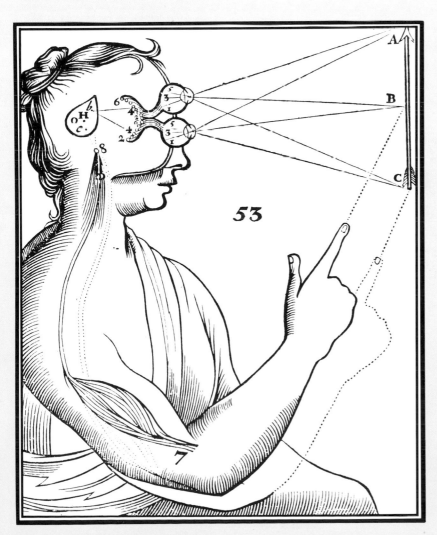

Debates about the tests for intelligence
The scientific study of intelligence was pioneered by the British scientist Sir Francis Galton (1822-1911). He believed that mental and physical attributes were inherited, an idea endorsed by his cousin Charles Darwin (1809-1882). The issue remains contentious – those who believe that intelligence is largely inherited point to studies on identical twins raised separately, which suggest that heredity accounts for as much as 80 percent of intelligence. Against this, the Swiss psychologist Jean Piaget (1896-1980) regarded intelligence as stimulated by environment: information-processing skills adapt an individual to an ever-changing environment. A third view is that intelligence consists of skills in a particular culture; technological societies require abstract reasoning, learned during formal schooling. Hence it is increased by motivation and reduced by poverty – children brought up in a "culture of failure" have feelings that limit their educational goals. Selection of tasks favor groups arbitrarily – girls are supposed to be better at language, boys at mechanical skills; other differences are found if races are compared.

Sir Cyril Burt (1883-1971), the most respected British psychologist of his time, "proved" that identical twins reared separately had almost identical IQs, regardless of widely differing environments. This was taken as showing that ability is innate, and cannot be improved by education. During the middle of this century the British education system, with examination at age 11 directing high scorers to grammar schools and average or low scorers to academically inferior schools, was based on Burt's published reports. After Burt's death his biographer recognized grave faults in his work, and in 1972 US psychologist Leo Kamin re-read Burt's work and immediately decided he was a fraud. Investigation strongly suggested that Burt had invented his data on twins, and that Burt's two alleged research co-workers never existed. US psychologist Arthur Jensen (b. 1923), Burt's disciple, still sees racial differences as proving a dominance of nature over nurture. He is supported by British psychologist Hans Eysenck (b. 1916), but strongly opposed by other scientists.

Some scientists believe that Japanese IQs have risen steadily since 1910 and in 1982 averaged 11 percent higher than Americans, with 10 percent having scores above 130, compared with only 2 percent of Americans. Others dispute the significance of these figures. Tests can be weighted to remove (or increase) differences of age, race and gender; as for instance when the IQs of children are calculated, their "mental age", revealed by the number of tests successfully completed, is divided by the actual age, then multiplied by 100 to give an IQ figure. Manipulation of the figures in a similar manner to take more contentious traits into account tends to lead to circular arguments as to the effect of environment on intelligence.

◀ *An illustration by René Descartes (1596-1650) of the pathways between sense organs, brain and motor muscles. Descartes saw the mind as a non-physical phenomenon independent of the essentially physical activity of the senses, nerves and brain. This view has dominated Western philosophy and is fundamental to most scientific research.*

The source of our emotions

The brain "feels" as well as thinks. Emotions, combined with reason, determine our reaction to people, objects and events. They forge bonds within families and between friends and colleagues. Centers in the hypothalamus and limbic system of the brain (◀ page 54), which were first discovered by Canadian neuropsychologist James Olds in 1953, are linked upward to the cortex (especially prefrontal) and have nerve connections to glands. Closely-grouped centers evoke pleasure, rage, and other emotions when stimulated. Emotions are difficult to conceal – although facial expressions can be controlled voluntarily, body changes such as dilation of pupils cannot. The blending of emotion and thought produces personality.

Describing the personality

Personality tests are often used to assess applicants for responsible positions. The 16PF test, devised by American psychologist R.B. Cattell (b. 1905), measures some 16 personality traits. A test devised by Hans Eysenck differentiates between extroverts and introverts – people with outgoing or inward-looking personalities – and between stable and neurotic personalities. It has been suggested that the qualities thus identified correlate closely with those suggested by the medieval notion of the four humors (◀ page 34). Another British psychologist, Liam Hudson (b. 1933), in *Contrary Imaginations* (1966), differentiates between convergers and divergers. Convergers tend to be conformist and do better at conventional intelligence tests; they approach problems logically and simplify them. They are less creative than divergers, who do better at open-ended tests that have no single answers, and are more likely to be independent-minded, self-reliant, and rebellious against authority.

Demonstrating the division of the brain

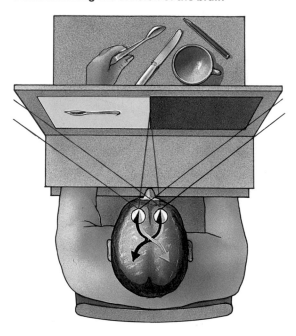

▲ *In a classic experiment, patients who had had the corpus callosum cut were asked to look through a screen allowing them to perceive an object for an instant with only the right side of the brain. Since this side of the brain cannot speak, the patient could not name the objects but could reach for the object shown with the left hand (which is controlled by the right side of the brain). The right hand could not pick up the object since the left side of the brain had not seen the object on the screen. The operation to sever the corpus callosum was done to cure a serious form of epilepsy.*

▶ *The right side of the brain is thought to be the center for activities needed for artistic skills and in particular the sense of patterns and design. It is claimed that by training this faculty, people can be taught to draw and paint more quickly than by conventional methods. The examples on the far right were drawn after only two or three months training by previously untutored students.*

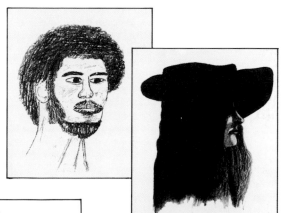

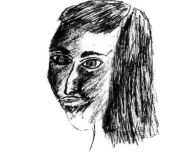

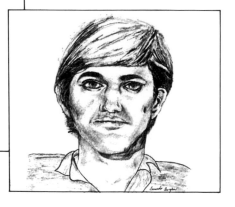

The two halves of the brain

The cerebral cortex is divided down the middle, with hundreds of thousands of nerve fibers – the corpus callosum – linking the two sides. The two hemispheres are equally important for determining motor functions and receiving sensory messages (◀ page 57). Over a century ago British neurologist Hughlings Jackson (1835-1911), studying brain-damaged people, discovered that injury to the right hemisphere caused relatively minor impairment of faculties. The left hemisphere is more important for speech and verbal comprehension, at least in most people; left-handed people sometimes have right-hemisphere dominance or no dominance at all.

In the 1950s it was found that cutting the corpus callosum helped many epileptic patients, preventing seizures from spreading across the brain. In the 1960s, the American Roger Sperry (b. 1913) found that, on recovery, these patients could read, write, sew, play the piano, ride a bicycle – their perceptions and skills seemed unimpaired. However, tests showed that, literally, the left hand did not know what the right hand was doing – a person could be buttoning a coat with the left hand and unbuttoning it with the right. A patient could describe by feel an object in the right hand, which sends fibers to the left (speech) side of the brain. When the same object was held in the left hand, the patient insisted nothing was there. Previously, Sperry had shown that normal cats could learn a

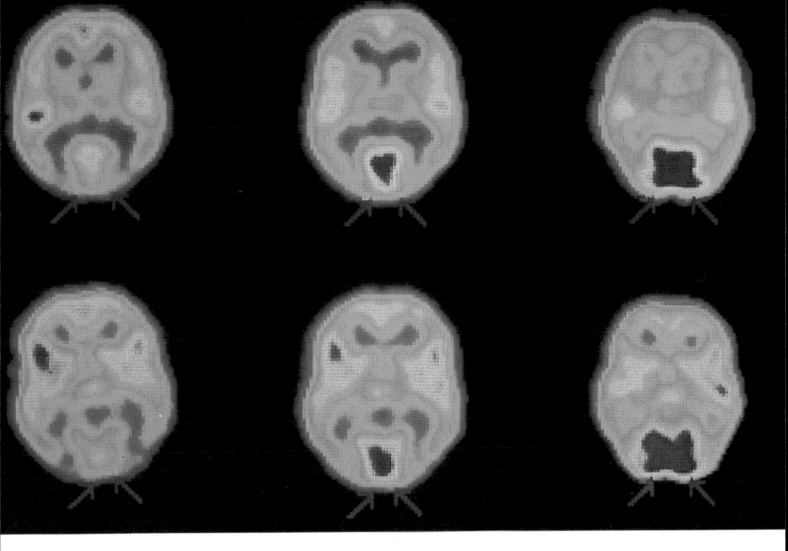

task with one eye masked and repeat it with the other eye masked, but when the corpus callosum was cut they could not. This indicates that a copy of information learned in one hemisphere is normally duplicated by the other, where it is accessible for comparison with new information.

In 1982 British neuropsychologists Donald and Valerie Mackay studied split-brain patients. The left eye was shown a number from 0 to 9, which was thus perceived by the right side of the brain. Then the patient was asked to guess the number. Since this requires speech, it meant using the brain's left hemisphere. The right side of the brain heard the guess and, although it could not make the patient speak, it did allow the patient to point at helpful cards saying "go up", "go down," or "OK." The game continued until the left side was correct. The pointing, of course, was seen by both sides of the brain. The two hemispheres played happily against each other; there were no stakes.

The Mackays then added another rule: for every incorrect guess, the left side had to pay the right side three tokens. For each correct guess, it received tokens from the Mackays. This game was "won" by the right side, which bankrupted the left. Next, the Mackays asked the left if it would drop its price to two tokens per wrong guess. They expected it to refuse (by pointing) but it did not – thus indicating that although there are effectively two independently-operating brains in such patients, there is only one will.

▲ Scans through the brain, showing the activity of parts of the brain at rest (left), with the eyes open (centre) and watching a complex scene (right). The visual cortex is at the base of the image. In this technique, radio-active "labels" are attached to the blood glucose; they therefore show on the scan the areas where glucose is required, indicating zones of high activity (red).

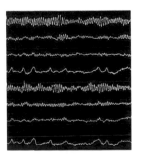

▲ ▶ Electroencephalography (EEG) records the brain's electrical activity through electrodes on the scalp. These reveal distinctive patterns of brain activity.

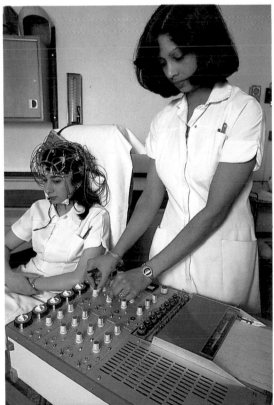

The larynx

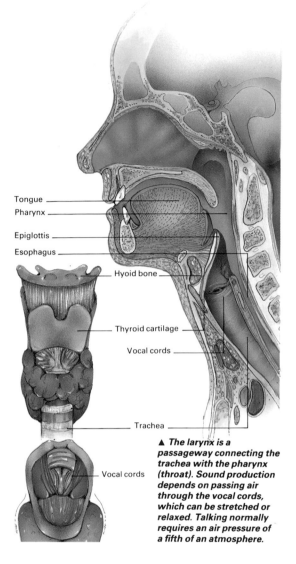

Tongue
Pharynx
Epiglottis
Esophagus
Hyoid bone
Thyroid cartilage
Vocal cords
Trachea
Vocal cords

▲ *The larynx is a passageway connecting the trachea with the pharynx (throat). Sound production depends on passing air through the vocal cords, which can be stretched or relaxed. Talking normally requires an air pressure of a fifth of an atmosphere.*

Speech is the only ability we do not share with animals. It is made possible by specialization of the brain and the larynx (voicebox). The larynx lies at the top of the windpipe. Its inner lining has two pairs of folds – the upper pair, present in all air-breathing vertebrates, are the valves allowing us to hold our breath under water. The lower pair, the vocal cords, are flat white bands, 13-18mm long in women and 17-25mm long in men. Sound originates from vibration of the cords, forced apart by air pressure. Other structures convert sounds into speech – pharynx, mouth, nasal cavity and nasal sinuses form resonating chambers that give voices their individual quality. We form vowels by moving muscles in the pharynx wall, and enunciate words using muscles of face, tongue and lips. Vocal range is determined by cord length and thickness. Voices are varied up and down the scale by muscle tension – when vocal cords are pulled taut they vibrate faster, and the pitch rises.

Speech and the brain

Two areas of cerebral cortex are necessary for speech. Broca's area, named after its discoverer, French neurologist Paul Broca (1824-1880), is in the frontal lobe, usually on the left, near the motor cortex controlling muscles of the lips, jaws, soft palate and vocal cords. When damaged by stroke or injury, comprehension is unaffected but speech is slow and labored and the sufferer will talk in "telegramese". Wernicke's area, discovered in 1874 by German neurologist Carl Wernicke (1848-1904), lies to the back of the temporal lobe, again, usually on the left, near the areas receiving auditory and visual information. Damage to it destroys comprehension – the sufferer speaks fluently but nonsensically.

American psycholinguist Noam Chomsky (b. 1928) has suggested that rules for meaning and grammar are inborn. This idea is supported by studies of children's speech. Their first negative statements consist of adding "no" or "not" to a positive statement: "no dog like it," instead of "dogs don't like it". Later they use the uncontracted form of will: "I will read you book," though they hear adults say "I'll read you a book." These habits are universal in young children, suggesting the idea of innate grammar.

Regions of the brain

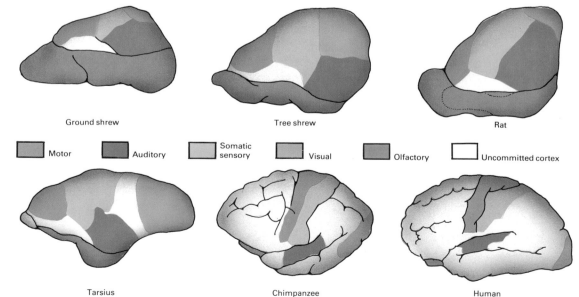

Ground shrew

Tree shrew

Rat

| Motor | Auditory | Somatic sensory | Visual | Olfactory | Uncommitted cortex |

► *A comparison of the regions of the cerebral cortexes of various mammals devoted to sensory perception shows a far lower proportion allocated in this way in humans. The uncommitted cortex allows language and reasoning in humans.*

Tarsius

Chimpanzee

Human

Expressing an idea

The brain forms an idea, as yet not put into words or defined grammatically

The idea is passed to the semantic component, where it is given a grammatical structure, and a decision is made on the type of the words required to express it

In the lexicon, suitable words are selected to express the components of the idea. These words may be stored in networks of association with each other, so that a search for a word in one particular field may give access to many others that relate to a similar context

The grammar or syntax of the sentence is firmed up, and the words chosen from the lexicon are given the appropriate endings and assembled in their correct order

The sentence is passed to the phonemic center, where the words are broken down into their individual sound components

The words in the lexicon are not stored complete, but broken into their component parts or morphemes. Thus prefixes, suffixes and word stems may be reassembled to form new arrangements as required

In the speech production center, the phonemes are converted into instructions to the vocal cords, and the idea is finally spoken

◄ *Speech production involves the assembly of the required sentence with words constructed and arranged according to grammatical rules. The sentence is then broken down once more into phonetic units and converted into speech.*

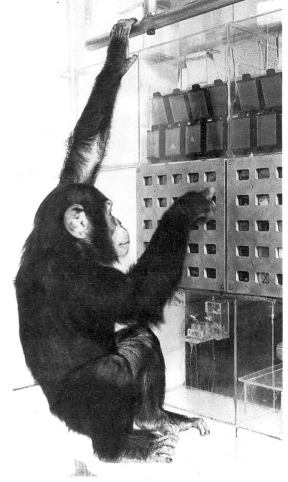

▲ *Experiments were carried out in Atlanta, Georgia, in the 1970s to use chimpanzees to assist in developing language-learning machines. This chimpanzee is seen using a computerized keyboard, on which individual keys stand for words. Combining keys allows the development of simple grammar. Such machines have proved to be of value in helping to teach language to severely disabled humans.*

Is language exclusive to humans?

Parrots, mynahs and budgerigars can learn and utter complex phrases, thanks to their well-developed syrinx (songbox) and an inbuilt tendency to mimickry. However, there is no evidence that they understand what they are "saying"; they cannot hold a conversation.

Stronger claims for language ability have been made for chimpanzees. In the 1960s and 70s American psychologists Robert and Beatrice Gardner taught deaf-and-dumb language to a young chimp, Washoe, and reported that she had learnt 132 words by age four, 180 by age eight. Later the experiment was repeated by US psychologist Herbert Terrace. His chimp, Nim, seemed to string words together ungrammatically: "give me orange give orange me eat orange give me eat orange give me you". But when Terrace watched videotapes of Nim and his teachers, he decided that Nim was actually responding to the subconscious prompting of his teachers. Although this interpretation was generally accepted, the debate about animal language is still unresolved.

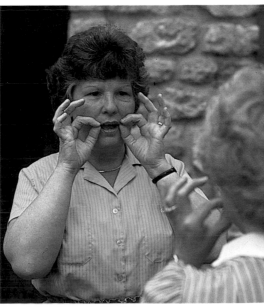

► *Sign language, as developed for use with deaf people, demonstrates the basic requirements of a proper language. Whereas most people use more or less eloquent gestures, perhaps with some to signify specific objects or actions, gesturing offers no possibility of constructing sentences. With genuine sign language, it is possible to use normal grammar.*

There is probably a limit to the number of stimuli we can sample at any one time

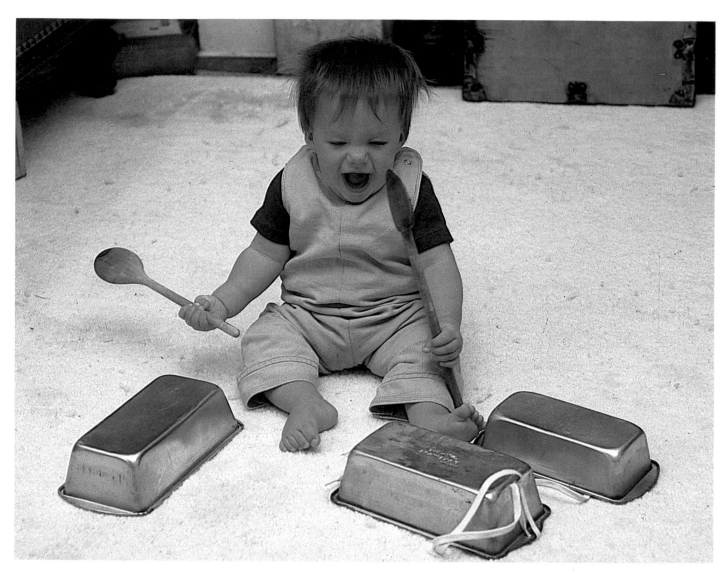

▲ *A young child, experimenting with the environment directly, sees everyday items as objects to be investigated for their intrinsic qualities as much as their use. This exemplifies Piaget's first "sensorimotor" phase of learning, when intelligence is non-verbal, and the child's interaction with the world is purely motor and sensory.*

Child development

Swiss psychologist Jean Piaget (b. 1896) believes that intellectual development moves through set stages. He claimed that for the first two years children use only muscles and senses to deal with objects and events. From ages two to seven they are in the "pre-operational" stage, using words for objects and feelings. They manipulate objects experimentally, using trial-and-error, intuition and experience. From seven to twelve they are in the "concrete-operational" stage, using logic for the first time and classifying objects; from twelve onward they have the mental operations of adults, thinking flexibly, making and understanding hypotheses. Piaget's views are challenged by British psychologists Barbara Tizard and Martin Hughes, who argue that children may use more complex ideas in conversations with their mothers than they reveal to teachers or researchers.

How do we learn?

Learning is the acquisition and storage of information in a way that allows its use to modify future behavior. It is distinguished from memory – the act of storage or the storage mechanism itself – and from remembering – the process of bringing the learned information out of storage. People vary in their approach to learning, some using visual imagery, others verbal skills, for example. Learning a new idea or skill is slow at the first attempt, followed by a prolonged acceleration but slowing again at a later stage. It is influenced by our physical state and environment – divers who learned lists of words when under water could recall them better during their next dive than they could on dry land, and stories heard after drinking alcohol are more easily recalled after a few drinks than when sober.

The simplest form of learning is habituation – pupils contract strongly if a light is shone once in the eyes, but contract less if it is shone repeatedly. Almost as simple is sensitization – we learn early in life to withdraw our hands from something hot, and react similarly when touching something that appears hot but is not, such as the sole of an electric iron that has cooled down. A more complicated learning – Pavlovian or "classical" conditioning (♦ page 121) – was identified by Russian physiologist Ivan Pavlov (1849-1936). Pavlov's work was

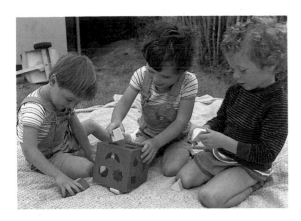

▲ *In Piaget's second phase, children manipulate objects in their minds as well as physically, and begin to use trial and error as a means of assembling knowledge.*

▼ *In the third phase, children learn to analyze situations with a basic logic and to see objects both in terms of similarities and differences.*

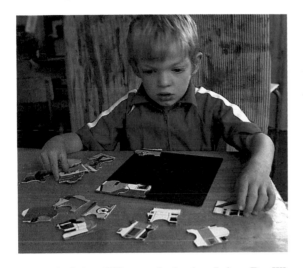

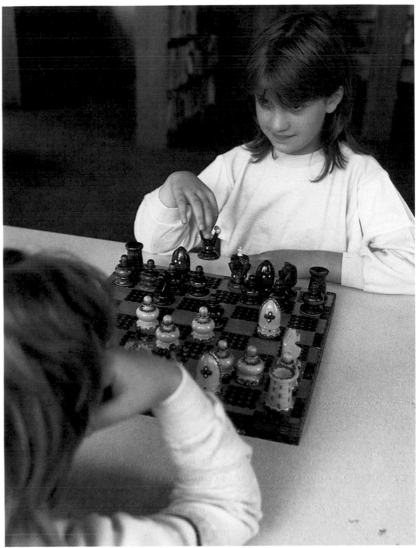

expanded by US psychologist John B. Watson (1878-1958), who identified a more active form of learning, operant ("instrumental") conditioning. An animal, on hearing or seeing a stimulus (in many experiments a bell or light) performs a response for which it is rewarded (or is punished if it does not perform). The studies based on this approach formed the basis of behaviorism, a branch of psychology explaining behavior in objective and purely physical terms, regarding thoughts as unspoken words. Led by US psychologist Burrhus F. Skinner (b. 1904), inventor of teaching machines, it concentrates on activities that are unambiguous, observable and preferably measurable. He regards humans as fundamentally the same as higher animals, although more complex, and sharing the same mechanisms of learning, perception and memory. The opposing school of thought, led by US psycholinguist Noam Chomsky, is mentalism – the idea that behavior results from our existing mental states and processes.

Effective learning requires attention, which consists of sensory focusing. Psychologists believe we can sample only a certain number of stimuli at a time – a greater range of input means less attention to each item. Attention to the outside world is consequently reduced when we are using our brains to think and solve problems.

▲ *As a child approaches adult capacity, new possibilities of flexible thinking become possible. Situations can be analyzed in the abstract, if necessary without recourse to sensory experience, and future scenarios can be envisaged and assessed. This corresponds to Piaget's final stage of intellectual development.*

The mystery of hypnosis

Hypnosis has probably been practised for centuries and was formally recognized in 1776 by Franz Anton Mesmer (1734-1828). He called it "animal magnetism"; later it was misnamed hypnosis, from the Greek for sleep. Brainwaves, heartbeat and respiration resemble those of wakefulness, and the knee jerk, absent in sleep, remains. Only about one person in 20 can be deeply hypnotized; rather more develop a light trance, and unwilling subjects are unaffected. On waking, the subject may not remember being hypnotized yet may continue to obey the instructions given under hypnosis. Hypnosis can be used to alter functions outside normal mental control, like secretion of digestive juices and glandular activity. Recently, hypnotherapy has produced dramatic cures in irritable bowel syndrome, a condition that does not respond to psychotherapy or placebo.

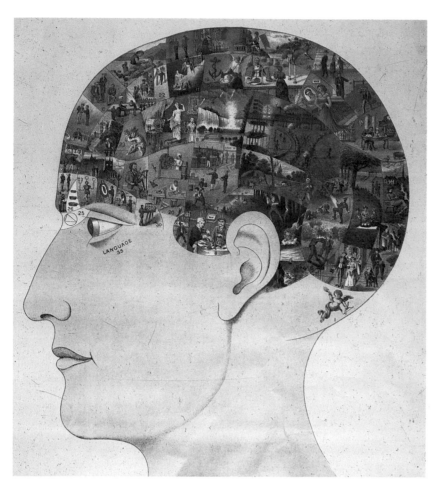

◄ Phrenologists thought romantic love was connected with the base of the skull, destructiveness with the area above the ears, constructiveness and ideality with the temples, cautiousness and friendship to the side towards the back, and benevolence, veneration, firmness and self-esteem along the top of the skull, from front to back.

Reading the bumps

Phrenology was the belief, propagated by the German physiologist Franz Gall (1758-1828), that the variable development of different faculties or aspects of a person's character affected the development of the skull's bones. The cerebellum, at the rear of the brain, was thought to hold the "instinct of propagation", and love of children was at the back of the head, below the area showing love of one's homeland. The presence of this "inhabitativeness" in both humans and animals showed that "faculties which are merely physical in brutes may become moral in Man". Intellectual functions were at the front of the head. Acquisitiveness was above the ears. A prominent acquisitive bulge, "being found very large in certain thieves", betrayed "a natural disposition to theft". The theory, based as it was on imagination, was wishful thinking, and "proved" that Caucasian people, with their steeper foreheads, had the "distinguishing marks of superior intellect", whereas the Negro race showed "an inferior intellect and a preponderating quality of animal force". However, it was admitted, of Whites, that "there is many a fool, and many a shallow-pated coxcomb, with a finely developed head".

Unusual mental powers

Parapsychology is the study of paranormal phenomena such as telepathy (the direct communication between minds), precognition (knowledge of the future) clairvoyance (perception of objects concealed from sight) and psychokinesis (movement of objects using mental energy). All are controversial. Telepathic experience, premonitory dreams and the like are part of folklore; in 1882 the Society for Psychical Research was founded in London to study them. However, a century later, orthodox science remains unconvinced by claims of this sort.

In 1927, Joseph Rhine (b. 1895) founded a parapsychology research laboratory at Duke University in North Carolina. For nearly 40 years his research team gathered evidence for extra-sensory perception, largely by using an immense series of controlled tests using illustrated cards or mechanically-thrown dice. However, experiments successful in parapsychology laboratories rarely, if ever, succeed in less sympathetic environments. Near the end of his career, Rhine learned that his protegé and intended successor, Walter Levy, had been discovered manipulating the recording equipment. The laboratory closed when Rhine retired in 1965.

In 1974 Israeli "psychokinetist" Yuri Geller convinced a few scientists that he could perform feats such as bending spoons using mental powers. This was later discredited, not by scientists but by a professional magician, James Randi, who showed he could duplicate all Geller's feats using simple conjuring.

The mystery of memory

Memory has three components – registration, retention and recall. There are at least two forms of memory – short-term (which, for example, allows us to retain a telephone number long enough to dial it), and long-term memory. Psychologists have recently come to believe that there is also a medium-term store, and that different categories such as tastes and smell, sights, physical abilities and abstract learning are stored in different ways or parts of the brain.

Canadian psychologist Donald Hebb (b. 1904) proposed a two-stage theory in 1947: electrical activity, vulnerable and impermanent, holds the memory in store; and later a structural alteration, perhaps involving synthesis of a protein or neurotransmitter, retains it securely. Karl Lashley (1890-1958) discovered that destruction of part of the cortex weakens memories but does not destroy them. US psychologist Karl Pribram (b. 1911) has compared memories with holograms. These give a three-dimensional image, and destruction of part of one leaves a complete but fuzzy image. Many psychologists now believe that new input is held in an immediate memory store for half a second. Selected items then go to the short-term memory, where they drive out what is already there. If they are sufficiently reinforced they go into long-term memory. US neurologist Eric Kandel has studied habituation, sensitization and classical conditioning in sea slugs. He finds that these forms of learning are accompanied by specific permanent chemical changes controlling neurotransmitter release – transmission becomes weaker after habituation, but stronger after sensitization. The human brain may store memories similarly.

The interaction of body and mind...The effect of the mind on disease...Stress and disease...Positive thinking to cure disease...Meditation...Biofeedback machines... PERSPECTIVE...Placebos...Illness during wars

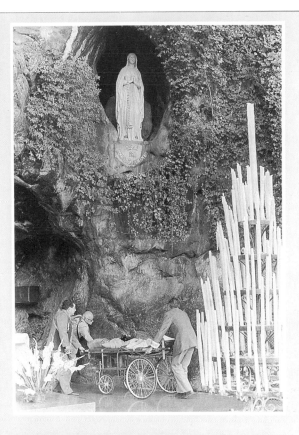

▲ *Lourdes, in southern France, has been a popular site for miraculous healing since St Bernadette saw visions of the Virgin Mary there in 1858. More than 60 miracles have been officially claimed.*

Mental states can have many physical influences, and affect susceptibility to a wide variety of ailments, from heart disease and peptic ulcers to common infections. Blushing with embarrassment is probably the clearest example of how mental processes can affect physiology involuntarily. Observations on "Beaumont's window" (♦ page 121) showed how readily gastric mucosa may be affected by emotion, and it has been known for some years that asthmatic attacks may be precipitated by anxiety and that response to this and other allergic conditions may be modified by hypnosis or relaxation techniques.

Physical disease triggered primarily by mental factors is called psychosomatic, from the Greek words *psyche*, meaning mind, and *soma*, body. In the past this word has been used in a derogatory sense to suggest that such diseases are "all in the mind". Psychoanalytic thinking in the 1930s tried to identify some conditions – including high blood pressure, rheumatic arthritis, ulcerative colitis and peptic ulcer – as being solely psychological in origin. In recent years the interaction between physical and emotional factors has been seen to be far more complex.

In part this has been the result of an increased awareness of the limitations of medicine based on a purely mechanistic view of Man. Anthropological studies have indicated some remarkable effects achieved by healing or harming rituals among "primitive" peoples, and have helped this change. However, a major part has also been played by the physiological research pioneered by Dr Hans Selye, who for many years directed the Institute of Experimental Medicine and Surgery at the University of Montreal, Canada. Here he developed his theory of stress as a physiological conditioner and was able to measure its effects in biochemical terms.

Mind, stress and illness

Stressful events (stressors, in Selye's terminology) induce a non-specific physiological response, regardless of whether the stressor is intrinsically a pleasant or unpleasant experience emotionally. Selye called this the generalized adaptation syndrome (GAS). A severe burn or a broken limb is the kind of traumatic physical event which Selye identified as a stressor. Psychological trauma has the same effect.

The basic effect of a stressor is to release hormones into the bloodstream from the adrenal cortex, the so-called "fight or flight" syndrome (♦ page 89). In addition to adrenaline, this includes the corticosteroids. In the short term, this response is beneficial, readying the body for improved performance. It increases alertness and diverts blood from stomach and bowels to muscles, making us better able to fight or flee. Stress-related disease today often derives from the inappropriateness of the "fight or flight" response, in a mismatch between lifestyle and instinct.

The placebo effect

One of the most convincing demonstrations of mind affecting matter is the placebo effect. When a new drug is tested on volunteers, some are given the drug and some an inert substance made to look the same. This is to enable the people conducting the trial to distinguish the real effects of the drug on test.

In the past, it has been found that where a drug recipient knows what its effect is supposed to be, he or she may show that effect even when they have received the placebo. Doctors now often prescribe harmless substances, knowing that patients, believing that the drug will cure them, will in fact be cured.

More than a third of patients suffering pain of one sort or another get relief from placebo analgesics. Placebos have been used to treat successfully such diverse conditions as headaches, seasickness, insomnia and epilepsy. In some cases, cures have been effective even when the patient has known that the drug is a placebo.

Some evidence suggests that a placebo's effectiveness may be related to the cost and unpleasantness of the treatment. Injected placebos seem to be more effective than oral ones, for example. A similarity between the difficulty of treatment and its effect is shown by some miracle cures. Visits to the shrine at Lourdes seem more effective among people who have had to travel a long distance than among those who live nearby.

Stress-related disease is more likely to occur in people with frustrated ambitions

Where the body shows a prolonged hormonal response as a result of unresolved stress, a number of disease states may result. The effect of the generalized adaptation syndrome on blood supply to stomach and bowels may cause gastrointestinal disorders such as peptic ulcers (◆ page 138) and diarrhea. Raised cardiac output and blood pressure result, which may be harmful (◆ page 166). Prolonged increases in cardiac output can lead to palpitations, for example. In a study of changes in pulse and blood pressure, using implanted electrodes, over the whole day, it was found that some events were particularly stressful. Driving is an example and overtaking, in particular, was accompanied by unhealthy heart behavior.

Personality and stress-related disease
Although stress-related diseases are often associated with executive positions, they actually occur through all levels of society. Boring, repetitive jobs lead to ulcers at least as often as managerial jobs. However, it may not be the job itself so much as the worker's attitude which affects health.

A number of studies have differentiated behavior into two groups. So-called Type A people are ambitious and forceful, as opposed to Type B who are not. A ten-year study of several thousand people in San Francisco showed that Type A people were twice as likely as Type B people to have a heart attack. Other research has suggested that the increased risk to Type A people is there only if they are frustrated. Ambitious and forceful people who achieve their goals may be no more at risk than Type B people.

Social isolation also seems to be a factor contributing to death soon after a heart attack. There may also be a correlation between survival and length of education, which could be related. Further evidence of the psychosomatic effects of such factors comes from research into unemployment. Unemployment tends to isolate men in particular from normal social contacts and is more prevalent at the lower end of the educational scale in developed countries. It seems to be causally linked to increased mortality.

Some "life events" are believed to be more likely to induce stress-related disease than others. Highest on the scale of such events is the death of a close relative or spouse, a type of stressor which one cannot either fight or flee. The stressfulness of events may be additive. In other words, two or three stressful events occurring within the same six-month period may have as strong an effect as a single, much more stessful event. There are many examples of such induced diseases. For example, research in several American laboratories indicates that stress impairs the body's immune response. Lymphocytes from individuals experiencing such adverse "life events" appear to be less efficient than usual in responding to foreign materials. This would account for the greater susceptibility of the body to both viruses and bacteria.

It may become possible in future to boost impaired immunity at critical times in a person's life by using substances called immune modulators. However, if mental outlook can affect physiology adversely, it is only reasonable that the reverse should also be true – that we should be able to affect our own physiology beneficially. Thus in looking at the reference groups, Type A and Type B, one study of Type A people who had had heart attacks showed a halving in the incidence of repeat attacks in a group which undertook a program aimed at converting them to Type B behavior.

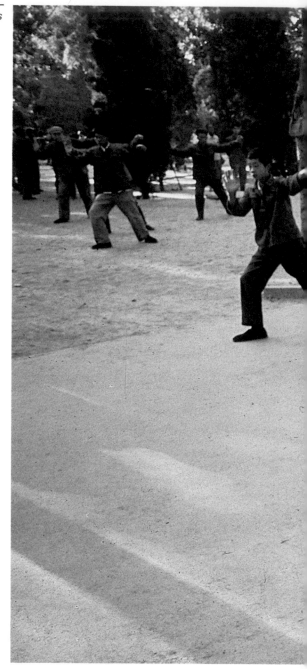

Event	USA	Japan
Death of spouse	1	1
Divorce	2	3
Marital separation	3	7
Marriage	4	6
Death of close family member	5	4
Detention in jail	6	2
Major illness or injury	7	5
Retirement from work	8	11
Losing job	9	8
Marital reconciliation	10	15
Sexual difficulties	11	10
Major change in health of family	12	9
New family member	13	23
Major business readjustment	14	12
Major change in financial state	15	21
Arguments with spouse	16	33
Death of close friend	17	16
Change to new line of work	18	13
Pregnancy	19	13
Mortgage foreclosure	20	19
Change in work responsibilities	21	22
Son or daughter leaving home	22	18

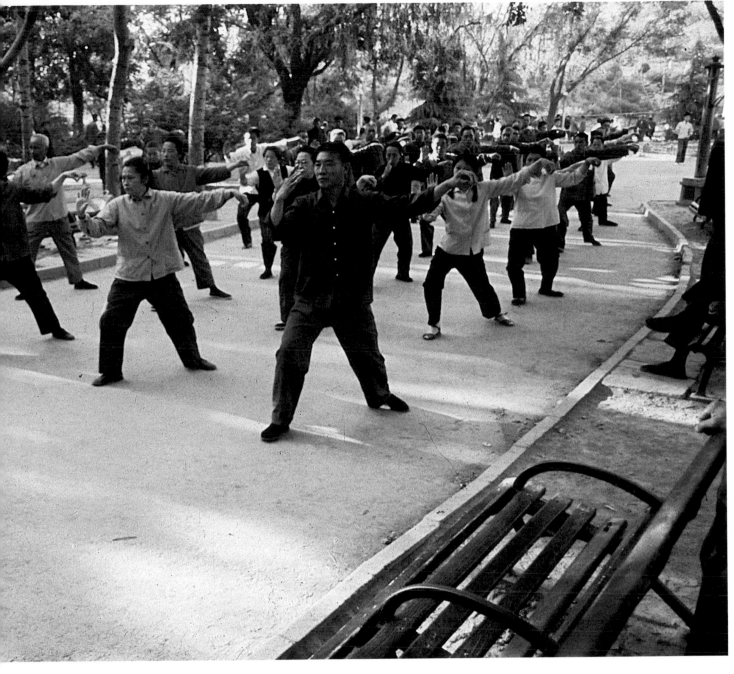

Event	USA	Japan
In-law trouble	23	20
Spouse starting or ending work	24	25
Start or finish of formal schooling	24	32
Troubles with superior at work	26	27
Outstanding personal achievement	27	24
Large mortgage loan	28	17
Major change in living conditions	29	26
Major change in working conditions	30	31
New school	31	34
Major revision of personal habits	32	29
New home	33	37
Major change in recreation	34	38
Major change in social activities	35	39
Major change in church activities	36	42
Major change in sleeping habits	37	35
Major change in eating habits	38	36
Small mortgage loan	38	30
Major change in family get-togethers	40	40
Vacation	41	41
Christmas	42	43
Minor violations of the law	43	28

▲ Body movement and meditation activities, such as Tai Chi, practised widely among the Chinese, can help relieve stress. The concentration and movement bring what is described as unification of body and mind.

▶ Shopping for bargains in the annual sales can be a highly stressful activity.

◀ A list of life events was evaluated by a group of Americans and Japanese according to how stressful they seemed. The answers were then assembled into a scale of relative stressfulness. The effect of these events is cumulative, so that a person undergoing three or four minor events may have similar stress to one suffering a major crisis.

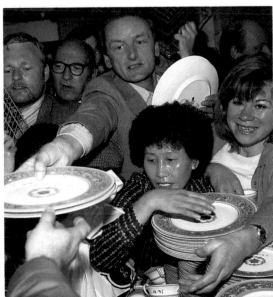

In recent years, certain relaxation techniques, such as meditation and biofeedback, have been promulgated as antidotes to stress. The common forms of meditation are yoga and transcendental meditation (TM). In TM, concentration on a very simple sound or thought leads to profound relaxation, accompanied by reduced metabolic rate and blood pressure. In biofeedback similar effects are produced with the aid of monitoring devices. It can clear migraine headaches, and reduce muscle tension during childbirth and anxiety attacks.

The evidence for the effects of mind on matter in more pathological conditions is more tenuous. It has been suggested that cancer can be precipitated by mental states. One view is that the immune system, which normally keeps cancer at bay, can be adversely affected by depression. Carl Simonton, in the USA, developed a visualization therapy based on this idea. He encouraged cancer patients to visualize an attack on their tumors. They did this in whatever terms they chose, not in scientific ones. Thus, they might see their body's defenses as a football team launching a concerted attack. Patients who were able to adopt this approach survived on average twice as long as "non-visualizers". Other studies have indicated that many patients diagnosed as having cancer often show no will to live. On the other hand, there is no doubt that some cancer sufferers do have a strong will to live and while many of them later die of the disease, it is also possible that their mental attitude affects the course of the illness (◗ page 228).

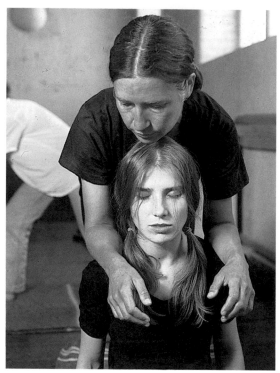

◀ A witch doctor in Indonesia; that they are able to induce both health and sickness in people by suggestion is a powerful example of the influence of the mind over bodily health.

▲ Practitioners of some forms of massage such as Japanese shiatsu claim to be able to prevent ill-health in many organs by relaxing muscles and manipulating pressure points.

Mind-induced diseases

The mind can also affect susceptibility to infection, as researchers at the Common Cold Unit near Salisbury in Britain have demonstrated. Of 48 volunteers given a common cold virus, half were told that later on in the experiment samples of their gastric juices would need to be crawn off with a stomach tube. When the volunteers' symptoms were afterwards assessed they were found to be significantly more severe in those who had the stomach-tube in prospect. Anxiety caused by the anticipated pain and discomfort had a marked effect on the course of the illness.

A striking example of the power of the mind is found in societies where people are aware and afraid of heart disease. Doctors often encounter patients with stabbing pains in their chest, which have no identifiable cause – known as Da Costa's syndrome after Jacob Da Costa, who first described it during the American Civil War.

When a war requires many men to fight who would not otherwise have joined the army, symptoms of heart disease are found in some of them, which have no cardiac origin. These are generated by fear and anxiety. Most frequently they show up as a physical incapacity to undergo training. Despite their non-cardiac origin they make the sufferer unfit for combat, removing him from the cause of his symptoms. During World War I, there were 60,000 cases among the British of whom more than two-thirds received disability pensions.

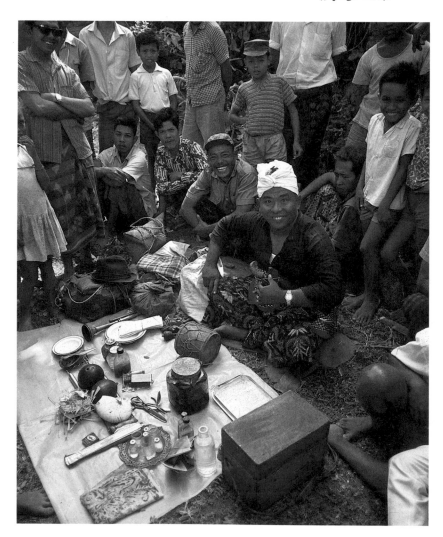

*The definition of mental illness...Neurosis...
Personality disorders...Psychosis...The treatment of
mental disorders...PERSPECTIVE...Freud and Jung...
Other founders of modern psychology...Munchausen's
syndrome...Redefining psychiatry*

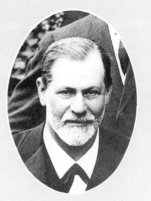

Sigmund Freud

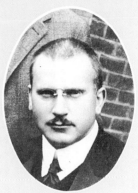

Carl Jung

Disorders of the mind, as opposed to disorders of the brain which have indisputably physical origins, are usually broken down into three main categories: neuroses, personality disorders and psychoses. Such disorders are, however, notoriously difficult to categorize, and behavior that is considered normal in some situations and at some periods may be regarded as abnormal in others.

Medical interest in mental illness developed in the 19th century, and the best-known attempt to explain the origins of mental disorders was that of Sigmund Freud, whose work as a psychoanalyst in Vienna at the turn of the 20th century led him to formulate the view that all such disorders were related to infant sexuality. Freud's view was challenged at the time, not least by Carl Jung and Alfred Adler, and is today generally considered to be too simplistic, failing to take other factors, including the social origins of psychological stress and society's expectations of normality, into account.

Mental illness is usually caused by a combination of factors, including the person's emotional disposition, emotional stress and sometimes physical stress. The symptoms may include disorders of perception, thought, memory, emotion, consciousness and the awareness of self. Neuroses, unlike psychoses, do not involve sharp breaks with reality or hallucinations; personality disorders involve set patterns of behavior that range from mild to behavior severe enough to resemble the pyschotic. Treatment of mental disorders may involve psychotherapy, group or art therapy, behavior therapy or treatment with drugs to alleviate the symptoms.

Freud – the founder of psychoanalysis

Sigmund Freud (1856-1939) developed the technique of free association – saying everything that enters the mind without attempting to make it logical or socially appropriate. This brings to consciousness repressed memories and drives. From this he formed the theory that human beings are controlled by powerful unconscious forces which frequently conflict with the demands of the conscious mind and are rarely subject to conscious control. He also realized that the whims and the desires of the unconscious are revealed in dreams.

Psychoanalysis, his system for understanding the mind and correcting its disorders, is based on the notion that the libido, the driving force present from birth, expresses itself as sexual energy and the will to live. If this is blocked or misdirected, however, it leads to conflicts later in life. He introduced the distinction between the id (that part of the mind concerned with instinctive desires), ego (conscious self) and superego (restraining forces).

Freud introduced the idea of the Oedipus complex (based on the mythical Greek king Oedipus who unwittingly killed his father and married his mother). The son becomes jealous of the place his father holds in his mother's affections and is consumed by feelings of aggression and hatred, which smoulder indefinitely. The tension between father and son is eradicated if the son marries someone (often physically like his mother).

Jung and the collective unconscious

Carl Gustav Jung (1875-1961), one of Freud's early colleagues, organized the first Psychoanalytic Congress in Salzburg in 1908 and was the first president of the International Psychoanalytic Association. He broke away from Freud in 1913 to form the school of "analytic psychology".

His ideas of a collective unconscious have been widely misunderstood. He was not proposing a "group mind", but saying that human behavior, conscious and unconscious, is affected by our evolutionary past and racial experience; that instincts are more subtle and fundamental than mere eyeblinks and knee jerks; and that evidence of these "intellectual instincts" is seen in the imagery of art and dreams.

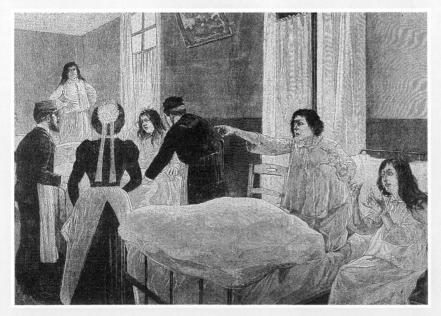

◄ *The French Hospice of St Anne for the mentally ill in 1901.*

Adler argued that the drive for power was a fundamental urge, expressed neurotically as the inferiority complex

Neurosis

The mildest psychological disorder is neurosis. All of us have reacted to stressful situations and felt depressed, anxious or fearful at some time. The neurotic person has similar feelings, the difference being that these feelings are central to their life and the conflicts arising from stress remain unresolved. The neurotic typically feels helpless and useless and acts in such a way as to lessen discomfort rather than strive for positive accomplishment. Unlike psychotics (◗ page 80), sufferers are fully in touch with reality but are handicapped by excessive emotional reactions. Classification of neurosis into various categories is fairly arbitrary but is based on the major symptom. The main neurotic states are hysteria, depression, anxiety and obsession.

Treatment for neuroses (◗ page 84) can involve psychotherapy or drugs, or both. Since many neuroses disappear spontaneously, psychotherapy (a scarce resource in most countries) is reserved for those cases in which the underlying cause is unlikely to heal itself. Phobias are treated with tranquillizers or desensitization – a form of behavior therapy where the patient is gradually exposed to the threatening situation or object. Anxiety and insomnia are usually treated with minor tranquillizers, and depression with antidepressives.

Charcot — the founder of modern psychiatry
Modern ideas of diagnosis and treatment start with French neurologist Jean-Martin Charcot (1825-1923), a flamboyant character, who founded the Paris school of psychotherapy at the Salpetrière Hospital. The first to describe many neurological diseases, he wrongly believed that hypnosis was a symptom of hysteria, but correctly believed that hypnosis resulted from suggestion and described its stages (lethargy, catalepsy and sleep-walking) in neurological terms. Freud was one of his pupils.

Adler and the inferiority complex
Alfred Adler (1887-1937), one of Freud's earliest supporters, was the first major disciple to break from him. Disagreeing with Freud's view that sexual conflicts lay at the root of all neuroses, Adler left the Viennese Psychoanalytic Society in 1911. He emigrated to the USA and founded the school of "individual psychology", convinced that the fundamental driving force was a desire for power, expressed neurotically as the inferiority complex. He also believed that men and women are fundamentally alike, differences being determined by social and cultural factors. Thus, in a male society, the female attempts to assert herself; her protest takes many forms and, where conflict arises, results in emotional disturbance.

Moniz and surgery on the mind
Egas Moniz (1874-1955), professor of neurology at Lisbon, is remembered for two major innovations, cerebral angiography and lobotomy. In 1935, at a neurological conference in London he learned that neuroses had been induced in normal healthy apes but could not be induced in apes whose frontal lobes were removed. Believing that mental illnesses had physical roots, he theorized that by severing the frontothalamic fibers, anxiety would be reduced. The first frontal lobotomies were performed in 1935. Of 20 patients, all survived; seven were declared cured and eight improved.

Hysteria
The condition of hysteria is one where subconscious motives produce physical symptoms that have psychological advantage or symbolic value. These include "conversion" symptoms such as paralysis, tremor, blindness, deafness or multiple allergy; and "dissociative" symptoms such as partial (and selective) amnesia, wandering around in a wraith-like state (fugue), madness (or rather the patient's idea of madness) and multiple personality. Frequently such symptoms vanish after a dramatic event.

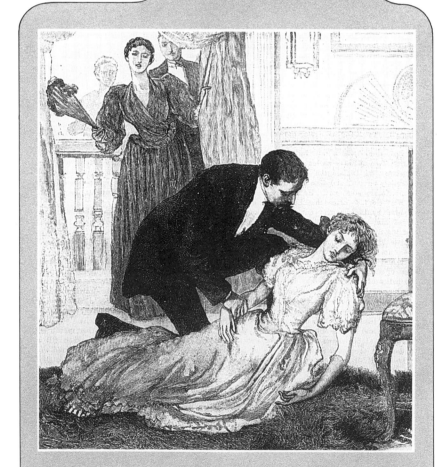

▲ *Fainting was a frequent reaction of women to emotional events in the 19th century. It was partly caused by tight corsetting impairing blood flow, but it was also a form of hysteria, made fashionable by the ethos of the day.*

STRESS

Depression
Neurotic depression is usually an overreaction or prolonged reaction to events, but may occur with little or no stimulus. Sufferers are preoccupied with the event that triggered the depression, and feel weighed down, inactive and unable to think rapidly. Depression is often mixed with anxiety.

▼ A Polish child, emotionally disturbed and depressed during the Second World War, scrawling wildly on the wall when requested to draw a picture of her home.

Anxiety
Neurotic anxiety develops when there is an overreaction to stressful events. Occurring in attacks or as a persisting state, its psychological symptoms include worry, dread and panic, and bodily symptoms include palpitations, shaking and diarrhea.

Obsession
In obsessive-compulsive disorders, sufferers feel subjectively compelled to perform an action or dwell on an idea, despite their own attempt to resist it. They recognize the compulsion as coming from within themselves but as being alien to their personality; attempts to dispel the unwanted thoughts or urges may lead to a severe inner struggle, with intense anxiety.

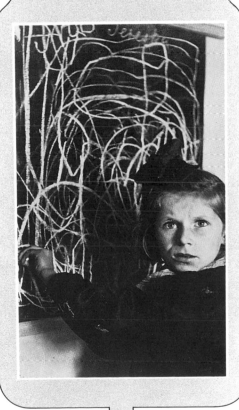

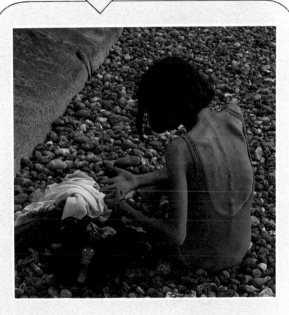

▲ Anorexia nervosa is an eating disorder classically found in emotionally immature girls with overprotective parents. Sufferers perceive themselves as fatter than they are, and starve or induce vomiting to stay thin. Bulimia nervosa, compulsive overeating found in young adult women, may be caused by ambivalence or aversion to male sexual advances.

Neurasthenia
Fatigue with irritability, headache, depression, insomnia or inability to concentrate on or enjoy things is called neurasthenia. It often follows infections, exhaustion or stress.

Phobia
Phobias are intense dread of things, frequently spiders and snakes, or situations, particularly crowds, enclosed spaces (claustrophobia), or open spaces (agoraphobia).

Hypochondria
Excessive concern with general health or some part of the body is hypochondria. Concern over mental health is rare in hypochondriacs, who usually feel mentally sound.

Münchausen patients may mutilate themselves to gain the attentions of the medical profession

Personality disorders

Maladaptive behaviors, which usually appear around adolescence and persist throughout life, can be personality disorders. They often resemble psychoses (♦ page 82) except that there are no delusions. The sufferer is less "ill" than abnormally developed – in the same way that a physically handicapped individual is not ill but has an abnormal physical constitution. Personality disorders can be categorized into two main areas. The first, known as organic, relates to disorders caused by some physical ailment, such as faulty brain development resulting from genetic make-up, infection or drug poisoning. The second, known as functional, relates to a breakdown in behavior resulting from environmental factors, such as childhood deprivation. Specific categories of functional disorder range from the paranoid to the psychopathic, and can include sexual deviations. Treatment (♦ page 84) often involves behavior therapy and major tranquillizers.

Affective disorders
Paranoid personalities take offence and defend their personal rights readily, never see themselves as being in the wrong but blame conspirators, and may be jealous and self-important. People with affective personality disorders may be elated, with enhanced zest and activity; or depressed, worried and pessimistic; or alternate between the two. Schizoid personalities are cold, hold back from social contact and affection, and avoid competitive situations. Explosive personalities are subject to outbursts of intense hate, anger, violence or affection. Anankastic personalities are meticulous perfectionists, rigid and cautious. Hysterical personalities are shallow, labile, dependent, suggestible and theatrical, needing constant attention and appreciation. Asthenic personalities appear passive, complying with the wishes of others and lacking intellectual or emotional vigor.

The most serious personality disorder is that of psychopaths, who disregard their social obligation, show impetuous violence or callous unconcern, and are cold, aggressive or irresponsible. They are often highly intelligent, do not respond to punishment, and are often adept at concealing or rationalizing their actions.

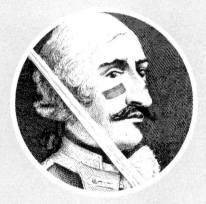

◄ *Baron von Münchausen in a classic portrait depicting his duelling scars.*

▼ *The view that the individual psyche is essentially social led to the development of group analytic psychotherapy. The theory builds on the Freudian theory and is therapy of the group, by the group, through the group, including the conductor as a member of the group.*

Münchausen's syndrome

Heironymus Karl Friedrich, Baron von Münchausen (1720-1797), a Hanoverian soldier, fought in the Russian army against the Turks and became notorious for his exaggerated accounts of his exploits. His name now is used to describe the uncommon syndrome of exaggerating or inventing symptoms.

Typically, Münchausen patients collapse outside police stations or doctors' offices, are pathological liars, have a "grid-iron" abdomen from operation scars, and are clingingly dependent on hospital staff, whom they thank profusely. Men slightly outnumber women; many have had extensive medical experience as patients, failed medical students, or in occupations such as nursing and radiography.

Examples include one patient with fictitious chest pain, who diverted an aeroplane to an unscheduled city; another injected feces into his joints to induce inflammation; others induced seizures or gynecological disease; eight patients are known to have had amputations after minor injuries – they seemed able to dictate their wishes for surgery to their doctors. Others have falsely claimed the death of a loved one in order to assume the role of distraught and suicidal bereavement. Often a mother has fabricated symptoms in her child; usually she chooses fits, though ex-nurses opt for more exotic disorders.

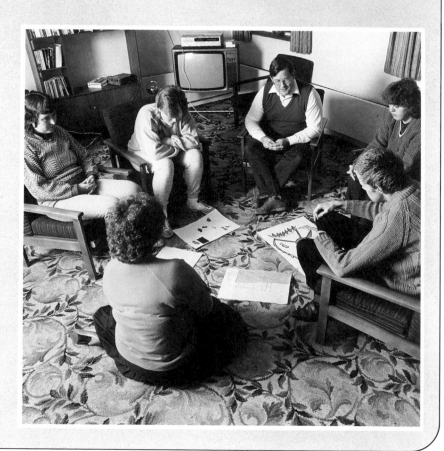

FUNCTIONAL

ORGANIC

Deviations of sexuality
Sexual activities are regarded as deviations when sexual gratification is derived in abnormal or unusual circumstances. Hence "deviation" is an ill-defined term. Sexual deviation usually is understood to include bestiality (intercourse with animals), pedophilia (sexual desire for children), sadism (desire to inflict pain or punishment during intercourse), masochism (desire to be hurt or punished during intercourse) and fetishism (sexual gratification from non-sexual objects, which frequently includes articles of clothing).

Exhibitionism is a compulsion to reveal the sex organs. In men this tends to be due to self-hatred or aggression to women; in women to emotional immaturity or hysteria.

Transsexuality is a fixed belief of having the wrong sex of body; transsexuals are not biologically of mixed or "wrong" sex. The only treatments are cross-dressing or a sex-change operation. Transvestism is pleasure, not necessarily sexual, from masquerading as the opposite sex. Transsexuals and transvestites are rarely homosexual.

Drugs
Regular consumption of alcohol, tobacco, glue vapor or certain drugs can lead to mental dependence (craving for the drug and compulsion to take it), and physical dependence (physical symptoms if the specific drug is withdrawn). Drugs causing dependence include narcotics (morphine, codeine, heroin and methadone), hypnotics and sedatives (barbiturates and tranquillizers), hallucinogens (LSD, mescaline and psilocybin) and stimulants (amphetamine and cocaine). Withdrawal of stimulant drugs causes lethargy, insomnia and restlessness; withdrawal of alcohol, or narcotic and sedative drugs, can cause excitement, tremor, insomnia and fits.

The mental symptoms of withdrawal are reduced by tranquillizers and the physical symptoms by beta-blockers (▶ page 84). There is no treatment that reduces the craving, which eventually fades but is readily reinstated if the habit is resumed. The most common addiction is to tobacco, but its seriousness is often disregarded because cigarettes can be bought legally and the habit is still relatively inexpensive and socially acceptable.

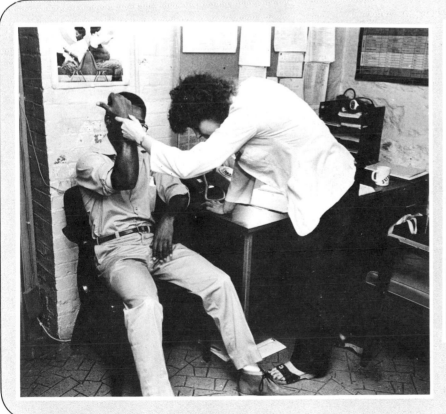

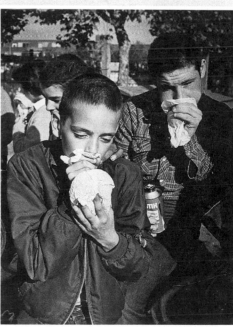

◀ ▲ *Drug addiction, from glue to heroin, can cause physical as well as mental disorders and requires treatment on both levels.*

Psychosis

A psychosis is not simply an extension of a neurotic illness or personality disorder – although some cases are indistinct, for the most part the difference is stark and dramatic. Psychotics lose touch with reality completely as they act out their fantasies in life. Like personality disorders, pyschoses can be divided between organic, caused by some physical ailment, and functional, which include two well known states – schizophrenic and affective reactions. Swiss psychiatrist Emil Kraepelin (1856-1926) devised the first classification of psychoses, dividing them into manic-depressive psychosis, paranoia and "dementia praecox" – renamed schizophrenia by his colleague Eugen Bleuler (1857-1939). Bleuler saw the essence of the condition as a splitting of the mind, not into two parts but into fragments; ideas are disconnected, emotions are inappropriate to thought and behavior to reality.

Schizophrenics often feel that their most intimate thoughts are known to others, and see themselves as the pivot of all that happens. Voices may address them, or comment on their behavior. Everyday objects may possess a special, often sinister, meaning, intended solely for the patient. Schizophrenics show little sign of holding to a train of thought, and may sit still in odd positions (catatonia) for hours.

Treatment for psychoses (◗ page 84) includes major tranquillizers, psychotherapy, or both. Mania or manic-depression is treated with the antidepressant lithium carbonate. Extreme cases of mood and behavior including catatonia, mania and paranoia are treated with electroconvulsive therapy (ECT).

ORGANIC
(◗ page 61)

▼ *The definition of schizophrenia varies enormously from one country to another; proportionately the diagnosis is twice as common in the USA as in Britain. In the USSR and South Africa the boundaries between penal and health-care systems are blurred. "Schizophrenia" is used as an excuse to denigrate intellectuals (such as Andrei Sakharov, below), who criticize the regime, and to deprive them of their liberty. Having committed no crime, they cannot be imprisoned; instead they are incarcerated in hospitals until they are "cured".*

Comparable cases are discovered from time to time elsewhere – in England in the 1970s, three elderly women were found languishing in mental hospitals 50 years after being sent there for having illegitimate babies, and two "mad" patients (a man and a woman) in Irish mental hospitals were found to have been committed on the say-so of their spouses, who wanted them removed.

Szasz and Laing – rethinking psychiatry

Thomas Szasz (b. 1920), psychiatry professor at the State University of New York, argues that since psychiatrists cannot agree on the causes, diagnosis or course of schizophrenia, it must be a bogus disease. Hence, psychiatrists are bogus doctors who think they are practising medicine but in fact are agents of social control, just as much in the West as in the Soviet Union. Szasz accepts that people have mental problems but does not regard these as diseases, and will only treat patients who come to him voluntarily. He also argues that, since mental illness is a myth, it also follows that insanity cannot be used as a defense in criminal actions. Only 10 percent of patients in British mental hospitals are detained compulsorily, compared with 90 percent in the USA. However, in Britain, "voluntary" detention can easily be replaced by compulsion if the patient does not cooperate and, in the USA, voluntary patients usually pay for themselves while compulsory patients need not. Szasz argues that, whatever the percentage, detention reflects an attitude; he condemns societies that lock up an individual who has broken no law.

British psychiatrist R.D. Laing (b. 1927) regards madness as a reasonable protective reaction against the stresses of the world in general, and family life in particular. He argues that families find an individual's withdrawal intolerable, calling the sufferer "disturbed", and that psychiatrists collude with the family.

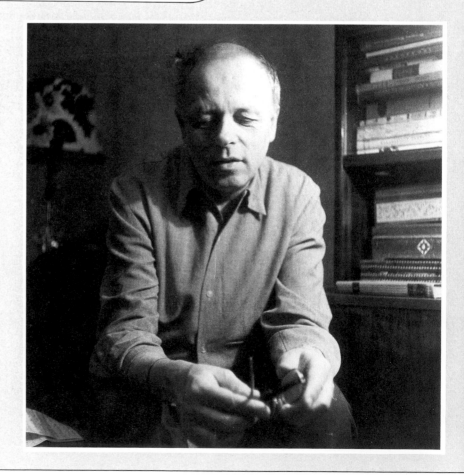

FUNCTIONAL

Schizophrenia

In hebephrenic schizophrenia the person's mood is variable and often inappropriate. They may be giggling, lofty, grimacing or smiling, making hypochondriacal complaints or continuously talking repetitively. Catatonic schizophrenics alternate between overactivity and stupor, or automatic obedience and negativism. Paranoid schizophrenics have long-lasting delusions and hallucinations, usually of persecution but sometimes of jealousy, exalted birth or Messianic mission. In acute schizophrenic episodes, a previously normal person experiences a dream-like state and a slight clouding of consciousness, with bewilderment; people, objects or things may become charged with personal significance. The condition usually remits spontaneously after a few weeks or months. Usually the cause is unknown; sometimes it is brought on by hallucinogenic drugs.

Autism

The form of schizophrenia beginning in infancy known as autism appears before 30 months. Autistic children respond abnormally to sounds and images, and have problems understanding speech. Their own speech is delayed, and is often a mere echo of what is said to them. Their grammar is immature and they cannot use abstract terms. The social problems of autistic children include poor eye-to-eye contact and cooperative play, and they may spend hours in repetitive or ritualistic behavior. Intelligence is usually low, and all but the brightest (about 15 percent) spend their entire lives in institutions.

Manic-depression

Affective disorders are recurrent psychoses consisting of either mania or depression, or alternating cycles of both. In manic psychosis (or the manic phase of manic-depressive psychosis), patients are excessively cheerful and active, speaking rapidly, shifting from one idea to another, teasing and joking. They may be overconfident, overoptimistic and overimportant, running up debts or endangering their social position by embarrassing behavior. In depressive psychosis (or the depressive phase of manic-depressive psychosis), patients feel their depression as a heavy physical blanket wrapped around them. They are unhappy with no apparent cause, find meeting people an ordeal, wake in the night, think slowly and indecisively, and feel unworthiness and guilt.

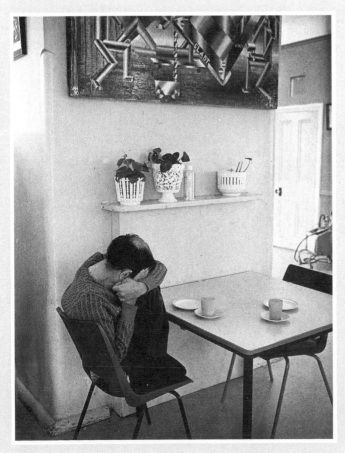

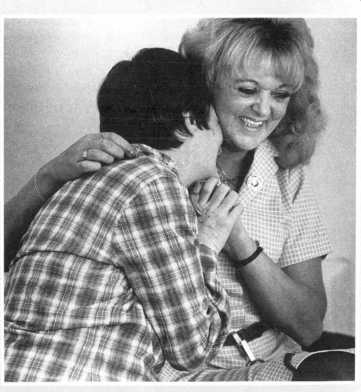

◄ ▲ Mental hospitals aim to provide an environment in which the patient can feel secure from external threats and from the danger of self-inflicted injury.

The treatment of mental disorders

Drugs treat the symptoms of mental disorder. Psychotherapy and group therapy aim to deal with the underlying cause. Psychotherapy encourages the patient to express spontaneous thoughts so that previous forgotten experiences and repressed feelings are brought to consciousness, giving insight into present behavior and feelings. Behavior therapy consists of rewards for desirable behavior.

"Major" tranquillizers include chlorpromazine (Largactil), and prochlorperazine (Stemetil). They impair aggression, fear responses, mania, paranoia, delusions and hallucinations, and halt the loss of self-care. "Minor" tranquillizers, such as diazepam (Valium), calm anxiety. They produce dependence if taken over a long period. Beta-blockers are also used to treat anxiety when symptoms are mainly physical, such as palpitations and tremor.

Antidepressives, which include dothiepen (Prothiaden) and trimi-pramine (Surmontil) work by gradually building up levels of certain brain chemicals. They do not produce a "high", and their effect is not felt until they have been taken for several days. Lithium carbonate is thought to work by replacing body sodium, which is involved in chemical reactions during mood changes. Adverse effects include fine tremor, which is relieved by a beta-blocker, and frequent urination.

With electroconvulsive therapy (ECT) the patient is anesthetized and given a muscle relaxant; then a small electrical current is briefly applied through terminals placed on each temple. Usually given in a three-week course of six treatments, it causes temporary memory loss.

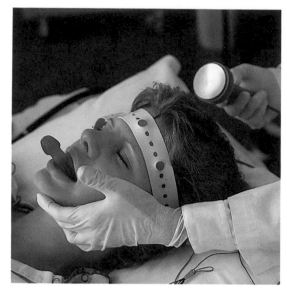

▲ Electric shock therapy involves passing a 100 volt current across the patient's head. Although its effect is still not fully understood, results show that it may prove life-saving for sufferers of affective psychoses and may help schizophrenics.

▼ The lunatic asylum of the 18th century, as seen by William Hogarth in his series of paintings the "Rake's Progress", was a place in which disturbed people were abandoned; whatever treatment they received was more sadistic than helpful.

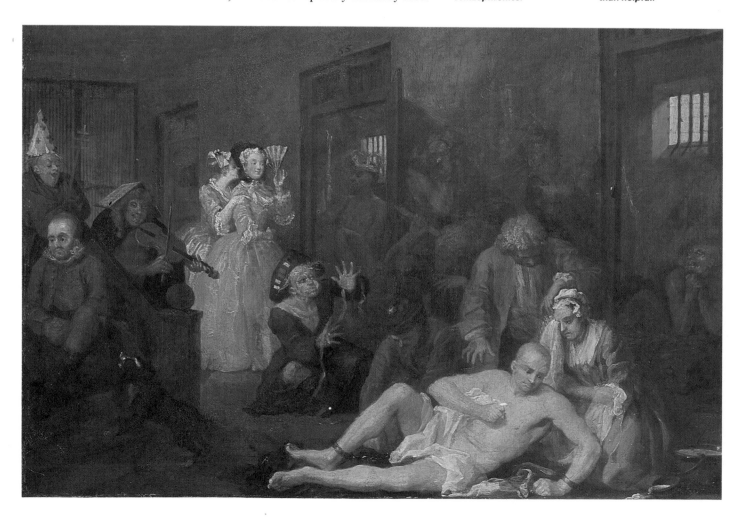

Hormones

Hormones and glands...The hypothalamus, controlling the endocrine system...Hormones of the pituitary gland...The adrenals and the stress reaction...Hormones of sex...Other hormone-producing glands... PERSPECTIVE...Studying hormones...The endocrine system...The race to find releasing factors

The body relies on two related systems for controlling various functions. The nervous system (◀ page 53) makes muscles contract and glands secrete, while the endocrine system – the ductless glands and the hormones they secrete – makes changes in the metabolic activities of tissues. The former provides the body's fast but short-lived communications. The latter produces messenger chemicals, known as hormones, which carry instructions that take longer to travel but are of prolonged influence. The word hormone means a substance that "sets in motion". Hormones are released through ductless glands when the body needs them and switched off when it does not. The nervous and endocrine systems coordinate their activities like an interlocking supersystem – parts of the nervous system stimulate or inhibit hormone release, and hormones are able to stimulate or inhibit nerve impulses. Hormones are controlled by that part of the brain called the hypothalamus; the few that seem not to be are secreted from sites very close to others that are.

Hormones cover a number of major functions. These include: enabling the body to cope with heat, cold, stress and starvation, and to counter dehydration, infection, trauma and bleeding; controlling reproduction, including egg and sperm production, pregnancy, birth and milk production; and controlling growth and development, the volume of the body fluids and their chemical composition.

The types of hormone

The endocrine glands make hormones, and are of two kinds. Most (including the hypothalamus, pituitary, parathyroids, adrenal medulla, and parts of the thyroid and pancreas) develop from ectoderm and endoderm (the layers of the embryo – developing baby – that make skin and gut linings). These glands produce water-soluble hormones – peptides, glycopeptides and amino-acids. Many or all of these attach themselves to specific proteins on their target-cell membranes and are transported inside, where they stimulate or dampen the system that converts ATP into energy (◀ page 158), thus activating the cell or shutting it down. The second kind of endocrine glands develop from mesoderm (the embryonic layer that makes muscle and bone). These include the thyroid, adrenal cortex, testicles, ovaries and, during pregnancy, placenta; these produce fat-soluble hormones, which pass through cell membranes and act directly on genes.

Prostaglandins (so-called because they were first found in prostate gland secretions) are produced and released into the bloodstream by cells everywhere in the body. They are potent but, because they are rapidly inactivated, their action is confined to nearby cells. Different prostaglandins fine-tune many life processes – they alter blood pressure, contract or relax smooth muscle, cause sedation, stupor or fever, reduce gastric secretion, and increase or block adrenaline release.

Insulin and glucagon

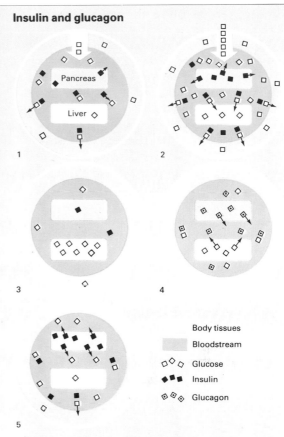

▲ The production of insulin and glucagon in the pancreas demonstrates the way in which the body's hormones maintain a steady internal state. The pancreas contains tiny clusters of cells known as islets of Langerhans which make two important hormones, insulin and glucagon. Insulin is produced when blood sugar levels are high (1) and lowers them by transporting glucose into body cells, particularly to the muscles (2). If blood glucose levels are low (3), glucagon is manufactured instead (4): this converts glycogen to glucose in the liver, restoring the blood sugar levels (5).

Body tissues
Bloodstream
Glucose
Insulin
Glucagon

Excessive hormone production

The American neurosurgeon Harvey Cushing (1869-1931) discovered that the disease now called Cushing's syndrome was caused by a tumor in the pituitary gland (◆ page 86). In 1901 he saw a 14-year old girl suffering from headaches and loss of vision. She was puny, obese and sexually immature – signs of excess production of corticosteroid hormones. Believing that her neurological symptoms were related to her abnormal development, he operated to see if she had a cerebellar tumor. She had not, and died six weeks later. Autopsy revealed a huge pituitary cyst. Shortly afterwards Cushing heard of a similar case in Vienna, and persuaded the surgeon to drain the cyst; the patient survived. The foremost surgeon of his day, Cushing performed over 2,000 operations and reduced the death rate from neurosurgery.

In 1984 a team of doctors and biochemists reported a case of Cushing's syndrome caused by corticotropin releasing factors (CRF) from tumor cells, some of which invaded the pituitary gland. Researchers may soon know whether Cushing's syndrome is always caused by excess CRF production.

The hypothalamus monitors and regulates production of most of the body's hormones

Control center of the endocrine system

The hypothalamus controls the endocrine system from the base of the brain by detecting the body's requirements for hormones, and then directly or indirectly stimulating their production. First, it receives messages from receptors which give the levels of hormones in the blood, or other indicators of the internal bodily environment. It then stimulates or inhibits the release of the appropriate hormones.

The hypothalamus does this by releasing various hormones into blood vessels that are connected directly to the anterior (front) pituitary lobe, so that they arrive there quickly and undiluted. These pituitary-regulating hormones are of two kinds – some release, and others inhibit, the specific pituitary hormones. The hypothalamus also releases two hormones – controlling blood pressure and uterine contractions at birth – into the general bloodstream, from the posterior pituitary gland.

The pituitary gland, which is only 1·3cm round, is embedded in bone above the roof of the mouth, and is attached directly to the hypothalamus. The anterior lobe, constituting three-quarters of it, develops from the embryo's mouth, whereas the posterior lobe is an outgrowth of the hypothalamus.

There are five types of gland cell in the anterior pituitary. These make growth hormone, prolactin, melanocyte-stimulating hormone (MSH), thyroid-stimulating hormone (TSH), follicle-stimulating hormone (FSH), luteinizing hormone (LH) and adrenocorticotropic hormone (ACTH). The last four are known as tropic hormones, and act on other endocrine glands, stimulating them into activity in their turn; the former act directly on the body.

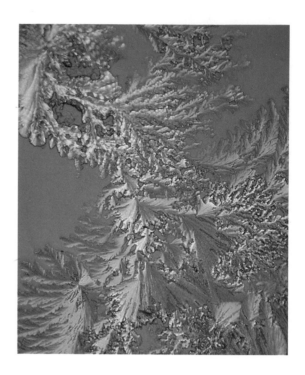

▲ *Crystals of adrenaline, also known as epinephrine, the hormone of the adrenal medulla that is released in time of stress to stimulate the body for quick reactions (♦ page 88).*

▼ *Computer-graphic reconstruction of the receptor-binding sites on a growth-hormone molecule. These sites lock onto the target cells, allowing the hormone to activate them.*

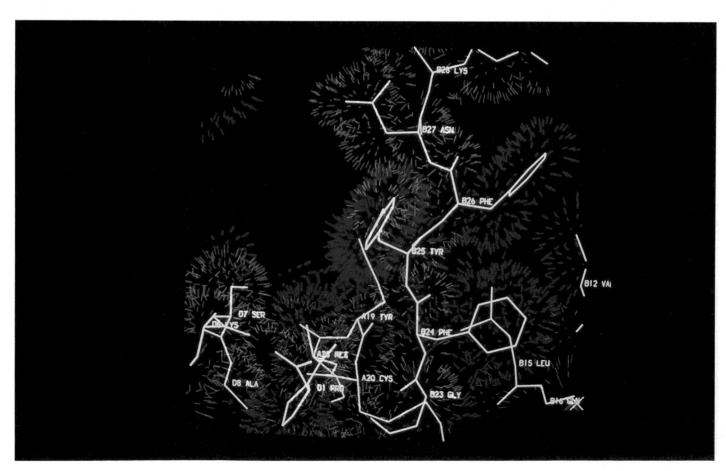

The anterior pituitary makes several hormones. Growth hormone (GH) stimulates growth, maintains cell size, and breaks down fat cells, converting fat into energy and raising blood glucose by making the liver manufacture peptides to promote growth. Melanocyte-stimulating hormone (MSH) darkens skin. Adrenocorticotropic hormone (ACTH) controls hormone secretion from the adrenal cortex. Prolactin makes the breasts produce milk. Other hormones of the anterior pituitary are thyroid-stimulating hormone (TSH), luteinizing hormone (LH) and follicle-stimulating hormone (FSH).

The skin manufactures Vitamin D, which acts as a hormone in controlling calcium levels in the blood, in association with PTH.

The thymus produces several hormones that stimulate the growth of B-lymphocytes.

The heart atria make peptides that inhibit the production of angiotensin and ACTH, thus helping to control blood pressure.

The stomach releases several hormones that stimulate or inhibit the release of gastric juices and the activity of the digestive system.

The adrenal cortex is stimulated by ACTH and produces aldosterone which makes the kidneys reabsorb salt and water; glucocorticoids, which promote metabolism and provide resistance to stress; androgens; and estrogens.

The placenta produces several hormones related with pregnancy, including estrogen, progesterone and relaxin.

The ovaries produce estrogen and progesterone which regulate the menstrual cycle and pregnancy, controlled by FSH and LH.

The brain's neurotransmitters may act as hormones elsewhere in the body; the pineal gland secretes melatonin, which seems to inhibit sexual activity.

The posterior pituitary secretes vasopressin (also known as antidiuretic hormone - ADH), which raises blood pressure by making the kidneys absorb more water and making arterioles constrict. Oxytocin stimulates the smooth muscles of the uterus during pregnancy, produces contractions at birth.

The thyroid produces calcitonin when blood calcium levels are high, to deposit calcium and phosphate in bone. Thyroxine and triiodothyronine increase heart rate, blood flow, blood pressure, gut contractions and anxiety.

The parathyroid makes parathyroid hormone (PTH), which releases calcium from bone into blood when blood calcium levels are low. It also makes the kidneys excrete less calcium and magnesium, and increases their absorption in the gut when Vitamin D is short.

The pancreas releases insulin and glucagon, which together regulate blood glucose levels. The pancreas also makes growth hormone inhibiting factor (GHIF) which controls the production of insulin and glucagon.

The adrenal medulla releases adrenaline and noradrenaline, in response to stress or low blood glucose. They produce the fight-or-flight response, raising blood pressure, respiration rate, muscle efficiency and metabolic rates.

The kidneys make erythropoetin, which stimulates red blood cell manufacture, and renin which stimulates the production of aldosterone in the adrenal cortex.

The testes are stimulated by LH to produce testosterone which controls secondary sexual characteristics, and inhibin, which inhibits the secretion of FSH, cutting sperm production.

The adrenal glands produce hormones enabling the body to withstand both immediate crisis and long-term stress

Controlling normal metabolism

The adrenal glands, one above each kidney, consist of cortex and medulla – two different glands with interrelated functions. The cortex, on the outside, is stimulated by ACTH from the pituitary. It produces three different kinds of steroid hormones – mineralocorticoids, glucocorticoids and sex hormones, though these last are produced only in insignificant amounts. The main mineralocorticoid is aldosterone, which prevents blood from becoming acid by making the kidneys reabsorb salt and water and excrete potassium. Production of aldosterone is controlled partly by ACTH but mainly by angiotensin, a plasma protein whose production requires an enzyme, renin, which is made in kidneys in response to low blood pressure or potassium excess. Thus when low blood pressure stimulates the kidneys to secrete renin, the angiotensin which is produced stimulates the adrenal cortex to produce aldosterone. The glucocorticoids consist of hydrocortisone, cortisone and corticosterone. Similar in action, they have three functions. First, they promote normal metabolism, providing energy by breaking down cells, especially of muscle, and transporting them to the liver to make new proteins. They also make glycogen and fat into glucose; if glycogen and fat are in short supply, the liver makes glucose from amino-acids. Second, they provide resistance to stress. Third, they reduce inflammation by strengthening the membrane of lysosomes, the cell structures that release inflammatory substances. An adverse side-effect of this is that they also retard wound-healing and microbe destruction. When high doses are given, they can make the lymph glands wither, which depresses immunity (◆ page 213).

Controlling stress

The adrenal medulla makes two chemically similar hormones, noradrenaline and adrenaline. They are released in response to stress or low blood glucose by nerve messages from the hypothalamus (not by hormones in the bloodstream). They enable the body to react to stress by producing the fight-or-flight response: raising blood pressure by increasing heart rate and constricting blood vessels, speeding respiration rate, dilating passageways in lungs, increasing the efficiency of muscle contractions, and raising blood sugar and metabolic rate.

In 1936 the Canadian endocrinologist Hans Selye discovered that certain unpleasant events trigger a set of bodily changes, known as the general adaptation syndrome. This raises blood pressure and blood glucose levels, gearing-up the body to meet emergencies. The hypothalamus reacts to stress by triggering two pathways – the alarm reaction for immediate effect and the resistance reaction for sustained effect. The hormones interact to adjust the response to the type of stress involved. The alarm reaction works mainly through adrenalines and glucocorticoids. The heart beats faster; blood clots more easily, is diverted to muscles and brain, and is released from storage in the spleen; sweating increases; saliva and digestive enzymes are reduced; glucose is made from glycogen in liver; breathing becomes faster and deeper. Metabolic rate rises, fats and then proteins are mobilized to make energy as the glucose supply is used up, blood vessels constrict more, and fibroblast cells (◆ page 212) inhibit inflammation. During the resistance stage, blood pressure remains high and metabolism is faster, allowing the body to deal with infection, emotional strain or physical effort. A state of exhaustion eventually sets in, as the glucocorticoids run short, and the sustained potassium loss causes widespread cell damage.

The adrenal glands

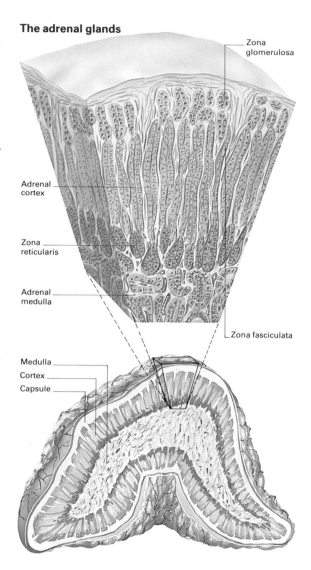

▲ *The adrenal glands, about 5 cm long and 3 cm wide, are placed on top of the kidneys like caps. The cortex and medulla are quite distinct, the cortex deriving from mesoderm and the medulla from ectoderm. There are three zones of the cortex, each producing different groups of steroid hormones. The hormone-producing cells of the medulla are known as chromaffin cells.*

The race for a Nobel Prize

In 1948 an English biologist, Geoffrey Harris, showed that the activity of the pituitary gland was controlled by 'releasing factors', of unknown nature, from the hypothalamus. The idea that the brain controlled hormones was at that time blasphemy to many scientists, including the scientific adviser to the British government, Lord Zuckerman (b. 1904). The two clashed violently at a conference in 1954. One observer, French scientist Claude Fortier, said, "What made it so disgraceful was the ferocity of Zuckerman's attack. He was almost blind with rage. It was one of the most embarrassing scenes I have witnessed".

Scenes and attacks were to be the keynote of ensuing research on releasing factors. It was a physiological problem, but required a chemist to identify the agent involved. Research was started by several teams including Harris in England, and

The fight-or-flight response

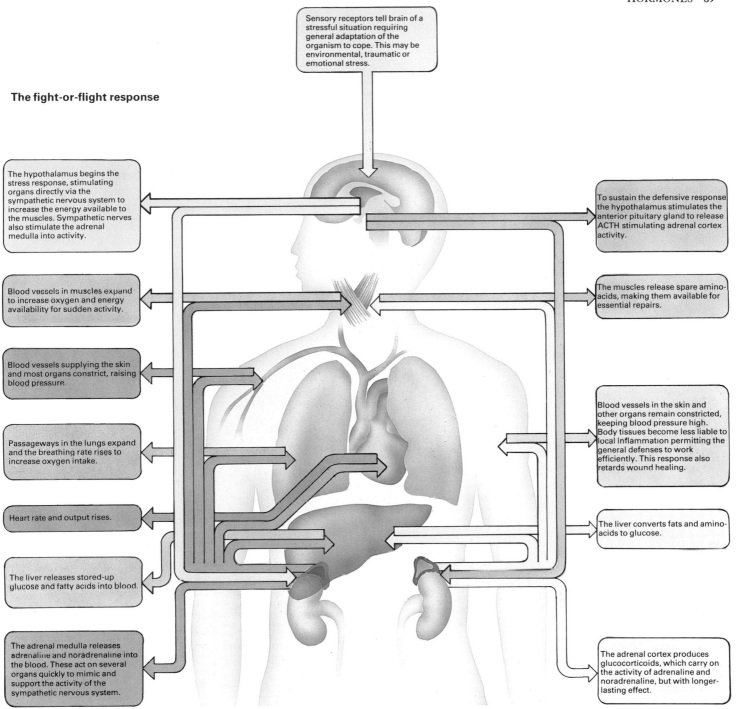

Sensory receptors tell brain of a stressful situation requiring general adaptation of the organism to cope. This may be environmental, traumatic or emotional stress.

The hypothalamus begins the stress response, stimulating organs directly via the sympathetic nervous system to increase the energy available to the muscles. Sympathetic nerves also stimulate the adrenal medulla into activity.

Blood vessels in muscles expand to increase oxygen and energy availability for sudden activity.

Blood vessels supplying the skin and most organs constrict, raising blood pressure.

Passageways in the lungs expand and the breathing rate rises to increase oxygen intake.

Heart rate and output rises.

The liver releases stored-up glucose and fatty acids into blood.

The adrenal medulla releases adrenaline and noradrenaline into the blood. These act on several organs quickly to mimic and support the activity of the sympathetic nervous system.

To sustain the defensive response the hypothalamus stimulates the anterior pituitary gland to release ACTH stimulating adrenal cortex activity.

The muscles release spare amino-acids, making them available for essential repairs.

Blood vessels in the skin and other organs remain constricted, keeping blood pressure high. Body tissues become less liable to local inflammation permitting the general defenses to work efficiently. This response also retards wound healing.

The liver converts fats and amino-acids to glucose.

The adrenal cortex produces glucocorticoids, which carry on the activity of adrenaline and noradrenaline, but with longer-lasting effect.

by physiologist Roger Guillemin and biochemist Andrew Schally in North America. From 1957 to 1962 Schally and Guillemin worked together but clashed, and Schally set up his own team. Their main contact after that was in public brawls at conferences. Finding the releasing factors required the tenacity to do exacting but boring work, dissecting brains, innumerable chemical procedures, purifying and analyzing minute quantities of chemicals. An army of research associates, students and technicians were involved, plus – for thyrotropin releasing factor (TRF) alone – the brains of five million sheep. The two teams worked separately, making the same mistakes and discoveries at remarkably similar times. In 1969 they reported the structure of TRF, with Schally six days ahead of Guillemin. Luteinizing hormone releasing factor (LRF) followed in 1971, again with Schally a few days ahead. Both of them owed their

discovery to their biochemists, especially Roger Burgus, Wylie Vale and Hisayuki Matsuo. Matsuo deserves particular credit: from his arrival in Schally's lab he took under five months to analyze LRF, working with antiquated machinery and chipped pipettes – Schally was unwilling to spend money that could be spent on pituitaries. Harris, who came near to identifying LRF, died in 1971.

Schally and Guillemin continued looking for other releasing factors while cultivating the people who decide Nobel prizes. Schally has been described as blunt and bombastic, interested in his work, sport and women; Guillemin as smooth and cultivated but devious; his papers regularly omit to mention relevant discoveries by Schally. The Nobel prize for the work on releasing factors was awarded in 1977 – half to Rosalyn Yalow, whose technique of radioimmunoassay made the discoveries possible, and a quarter each to Schally and Guillemin.

▲ *When faced with a stressful situation the body reacts with the "fight-or-flight" response, through the sympathetic nervous system and the sudden release of adrenaline and noradrenaline from the adrenal medulla. These instantly cause various changes that divert oxygen to the skeletal muscles. For a more sustained reaction, the pituitary stimulates the adrenal cortex to release glucocorticoids. These have the same general effect, but their effect lasts over a longer period.*

Two hormones enable the male to produce sperm according to the level of sexual activity

Controlling the sex organs

The testicles (like the ovaries) are controlled by follicle-stimulating hormone (FSH) and luteinizing hormone (LH), both secreted by the pituitary from puberty. Their release is controlled from the hypothalamus by gonadotropin releasing factor (GnRF). FSH stimulates sperm production and the development of sperm-nourishing cells. LH stimulates testicles to make testosterone, which promotes bone and muscle growth, sperm maturation, male sexual behavior and the physical attributes of maleness. GnRF (and hence FSH and LH) is switched on when testosterone levels fall, and off when levels rise. LH is often secreted on its own since FSH is also switched off by high levels of inhibin, a hormone produced by the sperm-nourishing cells. Inhibin governs the rate of sperm production according to the level of sexual activity. Because inhibin does not dampen production of LH, sexual activity does not affect production of testosterone.

FSH and LH also stimulate the ovaries. FSH makes the ovaries start the process of egg production and secrete estrogen, which promotes the development of the female reproductive system, especially lining the uterus (◆ page 180) and breasts, and is responsible for the general characteristics of femaleness. It also controls fluid and salt balance and stimulates growth. LH matures the egg-follicles, causes ovulation, enhances estrogen production and stimulates progesterone production, which prepares the uterus for implantation, and the breasts for milk-production. If implantation does not occur, the high estrogen and progesterone levels inhibit GnRF from the hypothalamus. This now inhibits LH secretion but restarts FSH. The lowered LH causes a fall in estrogen and progesterone, and menstruation occurs. If a fertilized egg is implanted, the placenta that it develops makes hormones that sustain the pregnancy (◆ page 184).

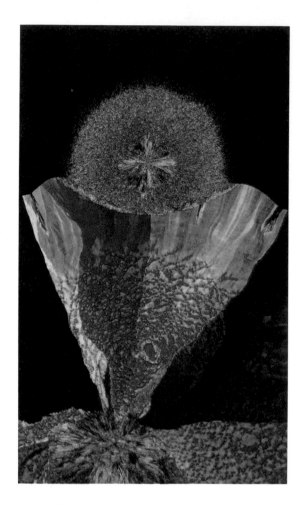

The hormones of pregnancy

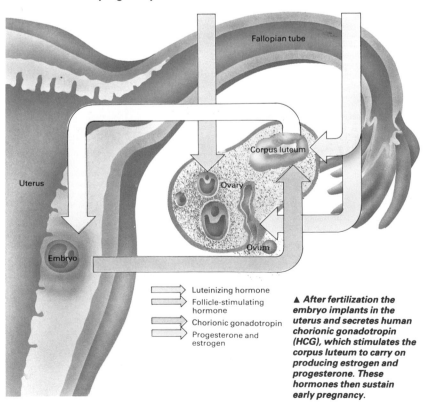

Luteinizing hormone
Follicle-stimulating hormone
Chorionic gonadotropin
Progesterone and estrogen

▲ *Progesterone, the hormone of maturation, works with estrogen to prepare the lining of the womb for the possible implantation of a fertilized ovum. Like estrogen, progesterone is made from cholesterol and acetyl coenzyme A in the ovaries.*

▼ *The Graafian follicles in the ovaries develop slowly and prepare the ovum for ovulation. During the maturation period, the Graafian follicle is stimulated by FSH to produce estrogen, but it also releases progesterone shortly before ovulation.*

▲ *After fertilization the embryo implants in the uterus and secretes human chorionic gonadotropin (HCG), which stimulates the corpus luteum to carry on producing estrogen and progesterone. These hormones then sustain early pregnancy.*

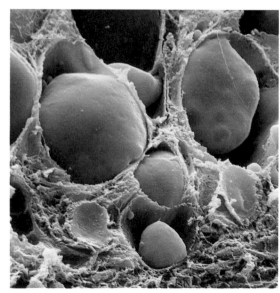

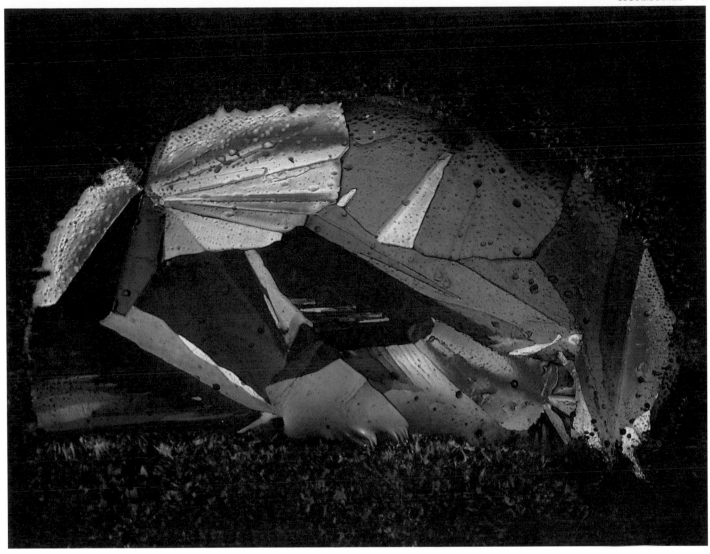

Why is one gland often inside another?

The thyroid gland, producer of thyroid hormone, is also host to the tissues (known as the parathyroid) producing calcitonin and parathyroid hormone. Embedded in the pancreas are the islets of Langerhans, which produce insulin, glucagon and growth hormone inhibiting factor (GHIF). The adrenal cortex surrounds the adrenal medulla. Is there any reason for this arrangement of hormone-producing glands?

The reasons for the structural arrangement of the thyroid gland are unknown, though it is noteworthy that all its three hormones affect nervous excitability – thyroid hormone does this by regulating calcium, whose level affects nerve conduction.

The pancreas's enzymes and hormones all affect digestion (GHIF inhibits the production of glucose) – but no one knows why they should lie so closely together in humans when they are separate in many lower animals.

In the adrenal glands of lower animals the cortex and the medulla are also separate, and their medullas make far more noradrenaline than adrenaline. The American biologist Julius Axelrod (winner of the Nobel Prize in 1970 for his work on nerve-transmitting substances) has shown that, in cases where the cortex surrounds the medulla, corticosteroids permeate the medulla and convert noradrenaline to the more potent adrenaline.

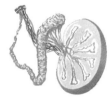

◄ Sperm are produced in the germinal cells within the testicle lobules, under the influence of FSH from the pituitary. The testicle also produces androgen hormones and inhibin, which inhibits FSH production when sexual activity is not high.

▲ Testosterone is one of the androgen hormones manufactured in the testicles and responsible for secondary male sexual characteristics.

▼ The maturation of sperm is also controlled by testosterone.

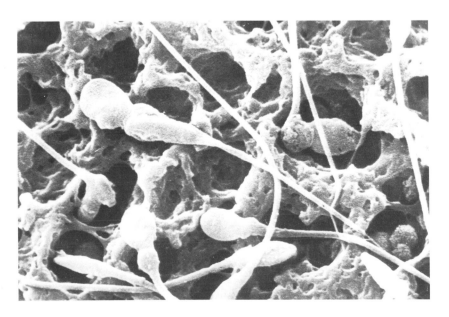

Controlling development

The thyroid gland, weighing 25g, lies below the voice box. Most of its cells are in groups – follicles – producing two similar thyroid hormones. These raise temperature and metabolic rate by stimulating fat and sugar metabolism and protein synthesis throughout the body. Along with growth hormone they regulate tissue growth and development, especially in children. Thyroid hormones increase heart rate, blood flow, blood pressure, gut contractions and anxiety. If the hypothalamus detects that their levels are low, or if the metabolic rate is low, or during stress, it stimulates the anterior pituitary to produce thyrotropin, which in turn stimulates the thyroid.

Calcitonin is made in cells between the thyroid follicles. Secreted when blood calcium levels are high, it removes calcium and phosphate from the blood and transfers them to bone – which acts as a reservoir – by activating bone-forming cells, inhibiting bone-destroying cells, and inhibiting production of parathyroid hormone.

Parathyroid hormone is produced in the two pairs of parathyroid glands, pea-sized masses of tissue embedded in the thyroid. When blood calcium levels are low, it releases a reserve of calcium by activating the cells that break down bone to release calcium and phosphate. It also makes the kidneys excrete less calcium and magnesium but more phosphate. When Vitamin D levels are low, parathyroid hormone increases gut absorption of calcium, phosphate and magnesium.

Other hormone-producing regions

The pineal (so-called because it is the shape of a pine cone) is a tiny gland above the cerebellum weighing 200mg. Though known for centuries, its function in humans remains obscure. It has been called the "third eye" as it is sensitive to light in lower animals. It is covered by layers of cerebral cortex but seems to play a part in night-and-day cycles, at least in animals. It produces melatonin, which dampens production of FSH and LH, and a hormone that may stimulate the adrenal cortex to secrete aldosterone. It may play a part in coping with stress. Rats deprived of pineals have more sexual appetite, and lizards deprived of pineals escape more easily from predators during daylight than intact lizards; at night there is no such difference.

The thymus is a two-lobed structure above and in front of the heart. Well-formed in babies, it reaches 40g at puberty and later diminishes. It has two functions: as master gland of the immune system (◗ page 213); and as an endocrine organ helping the immune system defend the body. It produces a range of similar hormones, of which the best-known are thymosins. These stimulate T- and B-cells and immunity against microbes and probably tumors; increase secretion of ACTH and LH, endorphins and glucocorticoids; and stimulate interferon production. The thyroid's output is highest in childhood and its decline may trigger the onset of puberty and the gradual process of aging.

The list of hormones known to be secreted in other body tissues grows yearly. The gut makes several hormones that regulate digestion. The placenta makes several hormones sustaining pregnancy and milk manufacture. The kidneys, when their oxygen supply is reduced, release renal erythropoetic factor. This converts a plasma protein into erythropoetin, a hormone stimulating red cell production. Skin makes Vitamin D. Heart atria make peptides inhibiting angiotensin and ACTH, and hence aldosterone. The brain contains at least 45 different kinds of neurotransmitters (◗ page 60), many of which function as hormones elsewhere in the body.

Growth of glands

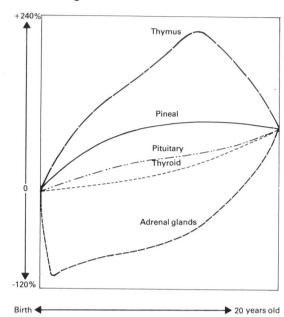

▲ Some glands develop at an even rate during childhood; the sex glands develop only at puberty. The thymus, which plays an important role in the development of the immune system, grows quickly in small children and begins to atrophy at puberty; by old age it is present only in residual form. The adrenals shrink in the first years of life but quickly regrow at puberty.

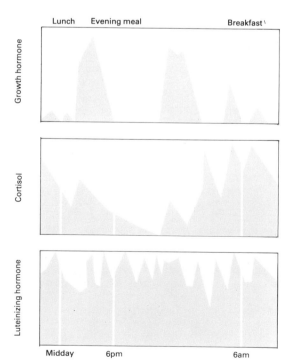

▲ The release of many hormones is not constant during the day. Growth hormone, which increases protein synthesis, promotes fat catabolism and releases glucose into the bloodstream, is intimately associated with exercise and sleep, as is cortisol, one of the glucocorticoids. LH, on the other hand, is released in small amounts regularly throughout the day.

The origins of hormonal disorders...Thyroid and parathyroid disorders...Growth hormone imbalance – gigantism and dwarfism...Addison's disease...Gout... Diabetes...PERSPECTIVE...Studying adrenal glands... The search for a cure for diabetes

The endocrine glands

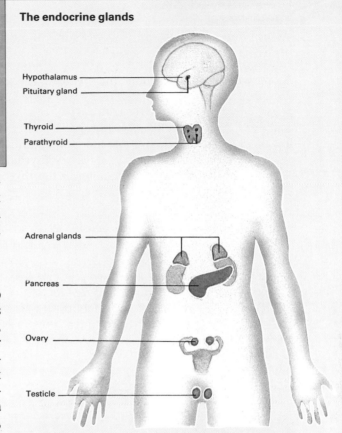

Hypothalamus
Pituitary gland
Thyroid
Parathyroid
Adrenal glands
Pancreas
Ovary
Testicle

When the body produces insufficient quantities of a particular hormone or enzyme, diseases result which doctors can usually treat successfully, normally by replacing the deficient substance. When a hormone is over-produced by a tumor, this can generally be found and reduced by operation or radiation.

Disorders of the thyroid gland

Hyperthyroidism, the excessive secretion of thyroid hormones (also known as thyrotoxicosis or Graves' disease), affects eight times as many women as men. Sufferers have increased appetite and anxiety, palpitations, sweaty hands and an inability to relax physically or mentally as they produce too much adrenaline. Often they have diarrhea, tremor, wasted limb muscles and (for reasons that are not understood) protruding eyeballs. In extreme cases this leads to thyrotoxic crisis – mental and physical exhaustion, delirium, fever, mania or delusions, and fast heartbeat. Immediate treatment is with cooling, sedatives and beta-blockers (◆ page 164). The disease sometimes ceases spontaneously. Longterm treatment is by antithyroid drugs, radioactive iodine to destroy part of the thyroid, or partial removal of the gland. Sometimes the remaining thyroid tissue diminishes some years after the operation, so patients are checked annually.

Hypothyroidism (myxedema) causes slow mental and physical acitivity, usually more obvious to relatives than to the patient. Its symptoms are often mistaken for aging. The sufferer is forgetful, tired and hypersensitive to cold, puts on weight, has dry skin and coarse hair. If the disease progresses, further symptoms may develop, including swollen face, puffy eyelids, thick skin and lips, large tongue, decreased sweating, slow monotonous nasal speech, and, occasionally, delusions. Children with thyroid deficiency are mentally retarded and babies become cretins with permanent mental impairment unless it is diagnosed and treated quickly. Treatment is with hormone replacement (thyroxine).

A goiter is an enlargement of the thyroid, usually from iodine deficiency, or very hard water which can interfere with iodine absorption. Goiters are common in mountainous areas because of the lack of fish – the main dietary source of iodine.

Hyperparathyroidism, overactivity of the parathyroid gland, removes calcium from bones, causing backache. The resulting high levels of calcium in the bloodstream cause weakness, loss of appetite, tiredness, and nausea. The kidney's attempts to excrete it can cause calcium stones. Treatment is by removing part of the overactive gland. Hypoparathyroidism – insufficiency of parathyroid hormone – causes tetany (spasm of hands, feet and glottis), convulsions and, sometimes, psychoses (◆ page 82). Treatment is with calcium injections in the acute phase, followed by Vitamin D.

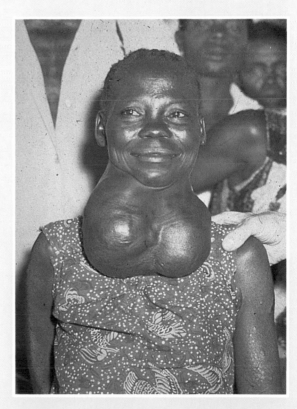

▲ *The swollen neck typical of goiter is a symptom of various thyroid disorders, often thyroid under-activity caused by lack of iodine in the diet. Iodine consumption may also be affected by exposure to cold, and a high fat and protein diet.*

The over-secretion of growth hormone can result in giants more than 2.5m tall

Growth hormone disorders

Oversecretion of growth hormone by the pituitary's secreting cells (hyperpituitarism) causes gigantism in children and acromegaly in adults. A patient with acromegaly has enlarged hands, jaw, sinuses, eyebrow ridges, tongue, lips, nose, ears, thyroid, heart and liver; thick, coarse skin; and sweats heavily. This condition is treated by a course of the drug bromocriptine; this has the same effect as dopamine, a neurotransmitter that reduces the output of the pituitary gland. Low output of growth hormone – known as hypopituitarism – causes dwarfism in children. In adults the effects are headache, partial loss of vision from pressure on optic fibers, loss of body hair, pallor from vasoconstriction, low blood sugar, low body temperature, and eventual coma and death from respiratory failure.

People whose pituitary produces insufficient vasopressin suffer from diabetes insipidus, a rare disease whose symptoms are thirst and excessive watery urine – 5 to 20 liters daily. Both hypopituitarism and diabetes insipidus are treated by hormone replacement.

Three to four percent of people over 40 suffer from Paget's disease. Increased formation and destruction of bone tissue enlarges affected bones but makes them painful, fragile and bendy. Increased blood supply to the bones makes them acutely feel warm. The pelvis, spine, tibia and skull are especially vulnerable. If the skull is affected headache and hearing loss occur. The cause of Paget's disease is unknown, but it may be a slow virus infection (◀ page 62). Treatment is concentrated on the symptoms: mithramycin (which slows cell division) or, if pain is severe, calcitonin.

Disorders of the adrenal glands

Overproduction of steroid hormones from the adrenal cortex may be caused by excessive adrenocorticotropic hormone (ACTH) secretion by the pituitary, and leads to Cushing's syndrome – moon face, distended abdomen, a "buffalo hump" of fat at the back of the neck, and depression. Women may produce noticeable quantities of androgen, and men of estrogen. Opinions about treatment vary, as do the symptoms. The usual methods are irradiation or partial removal of the pituitary. People suffering from over-production of aldosterone from the adrenal cortex notice constant thirst and an excessive urine production. Treatment for this is by operation or the drug spironolactone, which represses aldosterone.

The symptoms of Addison's disease – which is the shortage of adrenal cortex hormones – are weakness, weight loss and hyperpigmentation, especially in areas exposed to light or pressure, such as hands and knee creases. Athough old scars stay white, new ones go brown. Some patients, especially from dark-skinned races, develop vitiligo, in which areas of skin grow pale, while surrounded by excess pigment. There may also be hypotension, low blood sugar causing physical and mental tiredness, and loss of body hair, especially in women. Treatment is with cortisol (a glucocorticoid); some patients also need a mineralocorticoid. During periods of stress (as from a cold, injury or examinations), more cortisol is needed and any operation – even a dental extraction – needs special care.

Pheochromocytoma, a rare tumor of the cells of the adrenal medulla, causes the secretion of excess adrenaline and noradrenaline, with high blood pressure, pallor, sweating, palpitations and fear – in other words, a prolonged fight-or-flight response (◀ page 88). Treatment is by operation or beta-blockers are given.

Wilson's disease

In 1911, Dr Samuel Wilson (1878-1937), a US-born London neurologist, described an inherited disease. Excessive accumulations of copper damages various organs, especially the brain, liver and kidneys. It often starts with tremor or rigidity, then fever, spasticity, rigidity, and drooling develop; patients may develop schizophrenia, brain damage, dementia or other mental disorders. The sensory nerves are spared. Terminal patients are bedridden, mentally impaired and physically distorted. The incidence is 30 per million, of whom perhaps two-thirds are never properly diagnosed. The disease is inherited from both parents, but is rarely noticeable before adult life.

Treatment has been developed principally by British physician Dr John Walshe (b. 1920). He began with injections of dimercaptol, which sticks to copper and is then excreted. In 1956 he developed an oral treatment, penicilline, which "decoppers" patients, causing spectacular improvement. However, it sometimes causes sensitivity reactions requiring corticosteroids, and can cause skin diseases and optic neuritis. For those who cannot take penicilline, in 1982 Walshe developed another, trien.

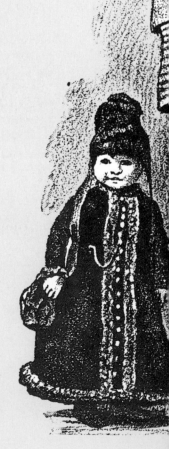

▶ A medical illustration of around 1900 showing a giant, a man of normal height and a pituitary dwarf. Gigantism is usually caused by over-secretion of growth hormone (GH) by the pituitary gland in childhood; this makes the long bones grow to an exceptional degree. Sufferers can be more than 2·44m (8ft) tall.

▶ Dwarfism is often the result of under-activity of the pituitary in childhood. The bones grow slowly, and the epiphyseal plates close abnormally early. Sufferers may have a low production of other hormones, and often do not reach sexual maturity.

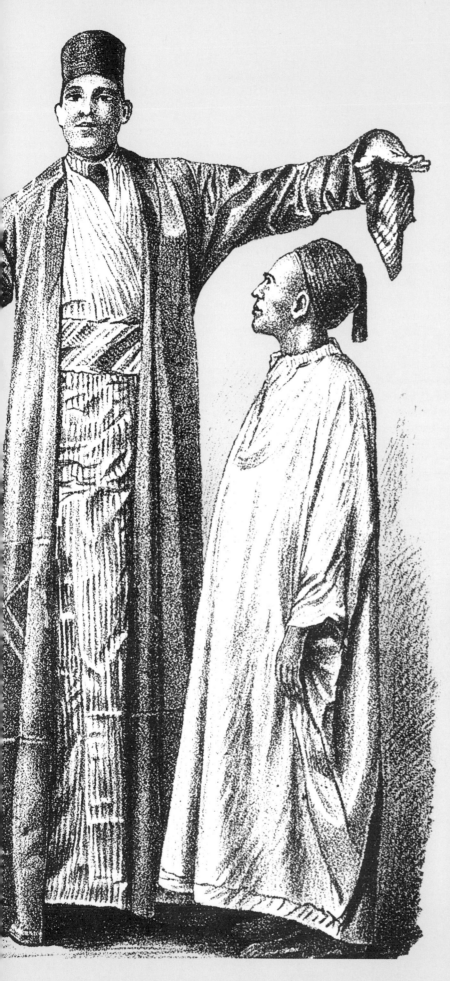

Hormonal changes in the menopause

The menopause, cessation of menstruation, may be abrupt or extend over many years. It is always abrupt in women whose ovaries are removed, otherwise trophic hormones from the pituitary try to stimulate the deteriorating ovaries, causing a variety of symptoms in 85 percent of women. Only a quarter of women are totally free from vasomotor symptoms – hot flushes and drenching sweats. Fifty percent suffer them for two to five years, and a quarter suffer for longer. Mental symptoms include palpitations, insomnia, fatigue, irritability, depression and emotional instability; most psychological illness in women in their 50s is hormonal. A few years after the menopause, women are susceptible to pain on intercourse and genital infections from loss of secretions, elasticity and tone. This is treated with estrogen cream. The menopause also heralds the onset of osteoporosis (loss of bone matrix and mineral with susceptibility to fractures and spinal curvature ♦ page 108). It is worst in thin women and the fair-skinned. Though rare in men, some osteoporosis is suffered by 15 percent of women aged 50, 30 percent at 60, 65 percent at 70 and 85 percent at 80. At 50 a woman is three times as susceptible to osteoporotic fractures as a man. This increases to four times at 60, and 5 times at 70. Treatment for menopausal symptoms consists of a daily dose of estrogen plus some progesterone for 12 days a month. This is reduced over two years to a minimal dose to keep the patient flush-free. A few women never cease treatment. Treatment, essential if the ovaries are removed before age 40, does not reverse osteoporosis but prevents it worsening.

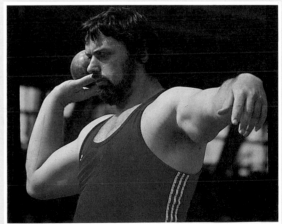

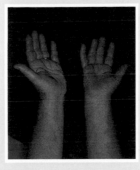

▲ *Shotputters and weightlifters are prominent among athletes who have taken anabolic steriods, synthetic hormones derived from testosterone, to promote muscular growth.*

◄ *Vitiligo, in which areas of unusually heavy pigmentation are mixed with areas of pale skin, may be a symptom of Addison's disease, caused by the shortage of glucocorticoids.*

96

Gout

Usually hereditary, gout is caused by over-production of uric acid, and is more common in men and the over-40s. Uric acid accumulates in the joints, causing recurrent bouts of swelling and pain. It often attacks a big toe first, later spreading to other joints. As the attack subsides, overlying skin becomes scaly and itchy. Chronic gout brings persistent pain and deformity, and the uric acid may form kidney stones. Gout can be precipitated by drinking too much alcohol, notably wines, and overindulging in certain foods, especially offal, fatty fish and fish roe. Attacks are treated with anti-inflammatory drugs.

Failure in insulin manufacture

Diabetes mellitus is caused by shortage of insulin, which is needed so that tissues can utilize sugar. A diabetic person's blood sugar rises after meals to higher levels than the kidneys can reabsorb, so it is excreted along with water to dilute it. This causes thirst. The loss of sugar causes skin eruptions, hunger and fatigue. The body burns fat for energy, producing a rise in ketones – partially burned fatty acids. At high levels, especially after stress or infection, this causes coma, requiring urgent hospital treatment. People whose diabetes started in childhood or early adult life require injections of insulin in doses that are tailored to fit the timing and content of their meals. The patient must follow a diet that aims at reducing day-to-day variation in insulin need, not at avoiding "bad" foods. People whose diabetes starts after middle age usually suffer less severely and can be treated successfully by drugs that reduce blood sugar. Diabetics need regular checkups to assess how well they are controlling their blood sugar and check for other symptoms. In most patients diabetes thickens the blood capillary walls throughout the body, damaging kidneys, the nervous system and eyes. Low blood sugar, caused by irregular meals or sudden exercise causes hunger, nausea and giddiness. It is relieved by eating sugar.

Isolating insulin

In 1893 it was discovered that partial removal of pancreas did not cause diabetes in humans but that complete removal did. In 1889 Oscar Minkowski (1858-1931) and Baron Joseph von Mehring (1849-1902) at Strasbourg also discovered that removal of a dog's pancreas caused diabetes. Minkowski was the first of many to try giving pancreatic extracts to restore diabetic animals or humans. It is surprising therefore that it was 30 years before insulin was successfully purified and used in treatment.

In 1905 French endocrinologist Eugène Gley (1857-1930) described experiments in which he injected pancreatic extracts into diabetic dogs, causing subjective improvement. Professor John Macleod (1876-1935), at Ohio, published a book in 1913 concluding that there was a secretion from the pancreas which could never be captured. In 1915 Israel Kleiner at the Rockefeller Institute started injecting pancreatic extractions into diabetic dogs, with good results.

The cure for diabetes

A Canadian, Fred Banting (1891-1941), qualified in medicine in 1916, served as a surgeon in the First World War and became a general practitioner with a part-time teaching job at Western Reserve University. After lecturing on diabetes he wanted to research on it for three months in the summer of 1921. Macleod, without enthusiasm, allowed him laboratory space, and an assistant, Charles Best (1899-1978). Best, a graduate biochemistry student, helped Banting to remove dog pancreases.

Many of the dogs died from postoperative infection; survivors were later given extracts of pancreas from other dogs which had been killed for the purpose. As the allotted ten dogs were soon used or lost from infections in the heat of the summer, several more dogs were bought from dealers. Banting and Best induced and cured diabetes in some of their dogs. Macleod, remembering others' failure, advised caution but made many helpful suggestions. Their extracts were often ineffective or toxic. Best made unsuccessful attempts to purify the extract; success came from James Collip (1892-1965), an experienced biochemist and friend of Macleod.

The first extract to be tried on a patient was Best's. Given to the 14-year old Leonard Thompson on 11 January 1914, it failed. He received Collip's extract on 23 January; that worked. Soon the world knew that diabetes could be cured but it was several years before insulin could be made on a sufficient scale for all; patients died knowing that cure was possible but unattainable.

Banting never got on with Macleod and conducted a permanent vendetta against him. He was furious at having to share the 1923 Nobel Prize with Macleod, and gave half his prize money to his colleague Best. Macleod, following suit, gave half of his to Collip.

Macleod, Best and Collip had distinguished careers; Best trained as a doctor but stayed in research, and Collip became highly successful at extracting and purifying hormones. Banting never made another discovery of note, and died in a plane crash in the Second World War.

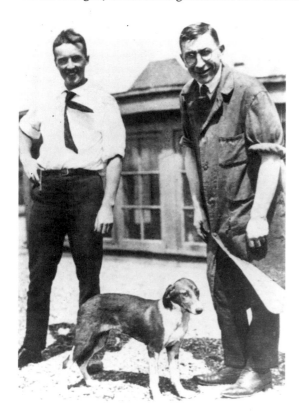

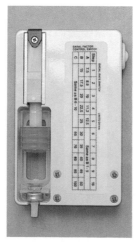

▲ An insulin pump can be attached to a patient and maintains an even supply of insulin in the bloodstream; such pumps need be refilled only once a year.

◄ Frederick Banting and Charles Best, photographed in 1921, with one of the dogs they used to help isolate insulin.

The skeleton, in infancy and adulthood...The body's joints...The muscles and their structure...Children's and adults' teeth......The composition of teeth... PERSPECTIVE...Collagen, the basis of bone...The marvel of the human hand...How muscles work...Early ideas of muscles and how they work

Without bones, teeth, cartilage and tendons we could not walk, move or eat, and the slightest jolt would damage the heart and brain. The skeleton gives support and, in conjunction with muscles, enables us to move; it also stores minerals and makes blood cells.

The infant and adult skeletons

Babies have about 350 bones, many of which fuse together during growth – for example the four "tail" vertebrae fuse to form the tailbone – so that there are only 206 in adults. Both numbers vary slightly: some people have 12 pairs of ribs but one person in 20 has 13 and mongols often have only 11. Some people possess extra fingers or toes. A baby's cranium has several bones that are not yet fused together. These overlap during birth like petals on a flowerbud, allowing the baby's large head to pass through the relatively narrow birth canal. This is why the head of a newborn baby (except one delivered by Caesarian section) is distorted and takes a few weeks to reach its normal shape. Fontanels are soft spots at the top of the newborn baby's head which cover gaps in the skull bones. They close up between the ages of six months and two years.

Of the 206 adult bones, there are 32 in each arm: collar bone, shoulder blade, upper arm (1), lower arm (2), wrist (8), palm (5), thumb (2), fingers (3 each). Each leg has 30: thigh, kneecap, lower leg (2), ankle (7), instep (5), big toe (2), other toes (3 each).

The skull contains 29: the cranium (8), face (13), lower jaw (1), ear bones (3 each side), and the throat (1). The backbone has 26: the neck (7), chest (12), lower back (5) and a tailbone. There are 24 ribs, a breastbone and two hip bones. Most of the vertebrae have very little capacity for movement against each other. The top two neck vertebrae are an exception. The first, the atlas, allows movement of the head back and forth and from side to side. The second, known as the axis, allows the head to rotate.

Collagen and the composition of bone

Adult bone is extremely solid and strong, due to its structure and composition. It is a lattice of about 70 percent mineral and 30 percent collagen (these proportions are reversed in babies, which is why babies' bones bend rather than break). Collagen is a protein; its amino-acids are crosslinked to give elasticity and strength. Its molecules are rod-shaped and arranged in three-strand ropelike structures (a "triple-helix"). The mineral is mainly calcium and phosphorus, and crystals of it lie in regular patterns in the collagen framework.

As collagen in the form of fine fibers (fibrils) can blend with other materials, it can produce a wide variety of connective tissue. Tendon is almost pure collagen, and because the fibrils are arranged in parallel it has great tensile strength. In skin the fibrils become cross-woven into sheets that can be stretched. In cartilage, collagen fibrils are embedded in a sugar polymer – an arrangement which provides shock-absorption.

The collagen is essential for holding mineral. If any collagen is lost (as in women after the menopause) it cannot be replaced, so mineral is lost too. All the minerals, including small amounts of magnesium, fluorine, chlorine and iron are constantly being removed and replaced. Around the bone shaft is a layer of cells called osteoblasts that deposit mineral, and osteoclasts that remove it. Some biologists believe the two types are the same and can reverse roles. Bone acts as "banker" to the rest of the body, foregoing minerals when they are needed, taking them back when there is enough.

Between the shaft and the epiphyses in growing bones is a section of cartilage which expands and is gradually replaced by bone. Cartilage also covers the end of the bone where it moves on the joint.

Section through long bone

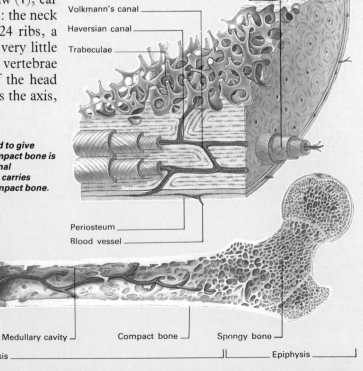

Concentric lamellae
Volkmann's canal
Haversian canal
Trabeculae

Periosteum
Blood vessel

▶ ▼ *Long bones such as the femur have evolved to give lightness with strength. The hollow shaft of compact bone is lined with spongy bone. A network of longitudinal (Haversian) and transverse (Volkmann's) canals carries blood, nerve and lymph vessels through the compact bone.*

Epiphysis

Articular cartilage

Blood vessel   Medullary cavity   Compact bone   Spongy bone

Diaphysis   Epiphysis

The complex bones, joints and muscles of the hand give both power and delicate movement

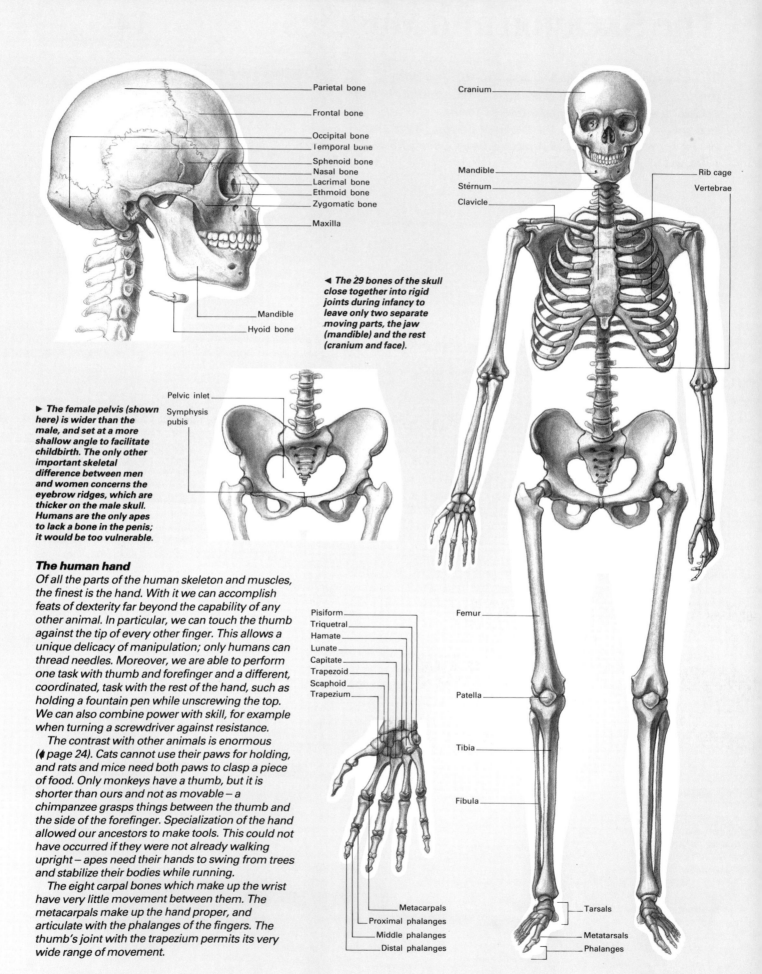

Parietal bone

Frontal bone

Occipital bone
Temporal bone
Sphenoid bone
Nasal bone
Lacrimal bone
Ethmoid bone
Zygomatic bone

Maxilla

Mandible
Hyoid bone

◄ *The 29 bones of the skull close together into rigid joints during infancy to leave only two separate moving parts, the jaw (mandible) and the rest (cranium and face).*

Cranium

Mandible
Sternum
Clavicle

Rib cage
Vertebrae

Pelvic inlet
Symphysis pubis

► *The female pelvis (shown here) is wider than the male, and set at a more shallow angle to facilitate childbirth. The only other important skeletal difference between men and women concerns the eyebrow ridges, which are thicker on the male skull. Humans are the only apes to lack a bone in the penis; it would be too vulnerable.*

The human hand

Of all the parts of the human skeleton and muscles, the finest is the hand. With it we can accomplish feats of dexterity far beyond the capability of any other animal. In particular, we can touch the thumb against the tip of every other finger. This allows a unique delicacy of manipulation; only humans can thread needles. Moreover, we are able to perform one task with thumb and forefinger and a different, coordinated, task with the rest of the hand, such as holding a fountain pen while unscrewing the top. We can also combine power with skill, for example when turning a screwdriver against resistance.

The contrast with other animals is enormous (◊ page 24). Cats cannot use their paws for holding, and rats and mice need both paws to clasp a piece of food. Only monkeys have a thumb, but it is shorter than ours and not as movable – a chimpanzee grasps things between the thumb and the side of the forefinger. Specialization of the hand allowed our ancestors to make tools. This could not have occurred if they were not already walking upright – apes need their hands to swing from trees and stabilize their bodies while running.

The eight carpal bones which make up the wrist have very little movement between them. The metacarpals make up the hand proper, and articulate with the phalanges of the fingers. The thumb's joint with the trapezium permits its very wide range of movement.

Pisiform
Triquetral
Hamate
Lunate
Capitate
Trapezoid
Scaphoid
Trapezium

Femur

Patella

Tibia

Fibula

Metacarpals
Proximal phalanges
Middle phalanges
Distal phalanges

Tarsals

Metatarsals

Phalanges

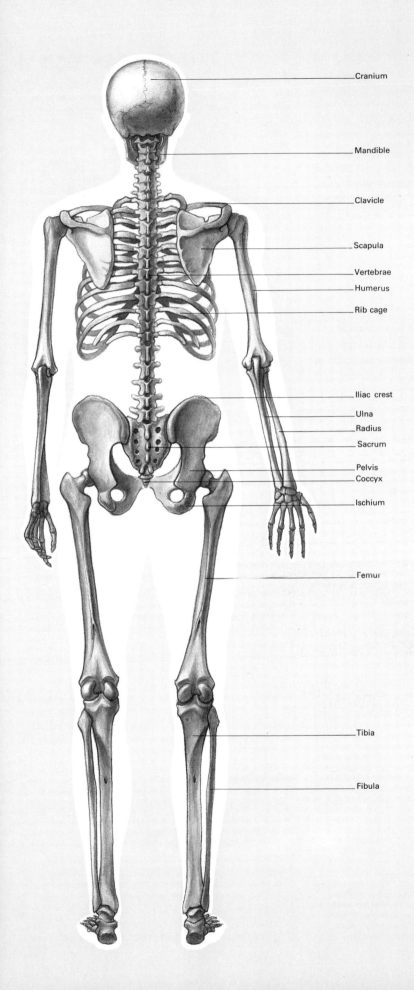

Cranium

Mandible

Clavicle

Scapula

Vertebrae

Humerus

Rib cage

Iliac crest

Ulna

Radius

Sacrum

Pelvis

Coccyx

Ischium

Femur

Tibia

Fibula

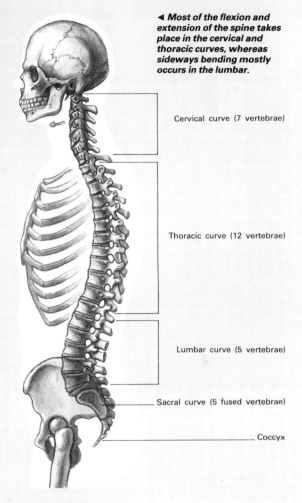

◄ Most of the flexion and extension of the spine takes place in the cervical and thoracic curves, whereas sideways bending mostly occurs in the lumbar.

Cervical curve (7 vertebrae)

Thoracic curve (12 vertebrae)

Lumbar curve (5 vertebrae)

Sacral curve (5 fused vertebrae)

Coccyx

The vertebral disks

The joints between adjacent vertebrae are responsible for the flexibility of the spinal column. Set between each pair of vertebrae is a collagenous disk. This acts as a shock absorber and most of the body load is transmitted through the disk. The disk has a central zone, the nucleus pulposus, which is encircled by concentric sheets of criss-crossed collagen fibers. The nucleus is gelatinous, consisting of randomly-oriented collagen fibers embedded in a matrix of water and sugar polymer. Because the nucleus can be deformed but not compressed, it redistributes any vertical pressures in a radial direction. However, under excessive loading, in disease or in old age the normally tough outer annulus may rupture with disastrous effect.

The smaller bones

Not every bone in the body can be shown in skeletal illustrations. The hyoid bone in the throat is the only bone not attached to any others; it supports the tongue muscles. The ear bones, given the quaint collective name of the ossicles, transmit and amplify vibrations of the eardrum, and are called hammer, anvil and stirrup because of their shapes (◊ page 45). Two parts of the skeleton that are not bones but are important parts of our shape are the ear lobe and the tip of the nose. As cartilage, these are flexible and can withstand knocks.

Every person has the same number of muscle fibers; physique depends on their development with use

Bones are too rigid to bend without damage, so they are hinged with joints. Though each joint is individually designed to give a particular angle and extent of movement, they can be grouped into three categories. In fibrous joints (such as where the skull bones meet or a tooth joins its socket) the bones' edges meet very closely with no gap between them. Such joints are very strong. Cartilaginous joints are the rarest. Found between the epiphyses and shafts of growing bone, and between the two pubic bones, they move only in exceptional circumstances: the pubic bones, for example, move apart slightly in childbirth. Synovial joints, like the knee and elbow, which are freely movable and contain fluid, are the most familiar kind. The cartilage-covered ends of the bones are lubricated by synovial fluid, made by its surrounding membrane. Bones lying side-by-side are bound together with ligaments, which are strong and fibrous, like tendons.

The body's musculature
The muscles of the skeleton have two mechanical functions: to maintain posture and to generate movement. At each end of a muscle is a tendon, also known as a sinew, which links it to a bone. Muscles produce movements by exerting force on tendons, which then pull on bones. A muscle has its "origin" on the stationary bone; its other end crosses a joint and has its "insertion" on the bone that is moved. Joints are levers – they consist of a rigid rod moving from a pivot and subject to two opposing forces, the effort exerted and the resistance encountered. Muscles work by pulling and are arranged in opposing pairs, since it is no use having a muscle to bend the arm if there is no muscle to straighten it. Isotonic contraction is the contraction that shortens a muscle, as when we lift an arm. Isometric contraction occurs when we keep the same position but encounter weight or resistance. Isometric contraction is essential to maintaining posture.

Skeletal muscles are composed of fibers up to 30cm long. Their total number is fixed by the first few weeks of life and is the same for everybody, whatever their physique. Muscle fibers increase in size with use, and make up about 36 percent of a woman's body weight, 42 percent of a man's. Each fiber works on an all-or-nothing principle and the degree of movement of a limb depends on how many fibers are contracting in the muscle. Contraction occurs when an electrical impulse reaches a fiber from a nerve. A muscle can contract more forcefully in response to the same strength of stimulus after it has already contracted several times – hence an athlete's need for a "warming-up" period before reaching peak performance.

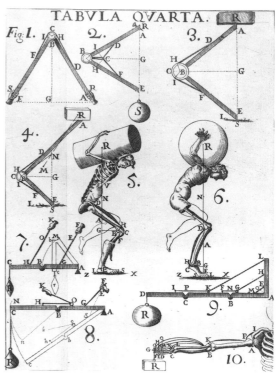

▲ Plate IV from Borelli's "De Motu Animalium".

Borelli's study of muscles as levers
Giovanni Alfonso Borelli (1608-1679), Italian physician, mathematician and astronomer, was the first man to apply mathematical principles to medicine. Educated in Naples and Rome, he became professor of mathematics at Messina, moving to Pisa in 1656. Here he studied animal functions, and anatomy.

In "De Motu Animalium" (1680-1681) he successfully applied the principles of mechanics to the active and passive movements of the body. He showed that bones are true levers, that their muscles power them, and that the distance of the muscle attachment from the joint determines the amount of force required for a movement to take place. In his book, Borelli also dealt with muscles and groups of muscles, interpreting their movements by geometry and mechanics as if they were levers. Then he examined the process of contraction. He recognized the contractile elements in muscle and deduced that contraction was triggered by a "physical reaction" traveling from the brain via the nerve.

How a muscle works
Each muscle has three layers of fibrous connective tissue: a thin layer around each fiber, a thicker layer enclosing each bundle of a dozen or so fibers, and a thick layer around the entire muscle.

When a muscle fiber contracts, individual filaments of actin slide like ratchets over fibers of another protein molecule, myosin. An individual fiber may contract for only a few thousandths of a second, and may need another fraction to regain its responsiveness to the nerve impulse; thus, to maintain an even contraction, nerves "fire" different fibers of a muscle in quick succession.

The structure of a muscle

Myofibril
Muscle fiber
Epimysium
Muscle

Fascicle

Perimysium

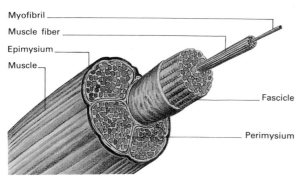

◄ *A muscle is covered in connective tissue known as epimysium and is made up of bundles (fascicles) of fibers, each one wrapped in perimysium. Epimysium and perimysium unite at the muscle's end to form the tendon. Each muscle fiber consists of a network of parallel myofibrils of actin and myosin. The myosin molecules are studded with "cross bridges"; when the muscle is stimulated to contract, these catch on the actin molecules and pull them along the myosin, thus shortening the fiber.*

The major joints

▶ *The most important pivot joint in the body is between the first and second vertebrae (atlas and axis). The axis has a projection on which the atlas moves; this allows the head to rotate.*

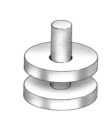

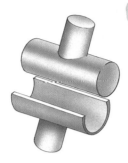

▲ *The hinge joint is found in elbow and fingers; it permits simple flexion and extension. The knee is a hinge joint modified with a twist that allows it to lock into place.*

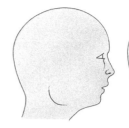

▲ *The human jaw can move freely in several planes. Movement forwards and back is called protraction and retraction; the jaw can also be moved up and down and from side to side.*

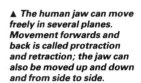

▲ *The saddle joint is found only where the thumb metacarpal articulates on the trapezium of the hand. As a modified ellipsoidal joint, it allows a wide range of movement.*

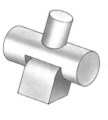

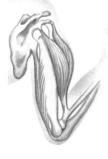

▲ *The muscles of a limb are paired into the flexors (which bend the limb) and extensors (which pull it straight). The main flexor of the arm is the biceps; the main extensor the triceps.*

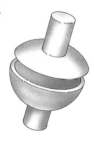

▲ *Ellipsoidal joints are found between the bones of the lower arm or leg and wrist or ankle; they permit flexion-extension as well as eversion-inversion (turning hand or foot to the side).*

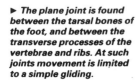

▶ *The plane joint is found between the tarsal bones of the foot, and between the transverse processes of the vertebrae and ribs. At such joints movement is limited to a simple gliding.*

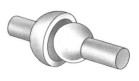

▲ *Ball-and-socket joints at shoulder and hip permit circular motion (circum-duction). Moving the limb out from the body is abduction; adduction is returning it to rest.*

Accurate measuring devices proved that muscles retain their original volume when they contract

Studying muscle contraction

The Dutch biologist John Swammerdam (1637-1681) was one of the earliest anatomists to rely on the microscope. He studied natural history and at first was mainly interested in insects, but in 1653 moved from Holland to France where, in 1664, he discovered the valves of the lymphatic vessels. Two years later he returned to Holland and was made doctor of medicine at Leiden. He discovered the red cells in frog blood and traced the development of frogs. He injected colored wax to demonstrate the blood vessels of animals and invented a method of making dry preparations of hollow organs such as the stomach. One of Swammerdam's most crucial contributions was to disprove the contemporary belief that fluid passes from the nerve into the muscle when it contracts. He carried out dissections under a microscope and discovered that a muscle contracted when the cut end of its nerve was stimulated. By dissecting, with nerve intact, a large muscle from a frog's leg, and transferring it to a glass cylinder containing water with a sensitive capillary tube to measure changes in volume, he established that a muscle does not increase in volume when it contracts.

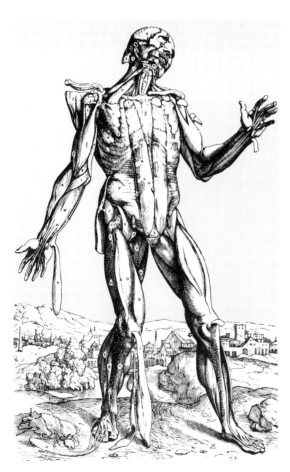

▲ **The Fifth Plate of the Muscles from "De Humani Corporis Fabrica" (1543), by the great Flemish anatomist Andreas Vesalius (1514-1564). As professor of anatomy at Padua from about 1537, his unprecedently scrupulous dissections and drawings conflicted with much received opinion about anatomy. His work, with its elegantly poised cadavers, is a masterpiece of Renaissance art as well as science.**

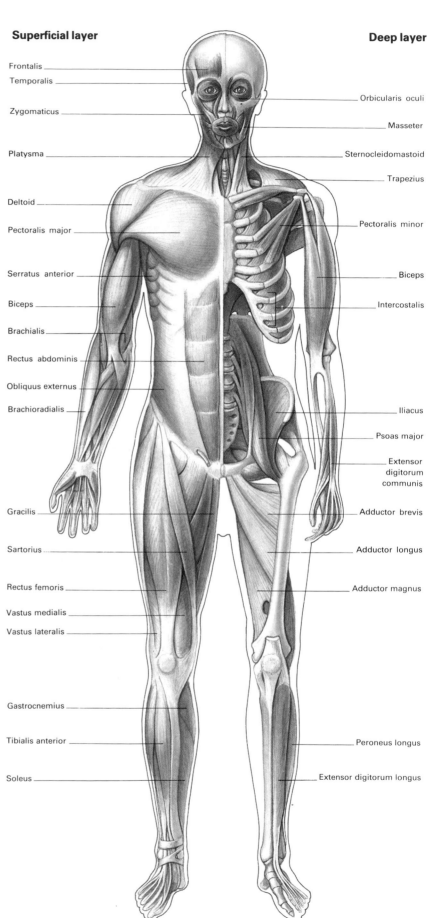

Superficial layer

Deep layer

- Frontalis
- Temporalis
- Zygomaticus
- Platysma
- Deltoid
- Pectoralis major
- Serratus anterior
- Biceps
- Brachialis
- Rectus abdominis
- Obliquus externus
- Brachioradialis
- Gracilis
- Sartorius
- Rectus femoris
- Vastus medialis
- Vastus lateralis
- Gastrocnemius
- Tibialis anterior
- Soleus

- Orbicularis oculi
- Masseter
- Sternocleidomastoid
- Trapezius
- Pectoralis minor
- Biceps
- Intercostalis
- Iliacus
- Psoas major
- Extensor digitorum communis
- Adductor brevis
- Adductor longus
- Adductor magnus
- Peroneus longus
- Extensor digitorum longus

Deep layer

Splenius capitis

Levator scapulae

Rhomboideus

Teres minor

Teres major

Semispinalis

Erector spinae

Gluteus minimus

Obturator internus

Vastus lateralis

Gracilis

Biceps femoris

Popliteus

Soleus

Tibialis posterior

Flexor digitorum longus

Peroneus longus

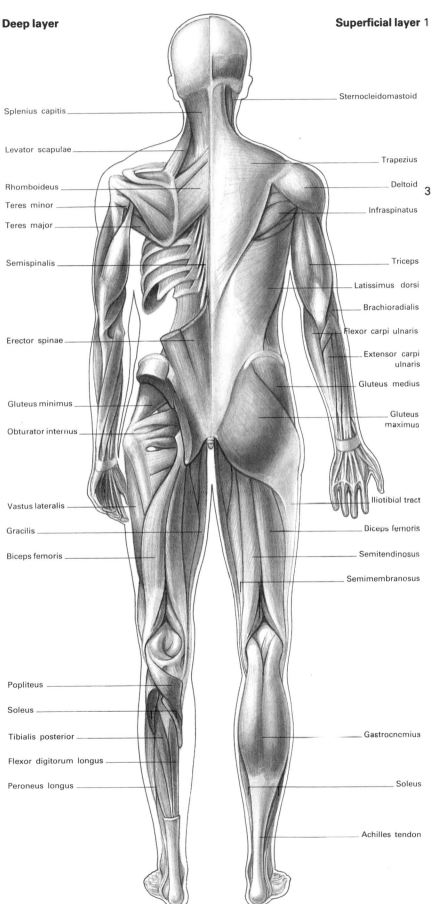

Superficial layer 1

Sternocleidomastoid

Trapezius

Deltoid

Infraspinatus

Triceps

Latissimus dorsi

Brachioradialis

Flexor carpi ulnaris

Extensor carpi ulnaris

Gluteus medius

Gluteus maximus

Iliotibial tract

Biceps femoris

Semitendinosus

Semimembranosus

Gastrocnemius

Soleus

Achilles tendon

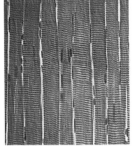
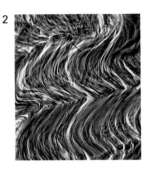

3

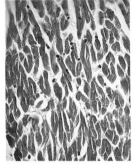

Voluntary muscle (1) can be controlled consciously and is striated or striped. It includes all the skeletal muscles, and those that control breathing. Involuntary or visceral muscle (2), which carries out automatic functions such as moving food through the gut, is smooth and unstriated. Cardiac muscle (3), found only in the heart, is involuntary but is also striated.

Muscle irritability

Albert von Haller (1708-1777) is universally regarded as the father of modern physiology. He was born in Switzerland, educated in Germany and Holland, and visited doctors and scholars in London, Oxford, Paris, and Berne before becoming professor of medicine, anatomy, botany and surgery at Göttingen in Germany. He used his knowledge of anatomy combined with his systematic experimental technique to discover the laws which govern the body. By examining muscle fibers he recognized what he termed irritability – the capacity to contract in response to a minutely small stimulus and then return to their former length. Haller thus distinguished between "inherent muscular force" and "nerve force". He saw each organ as having two properties, sensibility and irritability – for the action of each organ a specific stimulus is required. This view, though inaccurate, was a great step forward at the time.

The secret of muscle contraction

The fine structure of muscle and the way in which actin and myosin interlock in muscle contraction were revealed by Jean Hanson (1919-1973) and Hugh Huxley (b.1924), at King's College, London. Jean Hanson had become interested in muscle when she discovered marine worms had an unusual type of muscle fiber. Moving to mammalian muscle, she placed freshly-dissected samples in a solution that made the membrane leaky and examined it under the newly-developed phase-contrast microscope. She put a drop of adenosine triphosphate (ATP – the molecule produced in all living cells to store energy and produce work) at one end of the sample and drew it through to the other end using blotting paper. The muscle fibrils shortened, changing their pattern. Later, with physicist Hugh Huxley, she repeated the experiment with weaker ATP solutions, and reported the visible changes in muscle structure.

The teeth

No part of the body is harder or more resistant to destruction after death than the teeth. Yet none is as susceptible to decay during life. Most of us are born toothless, much to the relief of breastfeeding mothers. Human teeth grow to full size before they erupt through the gums. We start to produce the first "milk teeth" at around seven months, by which time we are likely to have been weaned. Thereafter we produce, on average, a tooth a month (with great individual variation) until we have 20: eight incisors for cutting, four canines for tearing and eight molars for crushing and grinding.

No more erupt until about six years, when the first of the 32 adult teeth appear. These, the molars, emerge further back in the jaw than the milk teeth. Later, the permanent incisors, canines and premolars emerge on the buccal (tongue) side of the milk teeth, which they should push right out of the jaw (if they do not succeed, they may be permanently crooked). The second set of molars emerge at around 13 and the third, the wisdom teeth, any time in the next ten years. Few of us have enough space for these in our jaws, so they are removed. Sometimes there is so little room that wisdom teeth remain impacted in the bone and have to be removed surgically. A few lucky people have no wisdom teeth, or dwarf-sized ones.

Like icebergs, teeth are mainly concealed under the surface. The root is up to three times as long as the crown and is embedded firmly in the jaw by a layer of hard membrane or ligament which acts as both anchor and shock-absorber. The main part of a tooth is dentine, a bone-like substance consisting of a similar mix of 70 percent mineral and 30 percent collagen. The crown has a thickish layer of enamel, an intensely hard substance made up of 4 percent organic matter and 96 percent calcium carbonate and calcium phosphate. Enamel stands up to the wear of cutting, tearing, crushing and grinding, and protects the dentine, which is very easily attacked by the acids that are produced by bacteria from sugar taken in the food.

Because enamel has no nerves, we cannot feel when it is attacked, but dentine has a rich network of blood, lymph vessels and nerves, which enter at the tip of the roots and penetrate the pulp cavity.

Deciduous and permanent teeth

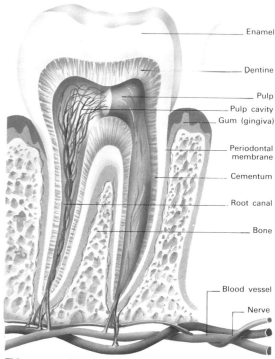

▲ This cross-section of a molar tooth indicates the typical relation of enamel to dentine. Although the fibrous joint between root and jaw is very strong and the root itself is surrounded by the hard cementum, the relatively soft periodontal membrane allows a modicum of movement for the tooth in the jaw. The enamel on teeth is the hardest substance in the human body.

▶ ▼ The 20 deciduous or milk teeth of a child and the 32 permanent teeth. The child's mouth contains no premolars, whereas the adult has two pairs in each jaw. The adult also has one more pair of molars (the wisdom teeth). The incisors are primarily for cutting; the canines (also known as cuspids) for tearing. The large, uneven surface of the premolars and molars makes them suitable for crushing and grinding.

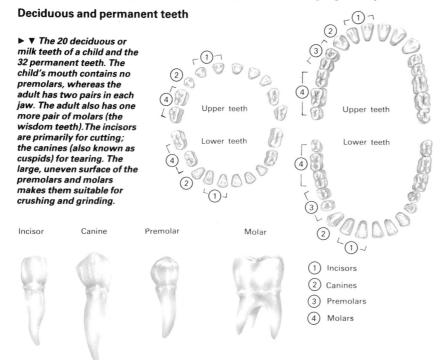

Upper teeth

Upper teeth

Lower teeth

Lower teeth

Incisor   Canine   Premolar   Molar

① Incisors
② Canines
③ Premolars
④ Molars

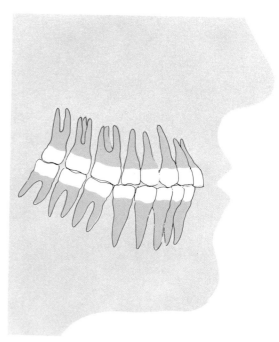

▲ In the ideal bite, the upper and lower rows of teeth should be symmetrically arranged, though the upper row should be slightly larger, so that when the premolars are biting, the upper incisors project slightly over the lower. Abnormalities in the bite, or in the evenness of teeth development, can often be corrected by means of various fixed orthodontic appliances, preferably during childhood.

The history of orthopedics...X-rays, transforming diagnosis...Fractures, sprains and pulled muscles... Spinal injuries and back pain...Dentistry and orthodontics...PERSPECTIVE...Accidental injuries... New techniques of orthopedics...Arthritis...Hip replacement, major surgery

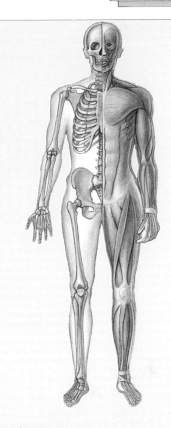

The skeletal remains of primitive Man often show signs of arthritis, bony tumours and tuberculosis. But they also show that our earliest ancestors distinguished themselves from the rest of the animal kingdom by attempting to do more than merely lick their wounds. Paleolithic Man made splints and attempted to cope with broken bones. Neolithic Man even attempted amputations and cut holes in skull bones (trepanning) with flint scrapers.

The tomb of the Egyptian King Hirkouf (2830 BC) has among the motifs at its entrance a crutch. Early Egyptian murals and pottery often depict hunchbacks, the lame, dwarfs and even such recognizable diseases as poliomyelitis. Equally, much of Hippocratic Greek medicine (*c.* 480 BC) relates to the treatment of deformities and injuries of limbs.

Nicholas André, professor of medicine in the University of Paris, coined the term "orthopedics" in the mid-18th century by taking the Greek stems orthos ("straight") and paidios ("child"). The term caught on and was soon being used to include not only children but also adults. Orthopedics is the study and treatments of diseases, deformities and injuries of the trunk and limbs. Besides bones and joints, it includes the related muscles, tendons, ligaments, bursae (the lubricating structure), nerves and blood vessels. As a subject, it became a speciality of surgery only in the last few decades of the 19th century.

An understanding of infectious disease, coupled with improved treatment, better diagnostic techniques (especially using X-rays) and the rise of chemotherapy and antibiotics, has greatly altered the pattern of orthopedics. Tuberculosis and poliomyelitis have now receded as important medical problems, to be replaced by a great increase in the number of injuries (trauma) incurred in a wide variety of ways both accidental and non-accidental, and by the untoward effects of changing diets and lifestyle.

Diagnosing and restoring broken bones

The X-rays that the German physicist Wilhelm Röntgen (1845-1923) discovered in November 1895 have completely transformed the diagnosis of broken limbs. Once the damage has been assessed it is possible to plan how best to restore a normal bone structure – the process of reduction. If there is an external wound this must first be cleansed and treated with antibiotic to prevent or halt any infection. The next step is to immobilize the limb or part of the body using splints or plaster of paris. Successful reduction requires that the broken ends of the bone be brought together. This can often be done by manipulation, but surgery may be required. Multiple breaks have to be opened usually to sort out the pieces. To achieve restoration, screws may be used, perhaps in conjunction with a metal plate.

Accidental injury

After cardiovascular disease and cancer, accidental injury is now one of the greatest causes of death. Traffic accidents play a significant part in accidental injuries, and such trauma, with increasing use of the automobile, motorbike and bicycle, is now approaching epidemic proportion.

Off the road, more than half of all accidents are caused by falls, and about 90 percent of such falls involve people over 65 years of age. As we become older our bones lose mass, especially bone tissue (collagen) rather than mineral, and this causes the bones to become more porous, brittle and rarefied ("osteoporosis"). Consequently a fall for an elderly person often causes severe damage.

Leisure pursuits, such as keep-fit, sport and do-it-yourself home improvement, are becoming responsible for an increasing number of accidental injuries. Injuries may consist of torn or stretched muscles, sprained or dislocated joints, "slipped" disks, hernias, pulled tendons and bone fractures. The cause is that the tissues are suddenly stressed beyond their intrinsic strength, or consistently stressed to their limits. Certainly they become loaded in a way for which they were not adapted. A fall can cause the weight of the body to be focused on a single bone, resulting in fracture, or on a joint, causing dislocation. Over-exertion may tear a cartilage or rupture muscle fibers, as happens in tennis elbow. Fracture, swelling or sudden stretching of the various components of the chassis may cause nerve injuries. Such damage may be only ephemeral (neurapraxia), long-lasting (axonotmesis) or even irreparable (neurotmesis). Likewise, blood vessels may become contused or compressed, causing local loss of blood circulation (ischemia) which can destroy vital tissues.

In the USA alone 1 million fractures annually lose an estimated $8 billion in working time

Classifying bone injuries

Fractures of living bone come in many forms. Simple fractures are those in which the adjacent soft tissues are not broken. When the tissues overlying the broken bone become wounded, and consequently often infected, the fracture is termed compound. If the bone is broken into more than two fragments, the fracture is said to be comminuted. Sometimes a bone becomes broken on only one side and bent on the other. These greenstick fractures occur in growing children when the bones tend to be springy. When one bone component is driven forcibly into another the resulting fracture is said to be impacted. Stress fractures in bone, as in metal, occur when the material becomes fatigued due to repeated strain. Pathological fractures are caused by abnormalities that may be in origin congenital, inflammatory, neoplastic (benign and malignant growths) or metabolic.

Injuries to joints are of three main types. In sprains, the ligaments that hold the joint together may become torn. In subluxations the articular surfaces remain in contact but they become displaced from their normal positions. In dislocations, the articular surfaces become completely displaced and part of one of the bones may also be fractured. Sprains need initial rest to allow the tear to heal, and cautious exercise not to tear the damaged ligament further. Subluxations can usually be treated by applying pressure in the reverse direction to the displacement. Treatment of dislocations is similar, but an anesthetic is often given to the patients while the components of the joint are forced back into their normal position. Typical dislocations can occur to the shoulder, the elbow, the fingers, the knee and the instep. Only with considerable violence is the normal healthy hip joint likely to become dislocated. However, with elderly people whose bones are becoming brittle, a fall or a blow to the hip may sever the femoral head (ball) of the main leg bone from its shaft, which in turn may shatter the hip socket. Treatment may be to nail the femoral head to its shaft or, in extreme cases, fit a total hip replacement (page 110).

Hernias

Abdominal muscle

Peritoneum

Hiatus

Epigastric

Umbilical

Inguinal

Femoral

Intestine

Strangulated hernia

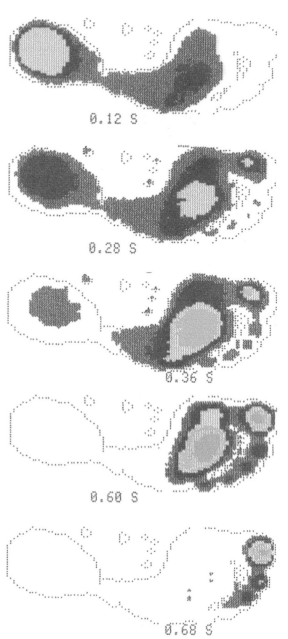

0.12 S

0.28 S

0.36 S

0.60 S

0.68 S

▲ *A pedobarograph records the pressure on each part of a foot through the stages of a single step. The foot shown here is healthy; the colors describe varying intensity in pressure. This technique, developed in the 1980s, can be used with the foot either stationary or walking to identify potential malformations at an early stage.*

Hernias
An organ or tissue may become protruded, or "herniated", from its normal cavity. The hernia may extend outside the body or between cavities within the body, as when a loop of intestine escapes from the abdominal cavity into the chest. Hernias may be congenital or acquired later in life. An acquired hernia is usually caused by overexertion. Soft tissue hernias most often occur in the groin, the thigh and the navel, and sometimes in the brain. A reducible hernia can be pushed back into its proper cavity; an irreducible hernia cannot. A strangulated hernia impedes blood circulation.

New techniques in orthopedics

Estimates suggest that the USA alone loses some $8 billion annually in working time through about one million fractures. If the disability time from these fractures could be cut by a half, the country would obviously save much money. Various physical techniques have been attempted in various countries to achieve just that.

The Russians have an ultrasonic tool which, they claim, can be used to join biological tissue, especially broken bones. To mend a broken bone, they bring the two halves together and treat them with a weak solution of acid to remove calcium salts and to make the collagen accessible. Next, they place a small plate of bone transplant over the join and bathe it in a polymerizable monomer mixed with bone shavings. The high-power, high-frequency vibrations (250 watts at a frequency of 26.5 kilohertz) cause the binder to penetrate deep into the bone parts and to harden sufficiently to hold them firm during the natural regeneration of bone tissue. German scientists have claimed similar effects using metal splints and alternating currents below 1 kilohertz.

US scientists assert that soft-tissue injuries, such as sprained ankles, strained shoulders and swollen joints, can be repaired in half the time by means of electromagnetism. They pulse the damaged tissues with high-frequency radiowaves at about 27 megahertz (just above the frequency of television). As yet there is still no satisfactory explanation as to how magnetic, electric or ultrasonic fields can actually affect living tissues.

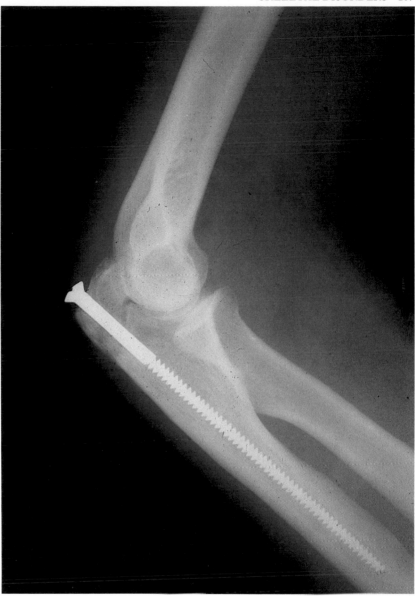

▶ *X-ray of a broken arm with a metal pin introduced into the marrow cavity in order to strengthen the bone. Wire may also be wound around the bone to assist it to set straight, and metal plates also may assist correct healing in the case of a spiral or a comminuted fracture.*

Fractures

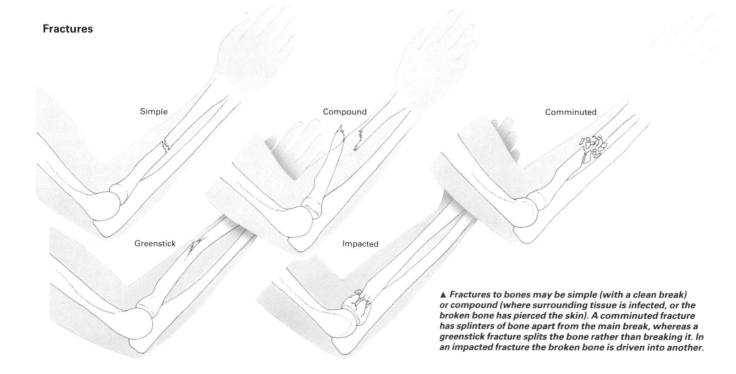

▲ *Fractures to bones may be simple (with a clean break) or compound (where surrounding tissue is infected, or the broken bone has pierced the skin). A comminuted fracture has splinters of bone apart from the main break, whereas a greenstick fracture splits the bone rather than breaking it. In an impacted fracture the broken bone is driven into another.*

Low back pain is responsible for more lost working days in one year than all industrial strikes added together

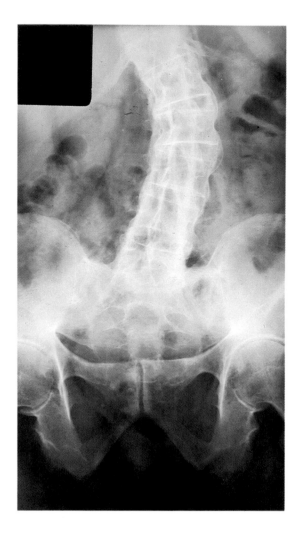

"Slipped" disks

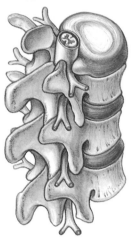

▲ **A prolapsed or slipped disk occurs when severe strain causes the pulpy nucleus pulposus of the intervertebral disk to be squeezed out and press on a nerve. The disorder may result from a flattening of the disks brought about by wear and reduction of mobility; it is cured only by lengthy rest.**

◄ **In the condition known as ankylosing spondylitis, the joints of the backbone become bony, and the spine grows rigid, with the patient typically locked into an extreme, forward-leaning posture.**

Arthritis

Arthritis is a general term that is used to describe damaged and painful joints. The inflammation and wear responsible for arthritis can arise from a multitude of effects. Treatment consists of rest, pain-relieving drugs and the control of symptoms (by antibiotics if relevant). Osteoarthritis is a degenerative disease in which joints become damaged and limited in their movement due to changes in tissue as they age. In extreme cases, where the joint surfaces become completely degraded, it may be necessary to replace the joint or part of it with artificial components. This has been achieved for the ankle, knee, elbow and hip.

Rheumatoid arthritis (◆ page 230) is a disease of unknown origin but which seems to involve the body's own immunological system turning against components of the joints. It is accompanied by disturbance of the normal body equilibrium, loss of weight and weakness. The joints become inflamed, and may be deformed, fused and immobilized (ankylosed). Typically the disease is first observed in the fingers and wrist. When it occurs in children it is termed Still's disease. Cortisone was for long used as an anti-inflammatory drug to relieve symptoms; it has largely been superseded by other related drugs, such as prednisolone, with less undesirable side effects.

Other joint infections

Ankylosing spondylitis is a disease of the spine in which the ligaments become bony (ossified) and the lateral joints become immobilized. The condition is aptly called poker-spine although it can result in a rigid deflexion of the spine and neck. It tends to affect young male adults, although it can also affect females. Its onset is associated with persistent low back pain and stiffness. It may spread to the shoulders, hips, knees and even jaw.

New growths, or neoplasms, affect bone and the soft tissues. A range of benign growths occur in bone, including osteoma, chondroma and cysts. Giant-cell bone tumors that sometimes develop in young people can be capricious. For the most part they are innocent but occasionally they invade the lung and become malignant. The truly malignant growths are a range of various sarcomas (◆ page 221); often they are secondary deposits from growths elsewhere. Soft-tissue neoplasms can involve fatty tissues, muscle, tendon, synovial tissues, nervous tissues and blood vessels.

A range of neuromuscular disorders can be responsible for spastic paralysis, muscular weakness (dystrophies) and limited reflexes. Many are incurable and supporting appliances can be used only to control the deformities.

In healthy people muscle, bone and tendon should develop in harmony. Obesity, the excessive accumulation of fat, stresses the normal working of limbs and joints, because muscles and tendons become overloaded. The effects of wasting diseases, as in beriberi, kwashiorkor, anorexia and sickle-cell anemia, can cause an imbalance through one set of muscles being stronger than their counterparts and lead to deformities. Deficiencies in the body intake of mineral salts and vitamins can also produce deformities of the skeleton.

Injures to the spine and back

The spine not only provides a "mast" for our body but it also protects and houses the spinal cord and its associated nerves. The collagenous disks that are interposed between the vertebrae of the spine act as shock absorbers and most of the body load is transmitted through them. If for any reason a disk ruptures (prolapses), it may come to press on a nerve, causing localized pain. (A common misconception is that disks can "slip" – in fact they burst and their gelatinous content is forced through the tough outer sheath that would normally contain it.) When the prolapse happens in the region of the neck the pain is referred (◆ page 48) and is felt in the arms. When the rupture occurs lower down the spine the pain seems to come from the back or legs.

Disk prolapse is common in the lower lumbar region, especially where the mobile lumbar spine joins the rigid sacrum and pelvis. It is a common cause of low back pain – responsible for more lost working days in one year than all the industrial strikes added together. Sciatica is a painful ailment in which the sciatic nerve, the largest nerve in the body, becomes constricted in either the lumbar or sacral regions. A prolapsed disk is only one of the possible causes of sciatica.

The intervertebral disk has no blood supply and in the adult the disk's healing power is virtually nil, leading to recurring pain. Treatment varies from rest, physiotherapy and pain-relieving analgesics to various forms of traction or external support. Sometimes an operation is used to remove the ruptured disk and fuse the affected vertebrae.

The founder of modern surgery

Ambroise Paré (1510-1590) was the greatest surgeon of the Renaisssance. Following an apprenticeship to a Paris barber surgeon, Paré gained a junior post at the city's largest hospital. Subsequently he became a military surgeon.

At first Paré treated gunshot wounds, as did other surgeons, by scalding them with hot oil of elders (sambucus). In one of the Italian campaigns, he ran out of oil and was forced to apply "a digestive of eggs, oil of roses and turpentine". He found that treatment with this ointment left his patients less feverish than did cauterization; certainly, their wounds were less swollen and less painful.

Paré was a considerable innovator, designing many surgical instruments, advocating the sterilization of wounds, and designing new ways of extracting teeth, filling cavities and making dentures. He found new uses for the jointed metalwork that was being fashioned for armor – he made artificial limbs, including an iron hand.

Lifting weights

The back bone is stabilized by a series of powerful muscles attached to its sides. When one lifts a heavy load the muscles automatically contract. However, bending forwards induces the muscles to relax so that lifting a weight from the floor can easily damage the spine. This accounts for the general good advice on lifting weights to bend the knees and keep the spine upright – the muscles then contract instead of relaxing so that spinal damage is prevented.

Pressure within the intervertebral disk is least when reclining but increases on standing, leaning forward and lifting heavy objects. Surprisingly, pressures are higher when sitting than standing.

Back pain is not always involved with injury and may be caused by inefficient muscles and abnormalities in the spine causing constriction (stenosis) of the canal. Sometimes the constriction can be relieved by the removal of part of the vertebral body.

Curvature of the spine (scoliosis) can be caused by abnormal development of the vertebrae, by the legs being of unequal length, or by weakness or paralysis. It is now rare in the developed world, but was probably responsible for many of the "hunchbacks" and deformed court jesters immortalized in fiction and plays. The most common type of scoliosis is of unknown (idopathic) origin – two children in every thousand suffer to some extent from it. The suggestion that heavy shoulder bags, bad diets or unsatisfactory beds can cause curvature of the spine is unfounded. Spinal braces may be required to correct the curvature and if the deformation increases, surgery; a metal rod along the vertebral column may be necessary.

A multiplicity of lesser postural ailments are also common, including knock knees, bow legs, rigid toes, hammer toes and flat feet and their converse, "raised" arches. Many of these deformities, if caught early, can be countered or controlled by special orthopedic shoes, or by surgery. The deformities may be congenital in origin, caused by some inherent error in the fetus, or by abnormal bone growth.

Many malformations affect joints. In congenital dislocation of the hip, the ball at the top of the major leg bone fails to become secure in a shallow socket. If the dislocation can be caught before the infant tries to walk, it is possible to hold the ball against the socket and thus encourage the latter to deepen its cavity.

Tuberculosis (♦ page 176) may spread to bones and joints when the bacilli are disseminated from their primary infection in the lungs. In osteomyelitis, the interior of the bone becomes inflamed. Infection may reach a joint to cause infective arthritis by way of the bloodstream, or spread from osteomyelitis or through a wound.

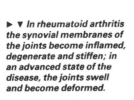

◄ *Thermograph of arthritic (top) and normal (below) knees, recording the heat difference between the healthy and infected joints. White and red areas denote unusual heat; blue and purple indicate cool skin.*

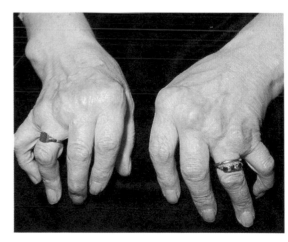

► ▼ *In rheumatoid arthritis the synovial membranes of the joints become inflamed, degenerate and stiffen; in an advanced state of the disease, the joints swell and become deformed.*

The onset of arthritis

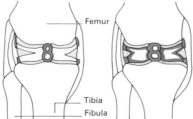
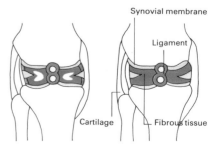
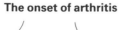

Femur
Synovial membrane
Ligament
Tibia
Fibula
Cartilage
Fibrous tissue

Major Surgery – Total Hip Replacement

The artificial hip

A marvel of modern surgery in the past 20 years is the replacement of arthritic and damaged hip joints with an artificial ball and socket fashioned out of metal and plastic. The procedure has freed millions of people from pain and enabled them to regain their mobility. In 1984 alone, throughout the world surgeons replaced about 425,000 hips, of which 120,000 were in the USA and 105,000 in Europe.

Such is the success of total hip replacement operations that the public views them now as run-of-the-mill. But total hip replacement, like heart surgery and kidney transplants (two other major operational successes of recent decades), depends critically on surgical technique and the general condition of the patient.

Hip surgery is major surgery. The artificial components must be made to high engineering specifications. They must be carefully inserted and aligned in their specific positions, and fixed to act normally in the human body. This they must do at 37°C in saline conditions, and with a host of biological processes and chemical materials produced by the body working against them. Few artificial materials can withstand such hostile conditions for many years, while being subjected to loadings of up to five times body weight.

Bone surgery is craft surgery; it is an art and not a science. The success of the operation depends on the skill of the surgeon to implant the artificial components correctly. It also depends on the patient's physician being able to control any adverse conditions, such as infection, even that of a tooth or of a toe, because implants are highly susceptible to infection.

Patients have to be selected carefully for this operation. Ideally the person must be free from infection, not overweight, and sufficiently fit to cope with the strain of an operation that can last between 1½ and 3 hours, or longer if there are complications. After the operation the patient must not expect to be too demanding on the joint or stress it in physical work. This favors someone of 60 upwards, in health that is otherwise reasonable. In special circumstances the operation may be performed on younger people, but with those under 20 the fact that they are still growing presents many problems.

Many surgeons take the attitude that every hip replacement is a potential problem for the years ahead and must be watched carefully and revised if necessary. Future implants could well be instrumented so that their performance under daily load can be telemetered out and monitored.

■ Antibiotic cover, aseptic techniques, careful handling of the tissues and the use of clean air operating theaters can help to reduce the infection rate to less than 2 percent (main illustration). Barrier gowns help to prevent the inadvertent flow of germs from the theater staff to the patient. Most hospitals insist that staff wear hoods in the operating theater to cover their head and hair. The surgical team consists of at least four people: the anesthetist, the surgeon, an assistant and a nurse. In teaching hospitals, there are often three surgeons – the consultant, the senior registrar and the house surgeon. It is sometimes necessary with complicated operations, to have another nurse to act as runner for special tools. The patient is positioned so as to give the surgeon the best way of approaching the hip joint. This may be from the front, the back or the side.

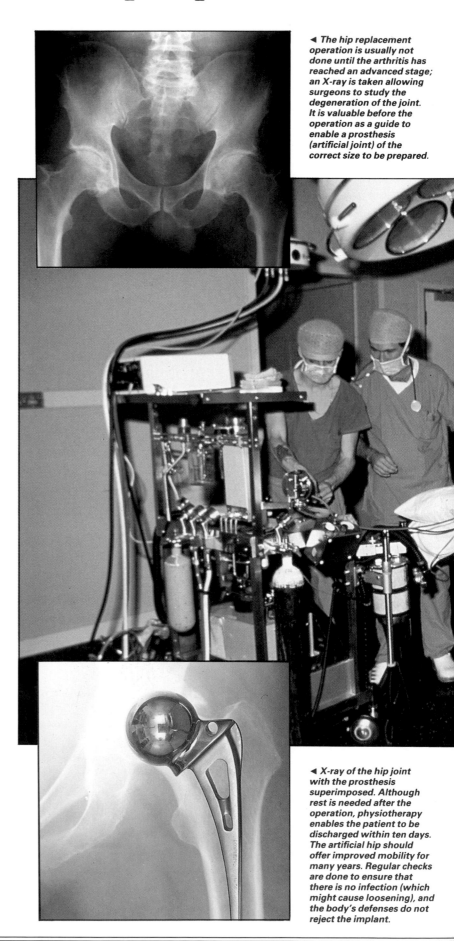

◄ The hip replacement operation is usually not done until the arthritis has reached an advanced stage; an X-ray is taken allowing surgeons to study the degeneration of the joint. It is valuable before the operation as a guide to enable a prosthesis (artificial joint) of the correct size to be prepared.

◄ X-ray of the hip joint with the prosthesis superimposed. Although rest is needed after the operation, physiotherapy enables the patient to be discharged within ten days. The artificial hip should offer improved mobility for many years. Regular checks are done to ensure that there is no infection (which might cause loosening), and the body's defenses do not reject the implant.

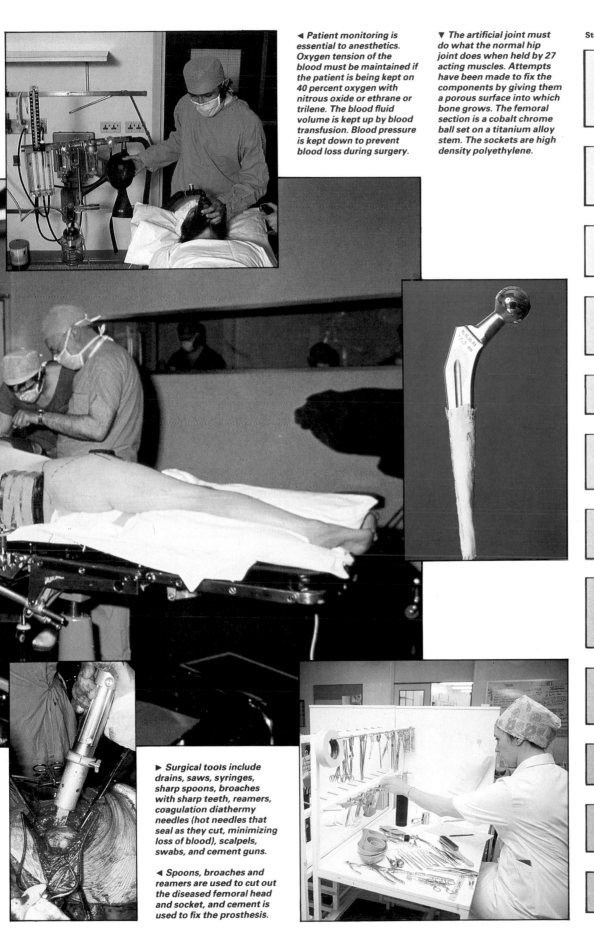

◄ Patient monitoring is essential to anesthetics. Oxygen tension of the blood must be maintained if the patient is being kept on 40 percent oxygen with nitrous oxide or ethrane or trilene. The blood fluid volume is kept up by blood transfusion. Blood pressure is kept down to prevent blood loss during surgery.

▼ The artificial joint must do what the normal hip joint does when held by 27 acting muscles. Attempts have been made to fix the components by giving them a porous surface into which bone grows. The femoral section is a cobalt chrome ball set on a titanium alloy stem. The sockets are high density polyethylene.

► Surgical tools include drains, saws, syringes, sharp spoons, broaches with sharp teeth, reamers, coagulation diathermy needles (hot needles that seal as they cut, minimizing loss of blood), scalpels, swabs, and cement guns.

◄ Spoons, broaches and reamers are used to cut out the diseased femoral head and socket, and cement is used to fix the prosthesis.

Stages in a typical operation

1 The patient is assessed for chances of success and recovery from the strain of the operation. X-ray taken; this serves as a guide for the surgeons.

2 Antibiotics given to minimize infection. Food prohibited for at least eight hours before surgery.

3 Washed, and dressed in a gown. Drug to relax given an hour before operating.

4 Taken to the anesthetic room; given anesthetic sufficient to subdue neurotransmitters for the estimated operation length.

5 Placed on the operating table in a suitable position.

6 Skin around the incision area swabbed, covered with a waterproof film, and surrounded with towels.

7 Incision made; muscles and other tissues clamped with minimal stretching.

8 Anesthetist continuously monitors blood pressure, heartbeat and breathing. Anesthetic, glucose or anti-clotting drips may be given.

9 Surgeon cuts away the diseased part. Prosthesis fitted. Hollow needle inserted to drain wound.

10 Wound closed, usually with dissolving sutures.

11 Returned to hospital ward and woken. Physio-therapy given.

12 Post-operative care may involve regular checkups.

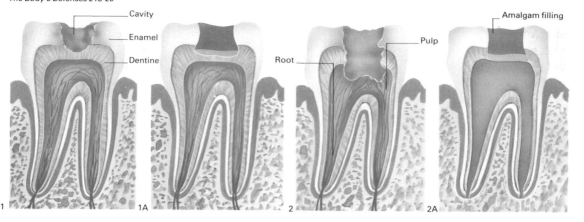

◄ *Tooth decay begins when the enamel is attacked by acid produced by plaque bacteria (1), and the decay may spread through into the softer dentine or the root, from where the infection may pass down the root canal (2) and form a painful abscess. To fill the cavity thus formed (1A, 2A), the dentist cuts away affected areas, lines the cavity and plugs the hole with a silver amalgam or a plastic filling.*

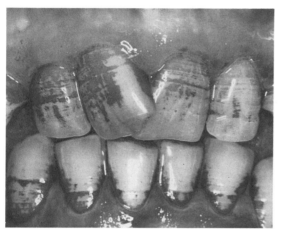

▲ *Plaque, a sticky covering of bacteria and food remains, builds up on teeth and is primarily responsible for the development of dental caries, as the acid produced by the bacteria eats into the tooth enamel. It is not usually possible to prevent plaque forming, but it can be removed by thorough brushing. Though usually hard to see, plaque can be revealed by taking a disclosing agent.*

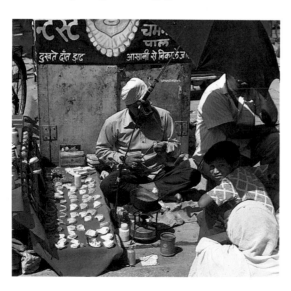

▲ *A dentist selling dentures on the streets of Jaipur, India; dentures may be required for cosmetic purposes, or because the teeth have fallen out through widespread caries or the spread of gum infections which loosen the roots. One of the most common forms of periodontal disease is caused by toxic organic chemicals produced by plaque bacteria, in addition to the acids which attack the teeth themselves.*

Dentistry

Much knowledge of how metals, plastics and cements can be used in the body comes from dentistry. Few "living" environments are more hostile to such materials than the mouth.

For many centuries various metals and cements have been used to make good the havoc caused by tooth decay (caries). Decay usually occurs in the presence of bacteria, such as *Streptococcus mutans*, which, in the "dental plaque" that builds up on the surface of the teeth, turn sugar into acids. These acids attack the protective enamel of the teeth, dissolving away some of the minerals, and eventually the infection destroys the dentine and nerves of the teeth. Various attempts have been made to develop vaccines against such disease, and to develop chemicals that block the activity of the bacterial enzymes that help acids to form. Dental researchers are also looking for chemicals to stop bacteria sticking to the teeth in the first place.

Caries sometimes occurs in the absence of detectable numbers of bacteria and thus may have other origins. The use of fluoride ions in fluoride toothpastes (and, controversially, in the addition of fluoride to water supplies) has certainly provided a way of strengthening tooth enamel. This and other conservation approaches, including the control of diets, have led to a 40-50 percent drop in tooth cavities in the developed world over the past 25 years.

The traditional approach to dealing with tooth decay is to remove the carious part, shape the cavity, sterilize it, line it with cement and to pack it with metal amalgam. Amalgams are made from a silver, tin, copper and zinc alloy mixed on a 50:50 basis, with mercury. Inlays, based on a carefully taken cast of the cavity, may be fashioned in gold or porcelain to fit the cavity. Teeth that are hopelessly decayed or irreparably loose are normally extracted.

Since the 1970s, dentists have used an increasing range of glass and plastic materials, including various acrylates such as methyl methacrylates and cyanoacrylates, to repair teeth. These materials often prove cosmetically more acceptable than metal amalgams, but have the disadvantage that they tend not to show up on subsequent X-rays. However, the new plastics have led to a revolution in tooth coatings and claddings. Thin plastic coatings can be used to seal off the enamel. Partial tooth replacements, or crowns, which hitherto had to be fashioned in gold or porcelain and pinned in place, can now be built up in plastics and cemented onto existing teeth.

Dentures and bridges are increasingly giving way to implanted artificial teeth and tooth roots. These can be fashioned from a wide range of materials including titanium, acrylic resins, ceramic-fired alumina, carbon fibers and even lignum vitae.

Skin, the body's largest organ...Functions of the skin...Structure of the skin...Skin coloration...Hair structure and growth...Sweat and oil glands...Fingertips and nails...PERSPECTIVE...The skin as an organ of communication...Skin parasites...Albinism... Fingerprints

The human skin is more than a bag to protect our outsides and prevent our organs from falling out. With its hair and nails, it forms what is known as the integumentary system, and is a complex structure performing functions, such as temperature control and excretion, which are essential for survival.

The skin is the largest organ of the body (20,000cm²) and the only one exposed to the outside world. It keeps out foreign substances (from bacteria and sharp objects to water), retains fluids, protects us from harmful rays, cools us when hot and keeps heat in when cold, and to a large degree determines our appearance. It makes Vitamin D, receives environmental stimuli and excretes water, salt and organic compounds. It envelops the whole body – even the eye is covered by a transparent layer of skin, known as the conjunctiva, which also lines the inside of the eyelids.

The structure of the skin

Skin is 0·4-3mm deep. It is usually thinner on under-surfaces. The hands and feet are exceptions to this, and they have the only skin that forms calluses in response to wear; feet develop thin calluses even without wear. On elbows and knees the skin is a little thicker than usual but it tends to graze easily. The only normal openings of the skin are at the mouth and anus, where it is continuous with the gut (though this originates in the endoderm, the layer of embryonic tissue from which epithelial cells of many internal organs derive, whereas the skin is ectoderm).

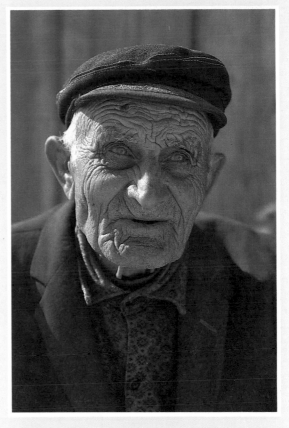

▲ Repeated exposure to sun and weather speeds the onset of permanent wrinkles, sagging, loss of elasticity, death of oil glands and increase of pigment cells.

Skin as an organ of communication
Whether or not the sebaceous glands in our skin are the source of pheromones (◀ page 47), there are many other ways in which we do communicate via our skin. A tan conveys a sense of health, vitality and even prestige. Conversely, acne can be a powerful barrier to social intercourse; children instinctively refuse to hold hands with other children having a facial rash, and relatively few people with skin diseases visit public beaches. Most societies use makeup and hairstyling to express personality, self-esteem and social rank.

Touching, stroking and grooming play a significant part in human relationships. Psychologists have discerned that apparently casual physical contact between strangers can be a powerful method of non-verbal communication. Kissing and other touching is one the most potent and sensitive means of strengthening the bond between people.

Creatures living on the skin
About half of us have a colony of mites inhabiting our eyelashes, living and breeding in the hair follicles and oil glands. These tiny relatives of the spider, 0·3mm long, are known as Demodex folliculorum. They are translucent, and have four pairs of stubby legs attached to the chest, with a grublike abdomen behind. Usually harmless, they sometimes cause scaling at the base of the lashes.

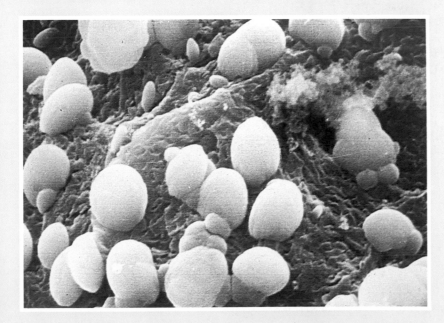

◀ A colony of yeast on the skin.

Millions of skin cells are shed every day and form a major component of household dust

Skin layers

The outer part of the skin, the epidermis, has four or five layers. At its base is a sheet of cube-shaped cells (the stratum basale). When these divide, the cells that split off are pushed upward, dying as they go. Above the stratum basale the cells become the stratum spinosum, with eight to ten sheets of many-sided cells that are still able to divide. Next are the three or four cell sheets of the stratum granulosum, which cannot divide. This layer contains a substance called kerato-hyalin, which is converted to a water-proofing material, hyalin, as it reaches the surface.

Next, especially in the thick skin of soles and palms, is the stratum lucidum, so-called because it is translucent. This layer is absent where the skin is covered by hair. Topmost is the stratum corneum, 25-30 sheets of flat dead cells that are shed and replaced constantly – the white dust that appears in bedrooms is mainly made up of human skin scales.

Below the epidermis is the dermis, which is a connective tissue containing a strong, fibrous protein called collagen (♦ page 97) and elastic fibers. These give the skin stretchability, strength and retractability. The dermis is thickest on palms and soles, and thinnest on the eyeballs and genital organs. In it are blood vessels, nerve endings, hair follicles, oil glands and sweat glands. Some nerve endings – notably Meissner's corpuscles, which are touch-sensitive (♦ page 41) – are in the upper corrugated layer of the dermis. Others – the Pacinian corpuscles, which are more sensitive to pressure – are in the thick lower reticular layer, alongside the elastic and collagen fibers.

The color of the skin

Skin is colored by three components: melanin, which is brown, in the epidermis (it is especially prevalent in Negro skin); carotene, which is carrot-colored and acts as a sun-filter, in the dermis (uncommon except in Orientals); and blood, in the dermal capillaries. Melanin, which absorbs ultra-violet rays, is made by specialized epidermal cells called melanocytes from an amino-acid called tyrosine. It is then taken up into other epidermal cells.

Manufacture and distribution of melanin is controlled within the brain by the anterior pituitary gland (♦ page 86), which produces the melanocyte-stimulating hormone. The number of melanocytes present in the body is the same in all races; it is their output of pigment which differs. Freckles are the result of the uneven distribution of melanin in skin cells. In general, children are fairer than adults, and women fairer than men.

Hair – the skin covering

Pigs and humans are the only common land mammals not to be enveloped in fur. From the fifth month of gestation the fetus is covered with delicate hair called lanugo. This is usually shed by the time we are born, and is replaced by fine down, called vellus, which is found everywhere except on the palms, soles, lips, tip of the penis and the labia. It is also absent wherever ordinary coarse hair grows.

There are two parts to a hair, the shaft and the root. Hairs grow from epidermal cells but, because the root is deep, it becomes embedded in the dermis where it lies at an angle. Hair is dead tissue, so its condition does not indicate our state of health, except to the extent that the presence of oil from the oil glands makes it glossier, and certain serious illnesses make us shed hair faster than usual.

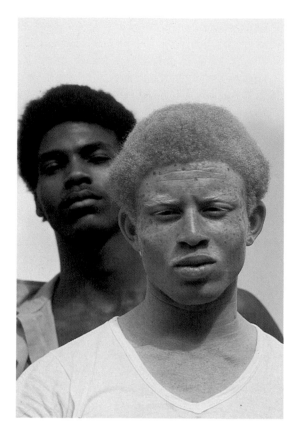

▲ *The albino stands out in many societies, and can be seen as an outcast, though albino animals are sometimes held as sacred.*

Life without skin pigment

Albinos are people who have no melanin because they lack the enzyme that makes it from tyrosine. Albinism is an inherited characteristic for which no treatment is possible. The eyesight is weak owing to the lack of pigment in the eye, which not only reduces vision but also prevents the nerve pathways from the eye to the brain from developing properly. Albinos have milk-white and pink skin, and snow-white hair. Their skin is inclined to scaliness, which protects it a little from the Sun. They sunburn easily and are dazzled by bright light.

In the British Medical Journal of January 1979, a 33-year-old man described what it is like to be albino. From an early age he was told that he could not do things such as playing football, for which eyesight is important. But, because he could kick a ball around with his friends until their ability, developed in lessons at school, outstripped his, he feels that he could have played adequately, given tuition. He is not allowed to drive because his eyesight fails the standard test, but he rides a bicycle in London without difficulty. He had no problems with classes at school or university, and can read normal print, though small print requires a magnifying glass. Sharing a music stand and reading train timetables posted on indicator boards are his only reading problems. He wears photochromatic glasses to correct his vision and protect him from sunlight.

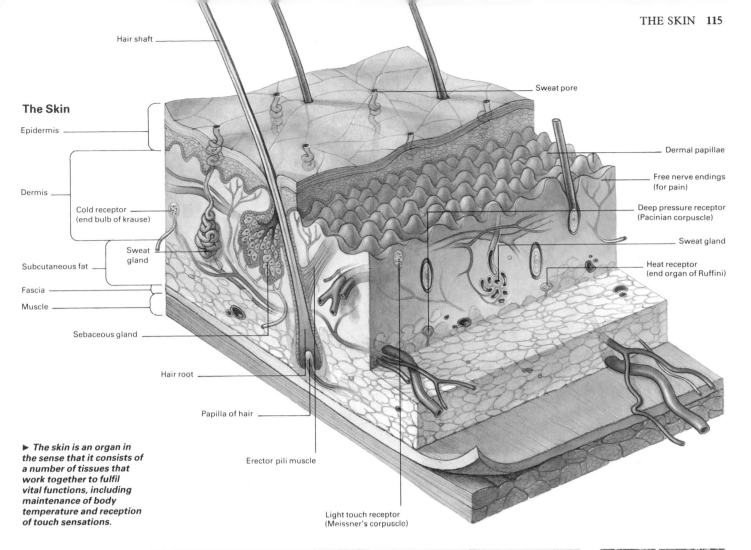

The Skin

Hair shaft

Epidermis

Dermis

Cold receptor
(end bulb of krause)

Sweat
gland

Subcutaneous fat

Fascia

Muscle

Sebaceous gland

Hair root

Papilla of hair

Erector pili muscle

Light touch receptor
(Meissner's corpuscle)

Sweat pore

Dermal papillae

Free nerve endings
(for pain)

Deep pressure receptor
(Pacinian corpuscle)

Sweat gland

Heat receptor
(end organ of Ruffini)

▶ The skin is an organ in the sense that it consists of a number of tissues that work together to fulfil vital functions, including maintenance of body temperature and reception of touch sensations.

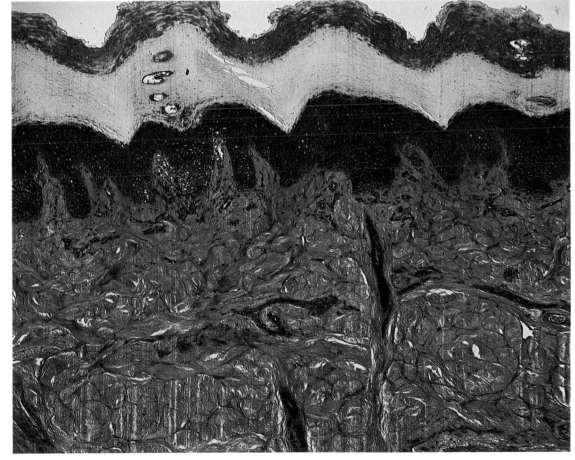

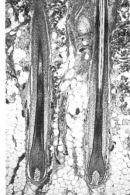

▲ Section through the scalp, showing two hair follicles. An average person is thought to have some five million hairs, of which about 100,000 are on the head.

◀ Section through the skin of a fingertip. The top layer makes up the skin ridges, and the white layer beneath is the stratum corneum, consisting of keratin. Beneath the three layers of the epidermis is the much thicker dermis, made up of connective tissue, blood vessels and sense organs.

The finger

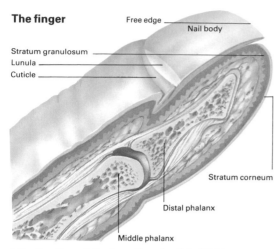

▲ *Section through the fingertip and nail. In 1984 it was reported that women have a higher degree of touch sensitivity in their fingertips than men; this is because their finger ridges are less prominent. Many women also find their fingertips and toes become cold more easily than men, since their blood vessels contract more.*

Fingertips and nails

Nails are modified epidermal structures similar to hairs. They consist of a root, a nail body and a free edge. Most of the nail is pink because the blood vessels in the nail bed or epithelium underneath show through. The white area at the base is called the lunula. Underneath is a layer of cells from which the nail grows, at the rate of about 1mm a week. The cuticle is the narrow band of skin around the edges of the nail.

Most of the skin is folded with diamond-shaped grooves. But over the palms, fingers, soles and toes, skin produces a series of narrow parallel ridges and grooves which form patterns made up of straight lines, arcs, whorls and loops. These increase the surface area, and hence the grip, of the hands and feet. Their arrangement is infinitely variable, and the pattern is unique to each person – even those of identical twins differ slightly. Sweat glands open onto the ridges so that fingerprints and footprints are left behind when a smooth object is touched. The creases of the palm do not foretell our life events, but they are abnormal in people suffering from Down's syndrome (◊ page 197) or in those who have been infected by rubella (German measles; ◊ page 243) before birth. This abnormality can be detected in the fetus well before birth.

The use of fingerprints to identify people for forensic purposes was pioneered in the 19th century by several scientists, notably Francis Galton (1822-1911), though the uniqueness of individual fingerprints was demonstrated by the Czech anatomist J.E. Purkinje (1787-1869) in 1823. The Chinese, however, had been using fingerprints for forensic purposes since at least AD 700. A different system of classification is used in some Spanish-speaking regions. Palm- and footprints are often taken to identify infants.

▶ *A human fingerprint. There are several systems of classification but the most common classes prints into loops (shown here), arches, whorls and composite.*

There are three layers to a hair shaft: a dense inner layer called the medulla (reduced or missing in fine hair); a cortex, which contains pigment granules in dark hair and air in white hair; and a scaly cuticle. The base of each follicle is an onion-shaped bulb, at the bottom of which is the papilla. This is the only living part of the hair and contains a germinal layer (the matrix) and blood vessels. On one side of the root is a sebaceous gland and a muscle, contraction of which causes gooseflesh. Around the follicle are nerve endings that respond when the hair is touched.

Hair that is round in cross-section grows straight, hair that is oval grows curly, and hair that is ribbon-shaped grows frizzy or woolly. Straight hair is the strongest type and least likely to break. Hair goes through cycles of growth, rest and replacement. That which is shed often remains in the follicle until pulled out or disturbed. Shaving and cutting does not make hair grow faster, thicker or coarser. The length of hair depends on time, growing at about 12mm a month. Scalp hair grows for two to six years, but eyelid hair for only about ten weeks before being shed. We normally lose 70-100 of our scalp hairs every day.

Skin glands

Skin contains glands that produce sweat and oil. Sebaceous (oil) glands, which are connected with hair follicles, are largest in the breasts, face, neck and upper chest. The oil they secrete keeps the hair and skin supple.

Sweating is the principal method of cooling the body, and sweat glands are of two kinds. Eccrine glands, though found over most of the body, are densest on the hands and feet. They also produce most of the sweat. Apocrine glands function from puberty in the armpits, pubic region and pigmented area of the breast, and secrete the sweat that gives individuality to our smell. Sweat consists of water, salt and waste products such as urea, uric acid, amino-acids, ammonia and lactic acid.

Ear wax is a blend of secretions from sweat glands and modified oil glands. This wax, together with hairs in the external ears, helps to prevent unwanted substances, especially water, from entering.

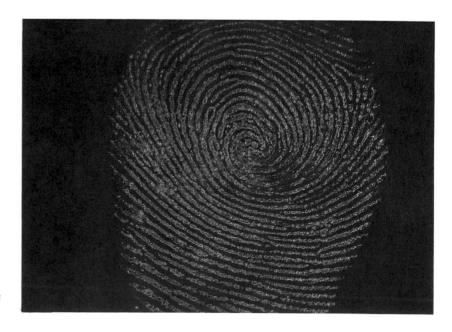

Burns...Plastic surgery...Skin grafting...Cosmetic surgery...PERSPECTIVE...The medicinal leech... Treatments for baldness...Dermabrasion...Moles and warts...Birthmarks and tattoos...Corns and calluses

Skin disorders and abnormalities are complicated by the fact that they are usually disfiguring. The bruises, burns and other blemishes that occur as part of the skin's normal function as the body's interface with the outside world also have cosmetic implications relating to the skin's role as an organ of communication and self-expression.

Bruises and burns

Bruises – dead blood cells resulting from damaged blood vessels – are absorbed by the body. They can migrate downwards under gavity, especially in old people whose skin is lax. Scarring, the skin's method of repairing severe damage, is more permanent.

Burns may be caused by chemicals, electricity, radiation, ice, flames or contact with hot liquids (scalds) or solids. The severity of burns depends on their thickness. Superficial or first-degree burns of the epidermis only are painful for hours or days but heal without scarring. Deep dermal (second-degree) burns destroy all but the deepest dermal structures such as sweat glands. These burns lead to scarring, with poor texture skin; their blood supply is often precarious and they can progress to deep burns if they become infected or inflamed. Full thickness (third-degree) burns destroy the entire dermis including the pain receptors. Chances of survival are poor if more than 50 percent of the skin is burnt or the patient is very young or old.

The transfer of partial or full-thickness skin grafts known as plastic surgery – is used to replace skin that is destroyed or badly scarred. Exposed surfaces are kept dry, and antiseptics are applied to skin flexures and face; dressings are applied in operating-theater conditions. Amniotic membrane (♦ page 184) may be used as a dressing. It fights infection, cuts fluid and protein losses and is readily available.

◄ *A leech feeding on a human forearm.*

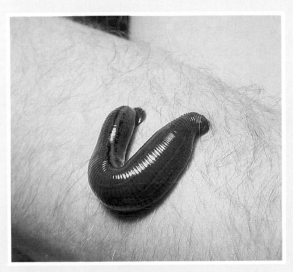

▶ *Leeches in medicinal use in the Middle Ages. At that time leeches were used indiscriminately for a wide variety of ailments, being intended to purge the system by reducing the amount of blood and so letting out noxious substances. Modern uses relate more specifically to reducing bruising or other cases where there is a build-up of blood beneath the surface of the skin.*

The medicinal leech

Leeches were originally collected from rivers by women who stood in the water and waited for the leeches to attach themselves. They were widely used in medicine until the late 19th century as a cure-all – it was thought they drew off "evil vapors". The medicinal leech was and still is a method of reducing bruises, inflammation and swelling.

Leeches feed by attaching themselves to the skin, making a three-sided cut. They are believed to inject an anesthetic – little pain is felt as the leech feeds – and an anticoagulant to prevent the collapse of the blood capillaries. As they suck blood, they add more anticoagulant while blood passes through their mouth. They feed rapidly, multiplying their weight eight-fold; they then dehydrate the blood and store it for long periods without putrefaction – red cells, antibodies and even bacteria can still be found six months after feeding.

Although largely superseded by new drugs, leeches are still applied today. Uses include reducing bruises around eyes that occlude vision, and encouraging blood flow in skin grafts after plastic surgery. Plastic surgeons in Nottingham, England, have now used them successfully in this way. A leech applied at once will feed for twenty minutes. Leeches live for six to twelve months without feeding and are at their best when hungry. If ravenous they start to digest themselves.

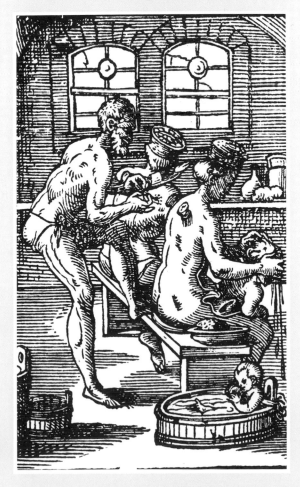

The amniotic sac in which a fetus develops is an ideal skin dressing

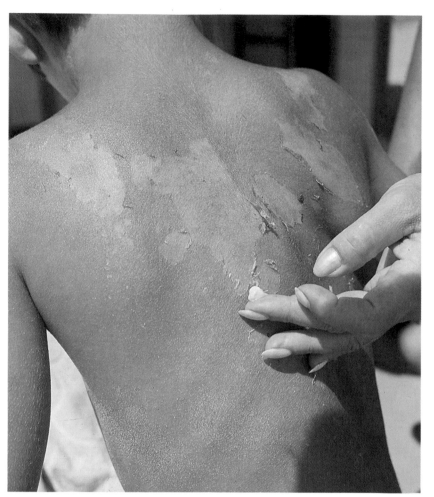

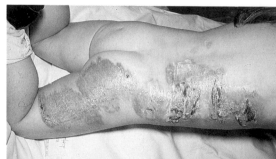

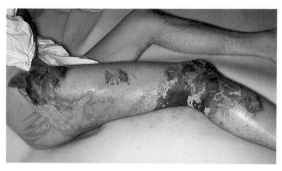

▲ *(Top) Second-degree of deep dermal burns, which often produce blistering but heal within seven to ten days; (above) third-degree of full thickness burns on a child's leg.*

◄ *Sunburn is the most common form of skin burning, caused by the sun's rays. The skin reacts by dividing faster and becoming thicker. Stronger exposure damages some of the epithelial cells and temporarily halts cell division. Thus cell division often stops, then restarts faster. When the growth has stopped, the outer, dead skin cells separate from the underlying skin and peel off painlessly.*

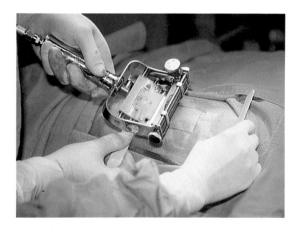

▲ *Skin for grafting is removed using a special knife allowing thin layers to be taken.*

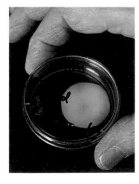

◄ *Human skin tissue grown in a culture. With this technique it has proved possible to grow skin to cover large areas and burns that are too extensive to be treated by grafting skin from other parts of the body may now be treated effectively in this way.*

Skin is grafted by taking a partial-thickness slice, usually from the thigh or buttock. Full-thickness skin is sometimes required, usually if the underlying tissues are lost to some depth; in these cases only small areas of skin can be taken. Skin from the side of the hand is used to cover deep wounds to fingertips. If large areas of skin are lost, dehydrated pig skin is used as a temporary graft, for periods of up to ten days. It must then be replaced by another temporary layer of pig skin in large sheets, or a graft from the patient's own body. Otherwise it becomes incorporated by the body, creating an antibody response and more scarring. In 1984 American scientists reported the possibility of growing a person's own skin in tissue culture. It takes about three weeks to grow a square meter from an original two square centimeters. Meanwhile the patient's skin is covered temporarily by human amnion or dehydrated pig skin. In punch grafting, circles of skin are taken from a healthy area, dotted around the wound, and allowed to spread. Flaps of full thickness are often moved in such a way that they retain some of their original position and are pivoted onto the exposed area. These "take" better because they retain some of their original blood supply. Cross-transfer grafts of skin (finger-to-finger or leg-to-leg) have the advantage of being similar to the original skin.

Skin grafts are taken with a Humby knife, which has a roller with replaceable blades and can be adjusted for depth of cut, or with a Silver knife, which uses ordinary razor blades and is adequate for small split-skin grafts. The donor area is flattened with two boards and a thin paring taken, spread on gauze, surface up; there is no need

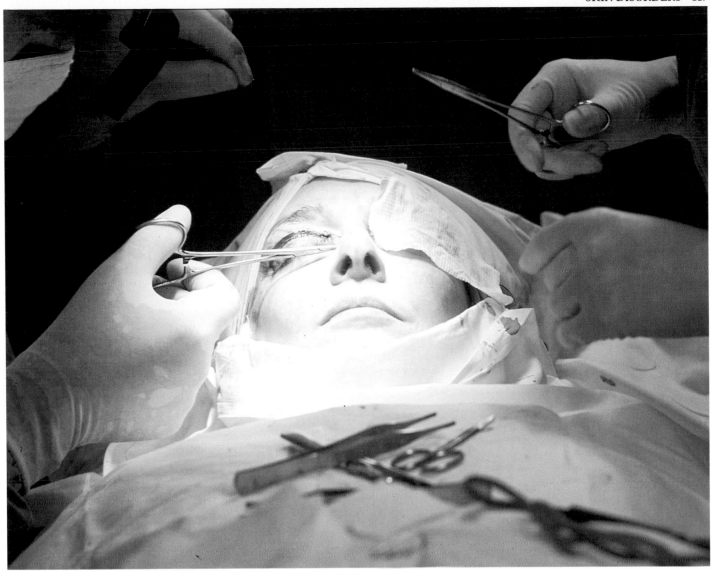

to cut the graft exactly to size. The donor and graft areas are then bandaged. Skin grafts are always surrounded by a scar and generally have a different color, texture and contour from the skin they replace. Skin wounds are closed by means of nylon stitches that are subsequently removed, or subcuticular stitches using absorbable thread made of polyglycolic acid. Dirty abrasions must be cleaned as a permanent tattoo may result. They therefore may need scrubbing under general anesthetic.

Cosmetic surgery

Modern surgery has introduced a range of options for conditions of disfigurement. Noses can be straightened, made smaller or – in cases where the bridge of the nose is flat – enlarged. For enlargement, a graft of cartilage, bone or plastic is used. Chin augmentation uses rubber or bone from the nose or thigh, and is done through an incision under the chin or within the mouth. Protruding ears can be made flatter by removing some cartilage behind the ear. For face-lifts, incisions are made in front of and behind the ears, extending to the neck hairline, and the skin is pulled up and back. Eyelids can be done with the face-lift or separately. Incisions are made along crease lines of the upper lid and directly below the lower lid.

Breast reduction requires incisions below the breasts or at the side. If a lot of tissue is removed the nipples are repositioned. Breast augmentation is done by implanting soft silicone gel between the breast tissue and the muscle, so that the breast drapes over the implant.

▲ *Cosmetic surgery offers the hope of restoring the youthfulness of aging skin by removing blemishes, wrinkles and bags under the eyes. This is done through stretching the skin and removing fat or excess liquid.*

Baldness treatments

Ordinary male baldness, an inherited condition, is the death of scalp hair follicles after exposure to male hormone. Other than by castration before puberty, baldness cannot be slowed, halted or reversed. There are three surgical treatments. Punch grafts or groups of one to 15 hair follicles are taken from elsewhere on the scalp and shared out over the bald area. Whole flaps of skin can be shifted round the scalp, leaving scars but hiding the bald areas. Finally, nylon fibers – artificial hair – can be implanted. However, this often leads to inflammation, infection and scarring.

Dermabrasion and peeling

"Sand paper" dermabrasion surgery improves the appearance of skin that has been pitted with acne. The improvement depends on the depth of pitting; about 60-80 percent of acne scars are improved. Chemical peeling is used to remove fine lines from skin. A solution of phenol and soap is applied to the face with a cotton swab. This produces a superficial burn and fibrosis. The skin then peels, removing fine lines as it goes. Pigmentation is also lost and so this is best used in pale-skinned people.

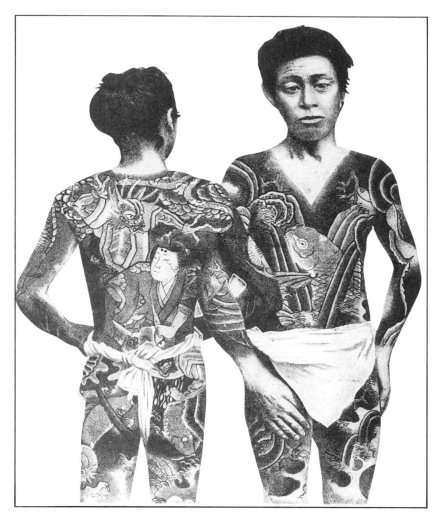

Natural blemishes

There are many natural growths on the skin, many of which can now be dealt with by modern medical techniques. Moles are harmless areas of raised skin, usually pigmented. They can be removed by shaving them flat or by cutting them out with a crescent of skin. Like the horny growths of hard skin known as warts or verrucas, they can also be removed by cryosurgery. In this technique, nitrous oxide at −70°C is applied with a cryoprobe for a few seconds – no anesthetic is needed. This freezes the cells, rapidly killing them. After thawing there is a watery discharge until a crust forms. Healing is complete within 14 days and scarring is minimal – leaving just a pale patch. More than one application may be necessary if the tissue to be removed is particularly thick.

Warts, which are caused by a virus, sometimes also disappear spontaneously. Those that persist can be removed by surgical incision, bloodless removal by freezing with liquid nitrogen or repeated applications of ointments.

Portwine marks are removed by argon laser, which penetrates the upper layer of skin without damaging it, and coagulates and kills the blood vessels causing the mark. These are replaced by transparent tissue and there is no scar.

Tattoos are permanent stains with ink injected under the skin but may be removed by carbon-dioxide or argon laser. Because of the thickness and depth of the tattoo there is always scarring but it is unpigmented.

Corns and calluses

These form in areas where the keratin layer of the skin is thickened. Calluses, uniform in thickness, are always present on the soles, even after prolonged bedrest. These become thicker after regular walking or running. Calluses also form on hands after rough work, and shrink or peel off when such work is stopped.

Corns are cones of keratinous skin. They form after repeated pressure on the sides or tops of toes; they can also form on tops or sides of fingers after work such as lathe-turning. They are tender when touched and may ache spontaneously.

Corns and calluses on hands can be prevented only by ceasing the activity that causes them. Corns on feet can be prevented by wearing comfortable shoes. All can be removed with a nail file or by dissolving with corn plasters.

▲ The ancient art form of tattooing was particularly highly developed in Japan and the Pacific.

◄ Argon lasers can be used to remove portwine stains, which result from blood capillaries bursting beneath the skin. These lasers can destroy and seal the blood vessels. They can also be used to remove tattoos, but leave a pale "negative" image on the skin.

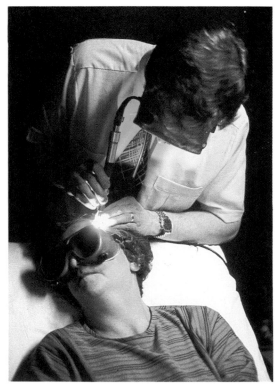

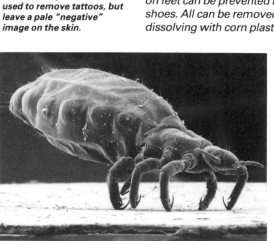

◄ A louse, the main parasite of the human hair. Head lice, body lice and pubic lice are distinct species. They are transmitted by close contact. Nits, the eggs of the head louse, stick firmly to the hair and must be removed by a special emulsion; they cannot be removed by regular washing with shampoo.

The digestive tract...Enzymes of digestion...Protein, fat and carbohydrates...Vitamins...Metabolism... The body's nutritional requirements... Identifying malnutrition...Vitamin deficiencies... PERSPECTIVE...Windows into the stomach...Starving to death...Studying metabolism...The discovery of vitamins...Nutrition around the world

Digestion times

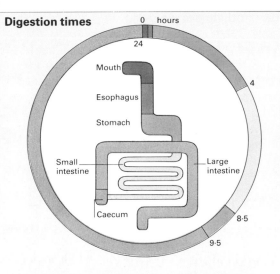

▲ *Food takes on average 24 hours to pass through the digestive system. It stays in the stomach for between 1 and 8 hours; then spends another 4 hours in the small intestine and 10 to 15 hours in the large intestine.*

One part of the body's "inside" is really "outside" – the alimentary canal which leads from mouth to anus (◀ page 113). The function of this long tube, with its various specialized regions, is to digest incoming food. Digestion is the process of breaking food down into simpler substances that can be assimilated as sources of energy and building materials for the body's maintenance and growth.

The metabolic process of digestion depends on enzymes – the body's chemical catalysts. Before this process begins, the teeth and tongue crush and grind the incoming food into small particles. To assist this mastication, saliva flows into the mouth from the parotid, submandibular and sublingual glands. Saliva is a lubricant and moistens food so that the tongue, working against the palate, can roll it into a soft bolus. Saliva also contains amylase, an enzyme that initiates digestion by converting some starch into maltose.

When food has been well homogenized, the tongue pushes it backwards to be swallowed into the pharynx. An involuntary transport system then takes over and carries it through the alimentary canal (◀ page 160). As the bolus approaches, the stomach lining and glands in its surface begin to produce digestive juices. Those from the lining contain enzymes, especially pepsin – which attacks proteins and converts them to polypeptides. The glands release hydrochloric acid to promote the action of the pepsin. (Mucus helps protect the stomach itself from the acid.) The stomach wall also produces intrinsic factor, which combines with Vitamin B12 to assist its absorption later in the small intestine. Some 1200-1500ml of gastric juices are secreted daily.

Beaumont's "window"
On 6 June 1822 a young French-Canadian soldier, Alexis St Martin, was shot by a musket which went off accidentally, piercing his stomach. US Army surgeon William Beaumont (1785-1853), quickly on the scene, pushed the protruding organ back into the wound. St Martin recovered well – except that his gaping orifice refused to heal, and all food and drink poured out unless the hole was plugged with a bandage. Because his patient refused an operation, Dr Beaumont was able to exploit this unique opportunity to study digestion as it happened. As well as observing how a fasting stomach contracted, he became the first researcher to identify hydrochloric acid in gastric juice. His "Experiments and Observations on Gastric Juice and the Physiology of Digestion" was a classic.

Pavlov's dogs
The Russian physiologist Ivan Pavlov (1849-1936) made many important contributions to the study of digestion – notably in discerning the nerves that control secretion by the pancreas. Pavlov made his most important discoveries by creating an opportunity for research like that which William Beaumont encountered by accident. He fashioned part of a dog's stomach into a tubular pouch, open to the outside and separated only by mucous membrane from the stomach itself. Because both reacted to stimuli in the same way, Pavlov could monitor the quantity and composition of gastric juices in various conditions.

His outstanding discovery was that of the conditioned reflex. Working with his dogs (though his results are applicable to humans too), Pavlov found that food placed in an animal's mouth triggered off the flow of gastric juices. This he termed an unconditioned response. When he rang a bell each time before feeding his dogs, however, he found that they began to respond in the same way even in the absence of food. This, the conditioned reflex, only develops if the cerebral cortex is intact and working normally.

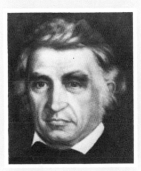
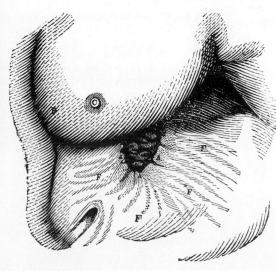

▲ ▶ *William Beaumont and his drawing of the "window" into Alexis St Martin's stomach, through which he was able to put weighed pieces of food directly into the stomach, and remove them after a timed period to monitor the rate of digestion. He showed that bile promoted the digestion of fats.*

Most of the digestive process takes place along the huge surface area of the small intestine

How food is broken down

Only 10-15 percent of protein, 30-50 percent of starch and little if any fat is digested in the stomach. That is why people can live even after their stomachs have been surgically removed. The principal stages of digestion begin as the semi-liquid "chyme" moves forward into the small intestine. Here the intestine secretes its own juice containing enzymes. These include trypsin to complete the breakdown of proteins into polypeptides, aminopeptidases which convert these into amino-acids, and several more which release glucose and other sugars from complex carbohydrates.

The second source of enzymes is the pancreas (another part of which makes insulin to regulate body sugar ◀ page 85). Pancreatic juice is secreted via a duct in the duodenum (the section of the small intestine nearest to the stomach). The juice contains the enzymes trypsin, the related chymotrypsin, and amylase to continue the attack on starch begun by the saliva. Its unique constituent is lipase, to digest fat. This splits each triglyceride into either a monoglyceride plus two fatty acids, or completely into fatty acids and glycerol.

The liver plays a role in digestion too, by producing bile. Stored in the gall bladder, this contains bile salts which emulsify the products of lipase action.

All the substances liberated by this powerful battery of enzymes are now ferried away for use by the body. Amino-acids from proteins, and sugars from carbohydrates, cross the intestinal wall into the blood. Vitamins (which, apart from B12, have not required chemical modification) also diffuse into the bloodstream. Glycerol, fatty acids and monoglycerides, in the emulsion released by the breakdown of fat, take a different route. They are united again in cells lining the intestine and become molecules of human fat. Aggregated into microspheres, they then pass into the lymphatic system (▶ page 154). Water and salts, including iron and calcium, are absorbed – water and sodium chloride continuing to be extracted as the digested material travels its remaining distance through the colon to the anus.

The small intestine – core of the digestive system

Until recently, biologists believed that most digestion of foodstuffs occurred in the space in the middle of the intestine. The wall was supposed to act as a simple filter, through which products diffused passively. It is now known that the surface cells themselves have digestive enzymes, plus active transport mechanisms for handling amino-acids and sugars, embedded in their membranes. Although the details are unclear, separate systems seem to move these substances first into the cells and then into the bloodstream.

The small intestine provides a huge area across which nutrients can be absorbed. Packed into the abdominal cavity, it consists of some six meters of tubing containing sets of projections that increase its internal surface still further. The most important of these projections are those known as the microvilli. These are finger-like fronds, 0·5-1mm high and several million in number, containing blood and lymphatic vessels into which the nutrients can be absorbed from the food. Their membranes contain arrays of enzymes and transport systems, and are the sites at which materials pass into the body. They contain, for example, enzymes that break down the disaccharides sucrose and maltose into their constituent sugars. There also seem to be four independent systems to mobilize four different classes of amino-acids.

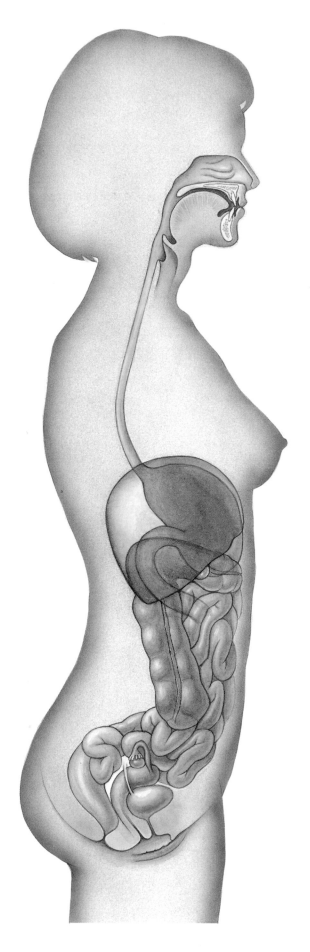

The digestive system

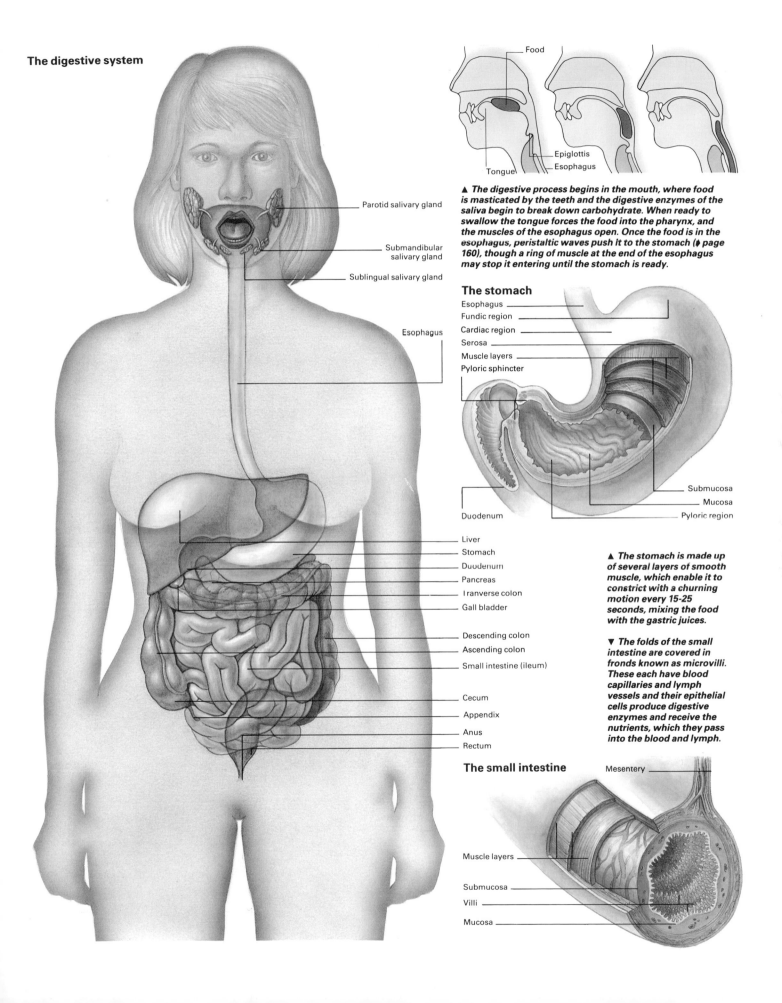

Food

Tongue

Epiglottis

Esophagus

▲ *The digestive process begins in the mouth, where food is masticated by the teeth and the digestive enzymes of the saliva begin to break down carbohydrate. When ready to swallow the tongue forces the food into the pharynx, and the muscles of the esophagus open. Once the food is in the esophagus, peristaltic waves push it to the stomach (*page 160*), though a ring of muscle at the end of the esophagus may stop it entering until the stomach is ready.*

The stomach

Esophagus

Fundic region

Cardiac region

Serosa

Muscle layers

Pyloric sphincter

Submucosa

Mucosa

Pyloric region

Duodenum

Parotid salivary gland

Submandibular salivary gland

Sublingual salivary gland

Esophagus

Liver

Stomach

Duodenum

Pancreas

Transverse colon

Gall bladder

Descending colon

Ascending colon

Small intestine (ileum)

Cecum

Appendix

Anus

Rectum

▲ *The stomach is made up of several layers of smooth muscle, which enable it to constrict with a churning motion every 15-25 seconds, mixing the food with the gastric juices.*

▼ *The folds of the small intestine are covered in fronds known as microvilli. These each have blood capillaries and lymph vessels and their epithelial cells produce digestive enzymes and receive the nutrients, which they pass into the blood and lymph.*

The small intestine

Mesentery

Muscle layers

Submucosa

Villi

Mucosa

The three essential types of food

In adults the average daily intake of protein is 50-70g. To replace that which is continuously being broken down they need 0·5-0·7g of protein per kilogram of body weight per day, or they will become depleted. Growing children require four or five times this quantity. Consumption of the other main dietary constituents varies more widely – from 300 to 600g of carbohydrate and from 50 to 100g of fat per day (three times more in cold climates). Within limits, the three food types can be interchanged as suppliers of energy. In the developed world, diets have around 12 percent in the form of protein, 48 percent as carbohydrate and 40 percent as fat. But in many Third World countries, the staple food of cereals, which comprise mainly carbohydrates, provides as much as 80 percent of energy.

Human protein is much closer in make-up to that of other animals than to the proteins in plants. So vegetarians, who avoid meat, must consume a wider range of vegetables and fruit than non-vegetarians if their digestive machinery is to receive protein containing an adequate range of amino-acids. Vegans, who also avoid animal products such as milk and eggs, have to take even greater care. They are also likely to be naturally deficient in Vitamin B12.

Measuring the energy content of food

Like a piece of coal, the energy content of a food item can be determined by burning in a calorimeter to see how much heat is generated. The energy is measured in calories, one calorie being the quantity required to raise the temperature of 1g of water by 1°C. Because this unit is unmanageably small, values are usually quoted in kilocalories – a thousand times larger and known as Calories. The energy an adult needs to ingest equals that used in physical activity plus that required for maintaining the tissues, including repair work necessitated by injury or disease. A child requires energy for growth too. Overall, the amount expended at rest (the basal metabolism) is about 1·25C per minute for a 65kg man and 0·90C per minute for a 55kg woman. Exercise such as walking briskly raises these figures about fourfold, while pursuits like tennis-playing demand a sixfold increase. A man expends on average 3,000C daily; a woman about 2,000C.

Breaking down the main food types

Three dietary constituents (water, salts and all vitamins except one) can be absorbed in their original state. The other main components – proteins, carbohydrate and fats – first need to be acted upon by natural catalysts known as enzymes. Proteins (from the Greek word for primary) are large molecules composed of chains of amino-acids. Digestive enzymes break these down, initially into shorter chains (polypeptides) and then into individual amino-acids, of which there are 20 different sorts. Much of the body's own fabric, including muscle and even the lining of the alimentary canal, is composed of proteins. But these are "self", in contrast to the "foreign" proteins which arrive in food. All proteins differ in the sequences of their amino-acids. A typical one contains around 150 of these building blocks. Digesting protein is like fragmenting the type used to print a book so that it may be reassembled as something else. The human body can change certain amino-acids into others; those it cannot synthesize are called essential amino-acids.

Carbohydrates (from the Latin for coal and the Greek for water) fall into two main groups. Monosaccharides are sugars such as glucose, which the body requires as sources of energy. Polysaccharides are more complex molecules, built out of monosaccharides. They include starch and cellulose in plants, as well as the glycogen used by animals as an energy store. Cane sugar (sucrose) and lactose in milk are disaccharides. Digestion involves breaking the larger molecules into their smallest monosaccharide units.

Fats are also made from simpler constituents. Most of those in food are triglycerides (one glycerol molecule linked to three fatty acids) which must be disassembled before being reassembled as human fats. They too provide both a source and stockpile of energy, as well as being important (though minor) ingredients in every cell. Like essential amino-acids, fatty acids the body cannot synthesize have to be consumed in the diet.

Death from starvation

Medical science often learns as much from the care and observation of the sick and dying as it does from laboratory experiments. This happened with the Irish Republican Army (IRA) hunger strikes in Northern Ireland in the late 1970s and early 1980s.

Until that time, biologists believed that to survive prolonged starvation the body needed to conserve protein while burning up fat. But the death of the hunger strikers in 1981 indicated that death is more likely to be precipitated by loss of fat than by depletion of protein. They appeared to be losing their lives at the moment at which they lost every last gram of their body fat.

The prisoners were all around 25 years of age and four of them weighed an average of 45·4kg when they died, following a period of some 60 days without food and after shedding approximately 23kg in weight each. At most the hunger strikers could have lost only 30 percent of their protein.

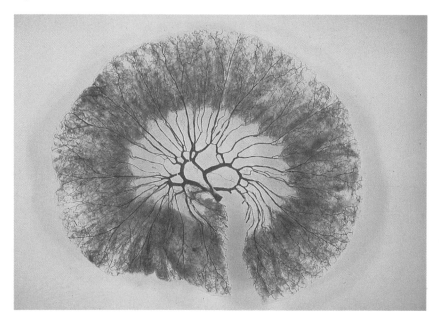

▶ **The blood supply to the small intestine.**

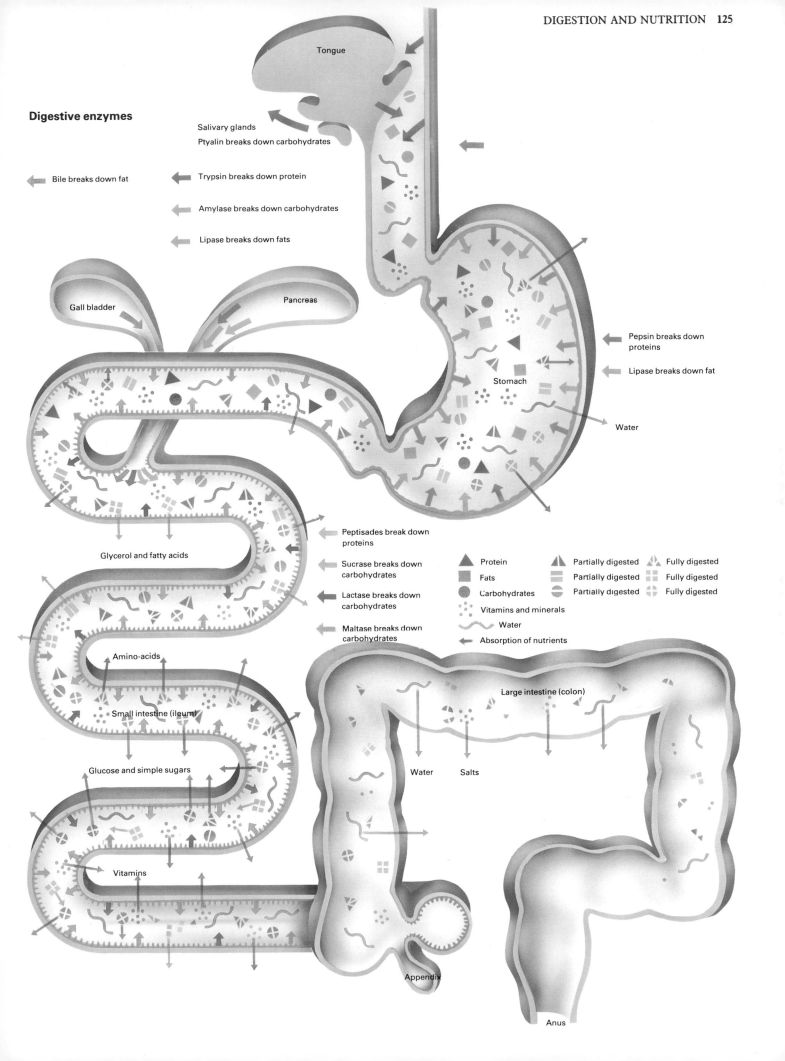

Digestive enzymes

Tongue

Salivary glands
Ptyalin breaks down carbohydrates

Bile breaks down fat

Trypsin breaks down protein

Amylase breaks down carbohydrates

Lipase breaks down fats

Gall bladder

Pancreas

Pepsin breaks down proteins

Lipase breaks down fat

Stomach

Water

Peptisades break down proteins

Sucrase breaks down carbohydrates

Glycerol and fatty acids

Lactase breaks down carbohydrates

Maltase breaks down carbohydrates

Amino-acids

Small intestine (ileum)

Large intestine (colon)

Glucose and simple sugars

Water

Salts

Vitamins

Appendix

Anus

▲ Protein
■ Fats
● Carbohydrates
⋮ Vitamins and minerals
〜 Water
← Absorption of nutrients

Partially digested
Partially digested
Partially digested

Fully digested
Fully digested
Fully digested

The body can absorb only a tiny fraction of the iron consumed in the diet

Minerals, vitamins, fiber and water

In addition to the three principal components of food, two other essential ingredients are minerals and vitamins. A person can receive sufficient calories yet become ill and even die due to a lack of these specific nutrients. Iron is a prime requirement, for the manufacture of hemoglobin (♦ page 158), but less than ten percent of that consumed in the diet can actually be absorbed. Calcium, needed for the growth and upkeep of bone and teeth, is invariably in good supply, though adequate amounts of Vitamin D are also vital for it to be absorbed. Iodine is necessary for the manufacture of thyroid hormones (♦ page 92). But it too (like salt, which is crucial to the maintenance of correct blood pressure and volume) is usually available in sufficient quantities. Selenium, zinc, copper and cobalt are among other elements needed in traces because they help enzymes to work or serve as parts of other key activities.

Vitamins are specific compounds the body cannot synthesize and which must therefore be secured through diet (or in some cases be partly manufactured by intestinal bacteria). Vitamin A, which is involved in producing the retina's light-sensitive pigments, comes from milk, fish-liver oils, butter, egg yolks, some vegetables and cheese. Vitamin D, formed in the skin when exposed to sunlight but also present in fish-liver oils, promotes the absorption of calcium. Vitamin C, found widely in nature (especially in citrus fruits and green plants) has several roles in maintaining tissues and fighting infection. Vitamin B12 and folic acid, required for the development of red blood cells, are synthesized by intestinal bacteria, though Vitamin B12 cannot be absorbed from this source and must be consumed in the diet. Vitamin K is essential for the production of prothrombin, part of the clotting mechanism (♦ page 153). It is rarely in short supply.

Of the B-complex of vitamins, a few are ill-understood or have indeterminate roles. The best characterized are Vitamin B1 (thiamine), found particularly in yeast and the germ of cereal grains, which is essential for certain enzymes to work; and Vitamins B2 (riboflavin) and B6 (pyridoxine), both of which also function in enzyme systems and are synthesized by bacteria in the gut. Nicotinic acid, active in enzyme systems that release energy from foodstuffs, is unusual in that the body can make it from trytophan (one of the amino-acids in protein) as well as acquiring it from meats and cereals. Vitamins C, B1 and folic acid are destroyed to a significant extent by food processing and cooking.

Fiber (roughage) and water are the remaining components of food. Although almost entirely indigestible, fiber is an important part of any prudent diet. Bran, though, can impair the digestion of other nutrients, by absorbing minerals like iron and calcium and removing them from the body. But this is significant only when these minerals are present in abnormally low concentrations. The fiber of cereals, vegetables and fruit is considered a healthy dietary constituent.

About half the weight of ordinary food is water. In a temperate climate, someone doing light work requires about two liters each day to replace that which is lost, so this leaves about one liter to be drunk as liquids. Considerably higher volumes apply in the tropics, where workers may have to consume as much as nine liters daily. Fortunately, because it needs a considerable amount of heat to evaporate, water is also a highly effective cooling agent. Its principal role, however, is as a "universal solvent", not only for digestion but also for the myriad other chemical reactions in the human body.

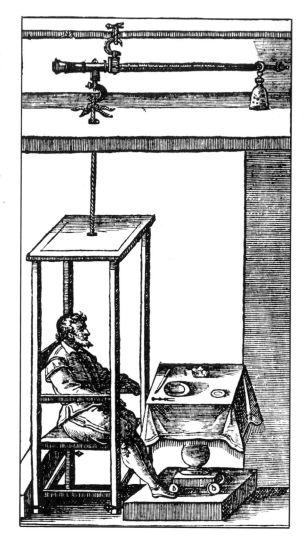

▲ *Sanctorius in his "Ballance".*

Measuring metabolism

Sanctorio Sanctorius (1561-1636) applied to medicine the principles of exact measurement preached by his Italian contemporary Galileo. His most far-reaching work was carried out in Padua, and involved monitoring the variations in his own body weight before and after eating and drinking.

A famous illustration shows Sanctorius sitting on his "Ballance", a chair suspended from the arm of a steelyard. Over a period of 30 years he spent as much time as possible in this device, weighing himself during various physiological states. He also weighed all the food and drink he consumed, as well as his excreta. The principal aim was to detect alterations in the "insensible perspiration" by which volatile substances were supposed to leave the body.

But Sanctorius's work was an important forerunner of much later research into the body's intake and use of energy. "That is the most proper time of Eating, wherein the Body comes to some healthful Standard, as it enjoyed the day before, when empty," he wrote. "But that Apollo himself cannot find out, without the Ballance."

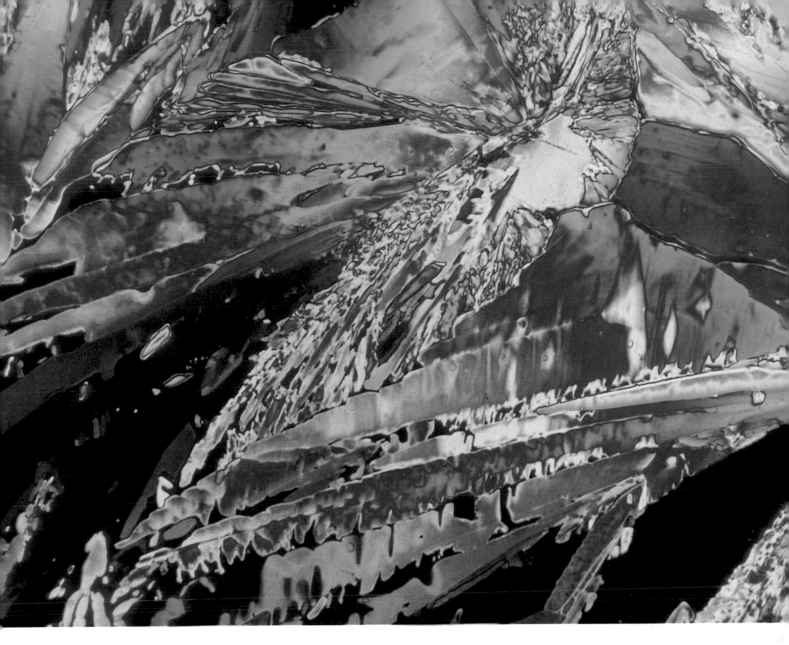

The discovery of vitamins

Disorders resulting from lack of vitamins were well-known long before vitamins themselves were discovered. Rickets, caused by the shortage of Vitamin D, was described in the 17th century and for centuries was cured by daily doses of cod-liver oil. Similarly, in 1753 a Scottish naval surgeon, James Lind, proved that sailors could avoid developing scurvy during long voyages by eating ample quantities of lemons or oranges. The discovery was taken up by the Royal Navy, whose emphasis on adequate supplies of citrus fruits for its sailors gave them the nickname Limeys. In scurvy, the small blood vessels rupture easily, causing swollen, bleeding gums, and red spots appear under the skin. But the substance responsible, ascorbic acid (Vitamin C), was not identified until 1907.

The physician who made the crucial break-through leading to our present understanding of vitamins and the disorders caused by their deficiency was a Dutchman, Christiaan Eijkman (1858-1930). He became director of a laboratory established to investigate outbreaks of beriberi in the colonies in Java and Sumatra. This disease is characterized by nerve malfunction (especially in the legs), edema and heart failure, and is now known to be caused by lack of Vitamin B1, and is associated with a monotonous diet of white rice.

By chance, chickens kept in the laboratory developed a condition, characterized by paralysis, which resembled beriberi in humans. There was no evidence that a microbe was responsible, but Eijkman noticed that his assistant had been feeding the birds on cooked rice from a nearby military hospital. When a new cook arrived – one who refused to allow the hospital's rice to be sent to the laboratory – the disease abated. Eijkman then found that he could precipitate the paralytic malady by feeding chickens on a diet consisting exclusively of polished rice, in place of unmilled rice. Moreover, bran removed during the milling would cure the condition, even if given together with polished rice.

Eijkman initially misinterpreted his findings, thinking that a poison and its antidote were responsible. Nevertheless, they led a few years later to the isolation from rice bran of thiamin, the first of the B group vitamins. Experiments in Cambridge during the first decade of this century by the British biochemist Frederick Gowland Hopkins (1861-1947) prompted the discovery of several other vitamins. In recognition of this work, he and Eijkman shared the Nobel Prize for Medicine and Physiology in 1929.

▲ Vitamin C, seen here in crystalline form. The effects of a shortage of this vitamin in the diet is well known. However, its exact role in metabolism is still not understood, though it is involved in the formation of connective tissue, neutralization of poisons and the healing of wounds.

Malnutrition is the lack of nutrients in the correct proportion, not simply of protein

Feeding the body

If the body fails to receive adequate nutrients from the diet, malnutrition results. As recently as the early 1970s, it seemed that the world's most widespread form of malnutrition stemmed from a shortage of protein. There was talk of a "protein gap", and of political initiatives to close that gulf between rich and poor countries. Today, nutritionists agree that the human body's protein needs were then grossly exaggerated. Although some underprivileged people do specifically require more protein, malnutrition far more frequently reflects a shortage of food in general.

Attention was focused on protein originally by Cicely Williams, the first woman medical officer appointed to the Gold Coast (now Ghana) in 1932. She described a deficiency disease among infants which she felt might be caused by a lack of protein or of some of its constituent amino-acids. Labeled "kwashiorkor", the condition was characterized by dryness of the skin and hair, reddening of hair, and a pot belly – resulting from edema (the accumulation of fluid) in the abdomen. Soon, biochemists found that victims also had unusually low levels of albumin proteins in their bloodstream. Recognition of kwashiorkor

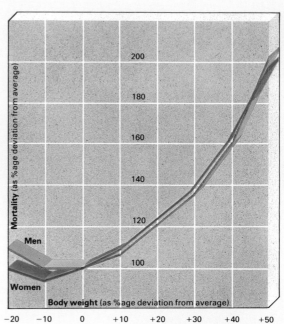

▲ ◄ ▼ *In the developed world, obesity, heart disease and dental caries are the most prevalent diet-related diseases. Obesity reduces the efficiency of the heart and lungs and increases the likelihood of coronary disease through excess of fat in the bloodstream, compounded by inactivity.*

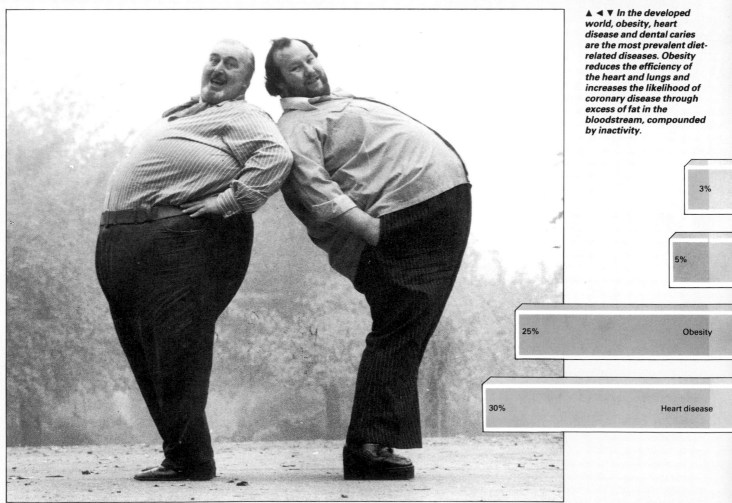

3%

5%

25%   Obesity

30%   Heart disease

99%   Dental caries

marked a major advance in the then confused scientific understanding of malnutrition. But while Dr Williams herself was cautious about generalizing from her findings, other scientists began to assume that insufficient protein was the hallmark of malnutrition everywhere. After the Second World War, UN agencies such as the Food and Agriculture Organization (FAO) devoted themselves to the task of boosting protein production as well as providing protein supplements for needy nations.

Redefining malnutrition

Kwashiorkor certainly existed, and still exists today. But biologists now realize that it is restricted to regions, such as the areas of Africa where Dr Williams worked, where most peoples' diet is based on the starchy root cassava – the only one of the world's principal staple crops that is truly deficient in protein. Populations dependent on yams can be at risk for the same reason. A key figure in this reassessment was the Indian nutritionist Professor P.V. Sukhatme who, during the late 1960s, reported that malnourished children in a village he was studying improved even when given foods such as beans and cereals, which are relatively low in protein. They had been suffering not from protein deficiency but from a shortage of both the protein required for growth and renewal and the carbohydrate required as a source of energy.

What is now termed "protein-energy malnutrition" (PEM) reflects the fact that the body needs *in the right ratio* foods providing protein and those providing energy. It is even possible for a poorly-fed child, given a disproportionate amount of protein, to develop symptoms of kwashiorkor – because its body breaks down the protein for energy. But with a balanced diet, energy foods "spare" any protein, even though it may be present in small amounts.

Malnutrition and health

Nutritionists are still reassessing the significance of the two extreme forms of PEM – kwashiorkor and marasmus. As well as dry skin and swollen belly, kwashiorkor is characterized by growth retardation, muscle wasting and mental changes such as apathy. In addition to growth retardation and muscle wasting, the cardinal features of marasmus are loss of subcutaneous tissue and the *absence* of edema. Because similar conditions can be produced by depriving experimental animals of protein and calories respectively, they have long been considered as the two extremes of PEM. But some experts now believe that both result from primary calorie inadequacy plus secondary protein deficiency, the outcomes and symptoms of which reflect an individual victim's capacity to adapt to these nutritional deprivations.

One result of PEM which is not in question is its severe influence on resistance to infectious disease. According to one survey, malnutrition increased the duration of diarrhea in underweight Nigerian children by 33 percent, and by 79 percent in children so malnourished that their growth had been stunted. The repercussions of a poor diet on microbial invasion are wholly bad, even though in some circumstances a poor diet can actually promote health – caries declined in Europe as a result of sugar shortage during the Second World War. But at the same time starvation conditions in German concentration camps caused many deaths from tuberculosis, broncho-pneumonia and other infections.

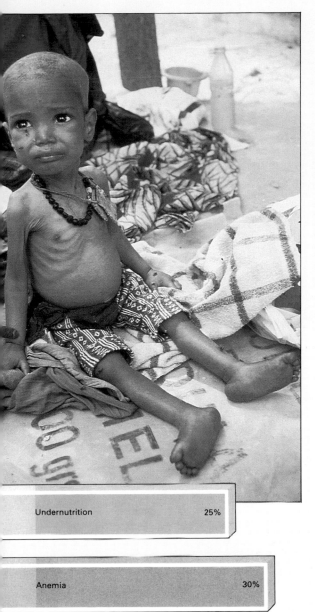

Undernutrition 25%

Anemia 30%

3%

2%

1% Eye conditions

10%

Developing world

◄ ▲ The developing world's nutritional disorders are primarily related to lack of nutrients, although the advent of a Western lifestyle has brought a slight rise in so-called "diseases of civilization", many dietary in origin, including obesity, heart disease and constipation.

The functioning of the human brain may be impaired by severe malnutrition in childhood

Protein and Calorie needs

As the realization grew in the 1970s that malnutrition was not so much caused by lack of protein, as of protein and Calories together, recommendations for the body's daily protein requirements were revised downwards, while those for Calories have remained fairly constant. In 1971, for example, the Food and Agriculture Organization (FAO) lowered its figure for protein per kilogram body weight per day for one-year-olds from 2·0g to 1·2g. But these guidelines disguise a second crucial aspect of protein, its quality. Although the distinction is not rigid, different types of protein can be divided into first-class (those providing amino-acids in roughly the correct ratio required by the body for synthesizing new proteins) and second-class (those deficient in certain amino-acids – such as cereal proteins, which contain little lysine). Although consuming enough total protein, therefore, a person can suffer from a lack of specific amino-acids – as with vegetarians or vegans who may not consume a sufficient variety of plant proteins to compensate for their shortage of particular amino-acids. Estimates for the adequacy of the Calories in the diet vary from those countries, such as the United States, Eire and Italy, in which daily energy supplies are on average between a third and a half more than is required, to Bhutan where the average supply is a mere 40 percent of the FAO recommendation.

The effect of malnutrition on intellectual performance is also being reassessed. Contrary to earlier beliefs that the adult brain is insensitive to even the most severe starvation, there are now indications that brain tissue is vulnerable at a certain period of growth. Rats given a drastically restricted diet immediately after birth develop fewer synapses per neuron in the cerebral cortex (◀ page 55). Extrapolated to human animals, such research implies that brain function might be impaired by severe malnutrition between mid-pregnancy and the second birthday. Whether this affects mental skills, and is partly responsible for the apathy that has been described as widespread in Third World countries, remains controversial.

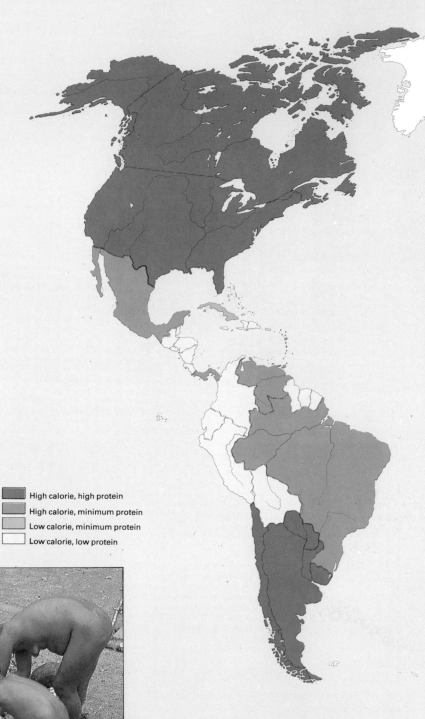

■ High calorie, high protein

■ High calorie, minimum protein

■ Low calorie, minimum protein

☐ Low calorie, low protein

◀ *Amazonian Indians cooking cassava; although poor in protein it is often supplemented by a wide range of other foods to provide sufficient nutrients.*

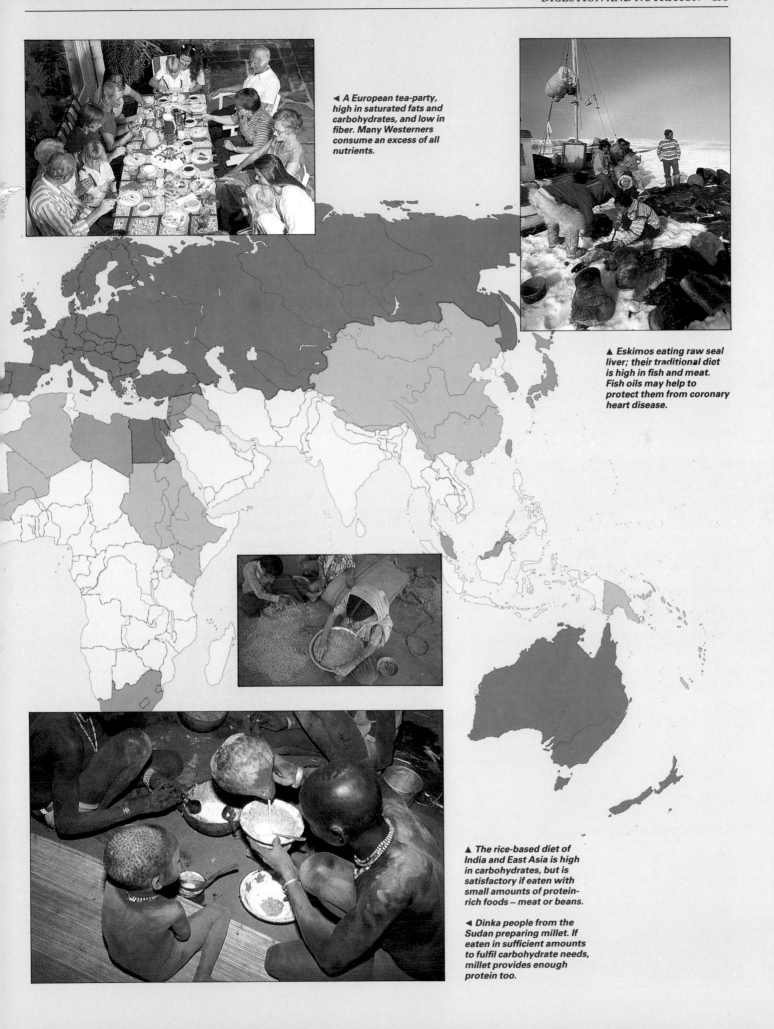

◄ A European tea-party, high in saturated fats and carbohydrates, and low in fiber. Many Westerners consume an excess of all nutrients.

▲ Eskimos eating raw seal liver; their traditional diet is high in fish and meat. Fish oils may help to protect them from coronary heart disease.

▲ The rice-based diet of India and East Asia is high in carbohydrates, but is satisfactory if eaten with small amounts of protein-rich foods – meat or beans.

◄ Dinka people from the Sudan preparing millet. If eaten in sufficient amounts to fulfil carbohydrate needs, millet provides enough protein too.

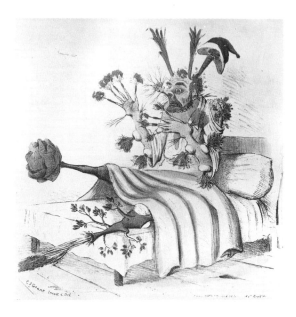

▲ *An 18th-century English vision of the dangers of a vegetarian diet. The British grew proud of their meat consumption in Tudor times, and meat remains a psychological, though not a nutritional, necessity for many.*

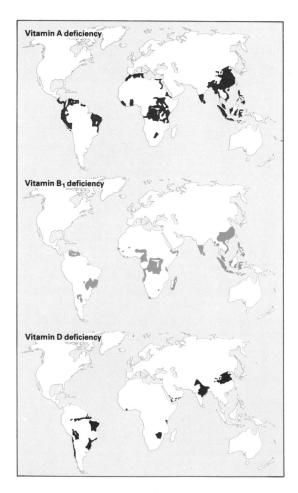

▲ *The distribution of the various avitominoses can be traced geographically, and can be used to predict the incidence of diseases, such as beriberi or rickets, that are known to be related to vitamin deficiencies.*

Even with adequate nutrition, the body may not always absorb food materials, particularly fats, completely. The outcome is steatorrhea – the passage of bulky, offensive, greasy stools. Among the causes are incomplete mixing of gastric secretions and failure by the pancreas to produce its digestive enzymes. Another is coeliac disease, in which the lining of the small intestine becomes thin and wasted. This results from sensitivity of the intestinal wall to the wheat protein known as gluten, and can be cured by eliminating this from the diet.

Vitamin deficiency diseases

Most Western diets contain adequate amounts of vitamins and mineral elements to satisfy our minuscule requirements. The body also stores such micronutrients as a hedge against temporary deprivation. But deficiency diseases develop quickly whenever food fails to provide enough of these substances to sustain the vital functions in which they play a part. Lack of Vitamin A, needed by the light-sensitive retina, causes first night-blindness and then total blindness. Some 250,000 people, mostly in Southeast Asia, lose their sight in this way each year. Because Vitamin A affects the regulation of cell growth, there are also suggestions that it prevents cancer, though this has not been proved. Just as beriberi is caused by lack of Vitamin B1 and often associated with a monotonous white rice diet, so an over-dependence on maize leads to pellagra, with its sore mouth and blisters of the hands, feet and face. This arises from shortage of nicotinic acid or of the amino-acid tryptophan.

Scurvy is the result of Vitamin C deficiency. It occurs even in well-fed nations among bottle-fed infants whose parents fail to supplement their diet with fruit juices or vegetables. Some specialists believe that mild forms of scurvy and deficiencies of B group vitamins are not uncommon among old people, particularly those living alone on grossly unbalanced diets. Vitamin C lack is also often related to smoking, which increases bodily requirements, as does infection.

Shortage of Vitamin D (produced in the skin by the action of sunlight, as well as being acquired from fish and other foods) leads to the childhood condition of rickets. Calcium is not absorbed properly, impairing the mineralization of bone, which becomes soft and may deform or fracture. Otherwise rare in the West, rickets appeared as a serious problem among Asian immigrants to Britain during the 1960s and 70s. Like the other "avitaminoses", it is preventible by ensuring a sufficient intake of the vitamin from appropriate foods. But the authorities rejected the option of fortifying chapatti flour, because this could have meant adults getting *too much* Vitamin D. Excessive doses of all vitamins can be harmful.

The best-documented deficits of individual elements concern iron and iodine. Although there are other forms of anemia, and other causes of iron-deficiency anemia in particular, that produced by a shortage of dietary iron is the commonest. It is curable and preventable by iron tablets, just as widespread use of iodized salt has virtually eradicated the thyroid gland enlargement known as simple goiter (◀ page 93). Although "health food" enthusiasts often overrate their significance, several other elements, needed only in minute traces, *can* be present in inadequate amounts. Zinc deficiency, little recognized until recently, impairs wound-healing and taste discrimination, as well as possibly retarding growth during childhood. Most trace elements are required for enzyme systems though some, like cobalt in Vitamin B12, form part of a complex compound.

Processing nutrients from food...Functions of the liver...How the liver works...Storing nutrients: fat cells and the liver...Processing waste: the colon...Excreting waste...The kidneys, cleansing the blood...How the kidney works...The body's liquid requirements... PERSPECTIVE...Studying the liver...Early investigations of the kidney

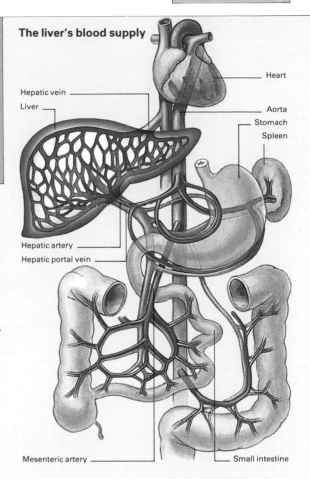

The liver's blood supply

Heart
Hepatic vein
Liver
Aorta
Stomach
Spleen
Hepatic artery
Hepatic portal vein
Mesenteric artery
Small intestine

As with a household or factory, raw materials entering the human body are needed for two main functions. Some act as sources of energy while others are required to repair the fabric and enlarge it when the structure is growing. Likewise, certain items delivered alongside essential supplies serve no useful purpose. Together with worn-out pieces of the fabric that have been replaced, these can be discarded as waste. Other parts of the intake, not wanted immediately, go into store to provide energy and materials for future use.

Fat, as external appearances suggest, provides a rich stockpile of Calories (◀ page 128) which can be drawn upon when needed. It is also the body's main energy reserve, with double the fuel value, weight for weight, of protein or carbohydrate. Adipose cells are the specialized repositories, capable of accepting and storing glucose and fatty acids from the blood and converting them to fat. Adipose tissue occurs throughout the human frame, with characteristically different distribution in males and females. It is laid down mainly beneath the skin, between layers of muscle fiber, and around the internal organs.

The liver – the center of metabolism

The body is much more complex than any theoretical model, however, and metabolic activities following the receipt of supplies are less easily separated – especially excretion and storage. The central role in animal metabolism is played by the liver, the largest internal organ of the body. A pyramid-shaped structure in the upper right abdomen, it has a double blood supply – the hepatic artery which provides its oxygen and the hepatic portal vein which brings absorbed food materials from the intestine. One function of the liver is as a depot. In addition to iron and vitamins, including B12, it husbands glucose and other sugars transported from the digestive tract. It converts them into glycogen and to a lesser degree fatty acids – which are also produced from the fat which arrives there from the small intestine. When glucose in the bloodstream becomes depleted the liver releases some from its store by breaking down glycogen or fatty acids.

As well as processing cholesterol absorbed from food, the liver synthesizes this substance, which is needed to make bile salts (and hormones including estrogen; ◀ page 90). Most of the bile salts left behind in the gut after helping to digest fat return to the liver from the ileum. Intestinal bacteria turn the rest into simpler compounds which are excreted in feces. The component responsible for bile's green-orange color is bilirubin, a breakdown product from hemoglobin. Together with the spleen and bone marrow, liver cells release this pigment by destroying old red blood cells. When it reaches the small intestine, bilirubin is also converted further by bacteria into substances which are eliminated in the feces (and which give them their characteristic smell).

▲ *The blood from the stomach and intestines, carrying the nutrients absorbed from the food, passes to the liver via the hepatic portal vein. The liver is also provided with oxygenated blood via the hepatic artery. Within the liver, these two blood supplies pass via the system of capillaries into the liver lobules. Blood finally leaves the liver in the hepatic veins.*

The liver performs more than 500 different functions, regulating the body's chemistry

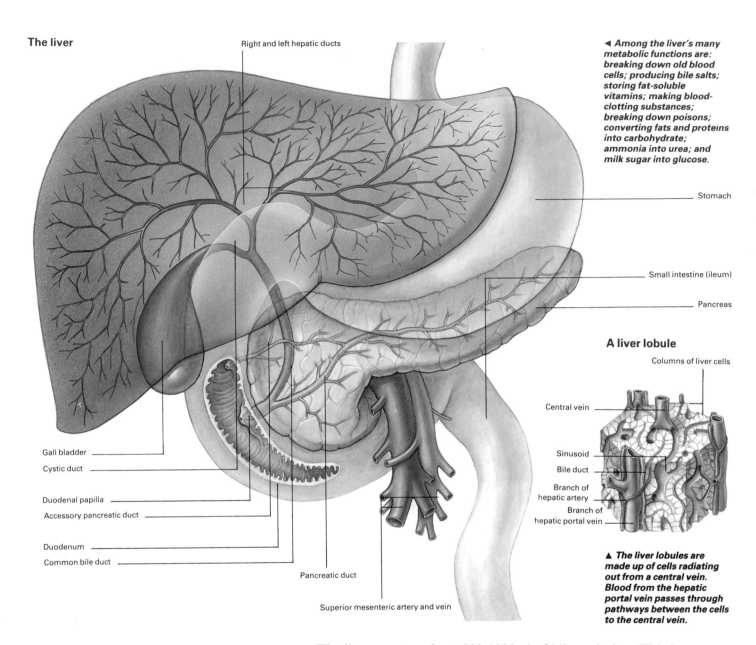

The liver

Right and left hepatic ducts

◄ *Among the liver's many metabolic functions are: breaking down old blood cells; producing bile salts; storing fat-soluble vitamins; making blood-clotting substances; breaking down poisons; converting fats and proteins into carbohydrate; ammonia into urea; and milk sugar into glucose.*

Stomach

Small intestine (ileum)

Pancreas

Gall bladder

Cystic duct

Duodenal papilla

Accessory pancreatic duct

Duodenum

Common bile duct

Pancreatic duct

Superior mesenteric artery and vein

A liver lobule

Columns of liver cells

Central vein

Sinusoid

Bile duct

Branch of hepatic artery

Branch of hepatic portal vein

▲ *The liver lobules are made up of cells radiating out from a central vein. Blood from the hepatic portal vein passes through pathways between the cells to the central vein.*

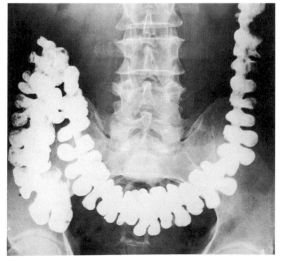

▲ *The colon, site of the final absorption of salts and water.*

The liver secretes about 800-1000ml of bile each day. This is concentrated and stored in the gall bladder, then discharged into the duodenum. The gall bladder can be removed without seriously impairing digestion. But the liver, although it has impressive powers of regeneration, is an essential organ, with some 500 different metabolic roles. In addition to storage and excretion, these include the manufacture of certain blood-clotting factors and the detoxification of poisons.

The body's waste products

Solid matter voided from the rectum as feces contains not only the breakdown products of bile salts and bilirubin but also a residue of indigestible and/or unabsorbable materials such as plant cellulose (roughage), remnants of cells sloughed off by the intestinal wall, and left-over enzymes and secretions. Although protein is usually digested completely, some fat is also present in the feces. The mixture provides ideal nourishment for the very different digestive systems of bacteria living in the colon. These proliferate vigorously and account for up to 20 percent by weight of the body's solid effluent. The colon

The kidney

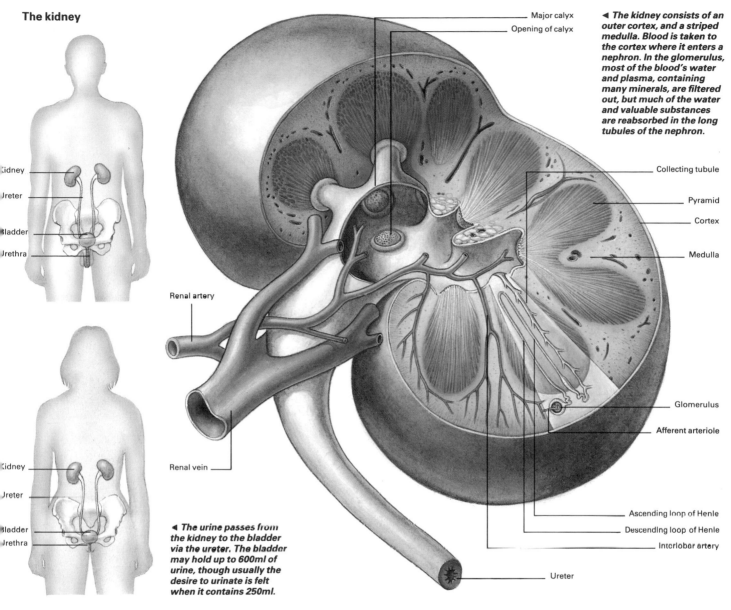

Major calyx
Opening of calyx

◄ *The kidney consists of an outer cortex, and a striped medulla. Blood is taken to the cortex where it enters a nephron. In the glomerulus, most of the blood's water and plasma, containing many minerals, are filtered out, but much of the water and valuable substances are reabsorbed in the long tubules of the nephron.*

Kidney
Ureter

Bladder
Urethra

Renal artery

Kidney
Ureter
Bladder
Urethra

Renal vein

Collecting tubule
Pyramid
Cortex
Medulla

Glomerulus
Afferent arteriole

Ascending loop of Henle
Descending loop of Henle
Interlobar artery

Ureter

◄ *The urine passes from the kidney to the bladder via the ureter. The bladder may hold up to 600ml of urine, though usually the desire to urinate is felt when it contains 250ml.*

also absorbs water, which nevertheless comprises about 65 percent of the 80-180g of feces excreted daily.

Gases also occur in the gut – two-thirds of them in the colon, where their movement causes the gurgling noises known as borborygmus. Air gulped down while eating is one source, but colon bacteria are responsible for the smelly and explosive mixture of gases (mainly hydrogen sulphide, methane and hydrogen) expelled as flatus.

When fats and carbohydrates serve as sources of energy, the end-products are carbon dioxide (removed through the lungs) and water, which leaves the body via the lungs and skin as well as via the kidneys. But when protein is broken down (as a last resort for energy but usually for the replacement of tissues) the principal left-over is urea. The kidneys eliminate this substance, while simultaneously limiting the loss of valuable substances such as glucose and maintaining the body's correct balance of water and the concentrations of salt and other chemicals. Working in harmony with other organs the kidneys thus help to maintain homeostasis – the constant composition of the tissues which is essential for efficient functioning of the body.

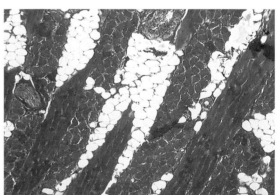

▲ *Adipose fat cells deposited in skeletal muscle tissue. A fat cell is a specialized form of connective tissue (♦ page 14) comprising a membrane, containing the nucleus, and otherwise entirely filled with fat. Some nutritionists believe that overeating in infancy may increase the number of adipose fat cells, and that this may cause a susceptibility to overweight in later life.*

Dual role of the kidney

The kidneys have a dual function. As well as serving as a principal organ of excretion they also regulate the body's salt and water content. These roles accompany each other because the kidney has evolved to enable animals to live on land, where water and salts must be conserved, effluents voided in concentrated form, and the tissue fluids strictly regulated. The lungs, bowel and skin also mediate between the outside world and the body's internal environment, but the kidneys play the key role.

The kidney's working units are nephrons – filters which remove waste products from circulating blood and turn them into urine. A nephron is a long, extremely fine tube, closed at one end and folded into a capsule containing a cluster of tiny blood vessels comprising the glomerulus. Each kidney contains a million or more nephrons. They extract most of the water and salts from blood, returning those needed by the body. Fluid filters out of blood in the glomerulus and into the tubule. Its composition then changes, as water and wanted constituents are selectively reabsorbed. The fluid left behind is urine, which passes along the ureters to the bladder, before being voided by micturition (◆ page 160).

Each day, a healthy kidney receives and processes about 1800l of blood – about 400 times the total amount in the body. During that same period it produces only about 1·5l of urine, returning the rest of the water to the bloodstream. Urinary output varies with work and climate, and can fall as low as half a liter per day in someone losing fluid by heavy sweating.

The kidney's performance as a concentrator is also vividly illustrated by the level of bodily wastes in urine as compared with blood plasma – 60 times more urea and 500 times more ammonia (a minor breakdown product of protein). It is no surprise that untreated kidney failure leads to early death.

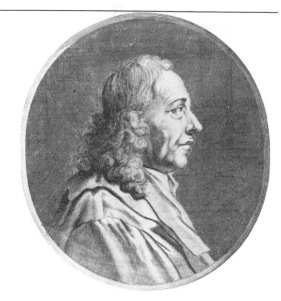

Marcello Malpighi

Glomeruli – the first look

The first person to see a glomerulus, the tiny coil in each of the kidney's nephrons, was an Italian anatomist and pioneer of the manufacture and use of the microscope, Marcello Malpighi (1628-1694). The professor of anatomy at Bologna from 1666 to 1691, he suspected that it played a part in the secretion of urine. We now know that this "Malpighian tuft" does the initial extracting. One of the earliest anatomists to be keenly interested not just in examining microscopically small parts of the body but also in working out how they function, Malpighi made many important discoveries. As well as revealing the blood capillaries which communicate between arteries and veins, he found that the liver releases bile through the bile duct, and that bile does not originate, as previously supposed, in the gall bladder. Among the other organs he studied were the lung, brain and spleen.

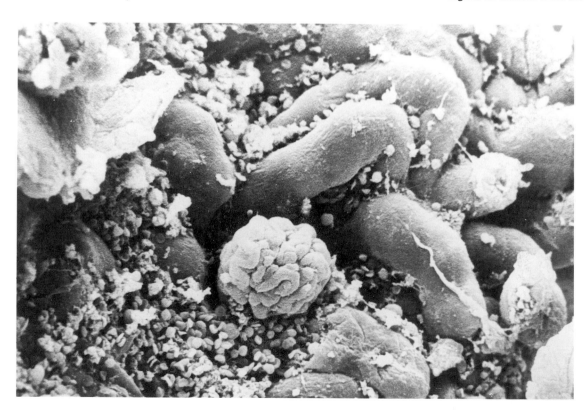

◀ *Scanning electron micrograph of a Bowman's capsule surrounding a glomerulus, the point at which waste products and water are filtered out of the blood in the kidney.*

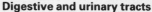

Colon disorders...Colitis and diverticulosis...
Appendicitis...Ulcers...Diarrhea and constipation...
Kidney and gall bladder stones...Prostate problems...
PERSPECTIVE...Living with a colostomy

Digestive and urinary tracts

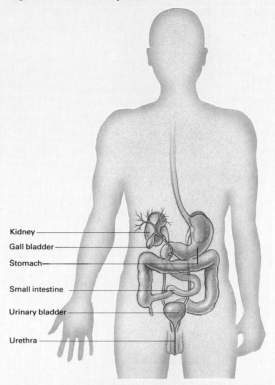

Kidney
Gall bladder
Stomach
Small intestine
Urinary bladder
Urethra

We are in direct contact with the outside world through our skin and its internal continuation, from mouth to rectum, which processes our food. A number of problems result from failures, malfunctions or imbalances in this system, all of them linked – to a greater or lesser extent – to diet.

Diseases of the colon

Colitis is characterized by inflammation of the mucous membrane of the large bowel, which causes bloody diarrhea. It usually strikes in adolescence or soon after. If severe, it can cause anemia, fever, tachycardia and weight-loss; if continuous, it needs surgical treatment. More usually, it is intermittent and the sufferer has only occasional attacks. These may be precipitated by various factors, including oral antibiotics. In addition to mouth ulcers, the side effects of colitis may include body rashes and conjunctivitis.

The incidence of colitis differs geographically and among different population groups. This has led to the idea that it may be diet-related. As with coronary heart disease, the incidence in Japan is substantially lower than in the USA, but among Japanese living in America, it is closer to the US than the Japanese level. Food allergy, notably allergy towards milk proteins, has been suggested as a cause. There is also some evidence that defects of immunity may be involved (⬦ page 230), and stressful events can cause sufferers to relapse.

Another disease which usually affects the colon is diverticulosis. This is the presence of one or more pouches, known as diverticula, in the gut wall which may cause pain and a change in bowel routine. The motility of the intestine may contribute to the formation of diverticula. Changes in collagen structure with aging may also play a part. However, the strongest influence could be the fiber content of the diet. In less-developed countries, where the disease is less common than in the West, the diet tends to be much higher in fiber. Similarly, vegetarians have a lower incidence of the disease than meat-eaters.

Diverticulosis can be treated simply by changes in diet and mild drugs to ease the pain and reduce intestinal motility. If the diverticula become inflamed, the condition is called diverticulitis. Diverticulitis arises in less than 10 percent of people with diverticula, when symptoms similar to appendicitis may appear. There is a danger of hemorrhage, and antibiotics and a water-only diet are required until the inflammation subsides. Recurrent diverticulitis may need surgery.

A diverticulum may become inflamed as a result of fecal matter lodging in it. Appendicitis can be caused in the same way. The appendix is a residual tube attached to the beginning of the colon and plays no part in human digestion. Its entrance into the intestine is easily blocked. If this is not diagnosed, the appendix perforates, causing peritonitis (inflammation of the peritoneum), which can be fatal.

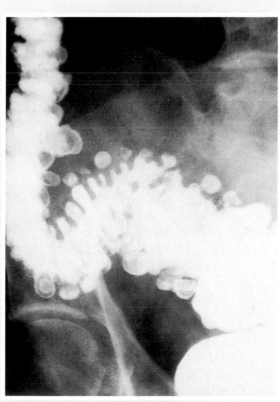

▲ *X-ray taken after a barium meal of diverticula, pouches appearing within the folds of the colon, which often develop after middle age. Diverticulosis is one of the so-called "diseases of civilization", a consequence of eating insufficient fiber, and the resulting unnatural bowel movements and constipation. Diverticula may become inflamed or perforated and lead to massive hemorrhage.*

Kidney stones have become more common in Western countries in this century

Peptic ulcers

Duodenal ulcers, breaks in the mucosal layer of the duodenum, are common. The immediate cause is an imbalance between the mucosal defenses and the amount of acid and pepsin (one of the digestive enzymes) in the duodenum. This is precipitated by factors which may include genetic predisposition, anti-inflammatory drugs such as aspirin, stress (◀ page 88) smoking and alcohol consumption.

The major symptom of a duodenal ulcer is pain, frequently after eating. If the ulcer perforates, so that the wall of the duodenum actually ruptures, the pain is very severe and the sufferer may collapse. In most cases ulcers heal spontaneously, but relapses are frequent. They can now be treated very successfully with drugs that reduce gastric acid production. Ulcer symptoms are also alleviated by avoiding any food which seems to cause pain – often fatty or spicy foods – and by eating small, frequent meals. Antacids (indigestion remedies) also alleviate pain but may cause constipation (if they contain aluminum salts) or diarrhea (if based on magnesium salts).

Ulcers also occur in the stomach, as a result of acidity and gastric reflux – the return of material from the duodenum into the stomach. Gastric ulcers are generally less severe than duodenal ulcers. Duodenal and gastric ulcers are known collectively as peptic ulcers.

The mouth and lips may also ulcerate, sometimes as a result of viral infections such as herpes. These ulcers may last up to two weeks, during which eating can be painful and difficult. Small mouth ulcers have a number of other causes. The tendency to ulceration seems to run in families and in women there is a relationship between ulcer formation and the menstrual cycle. Ulceration may also be an immune response to antigens in oral mucosa which cross-react with bacterial antigens (◆ page 221). Stress and colitis may also be a cause.

Diarrhea, constipation and stones

The two major gastro-intestinal complaints are diarrhea and constipation. Diarrhea may result from a number of causes including contaminated food or water, excess alcohol, food allergy and laxative abuse. Characterized by watery feces, it usually clears up spontaneously. It can be dangerous, particularly in infants and malnourished people, because of its dehydrating effect. The opposite is constipation – infrequent and difficult defecation, with the production of hard feces. Diet plays a major role, although it can also be caused by drugs, pregnancy and diseases including diabetes and parkinsonism. It is alleviated by a high fiber diet and by laxatives based on plants.

Problems arising in relation to the removal of waste may be directly connected with excretion (as with urinary stones) or have a secondary cause such as prostatic enlargement (◆ page 140). Urinary stone disease – the formation of mineral lumps in the kidneys and urinary tract – is another ailment which has risen in frequency in the developed countries during this century.

Urine contains many different mineral ions, some of which precipitate as solids at low concentrations. The predominant stone substances in the developed countries are calcium oxalate and calcium phosphate. Normal urine contains polymers which interfere with crystal growth, thus preventing stones from growing to a size where they are not naturally expelled in the urine stream. It is when stones become large enough to obstruct the urinary tract that they can cause trouble. This may show up as pains during urination, appendicitis-like pains (renal colic) or an increased incidence of urinary infections.

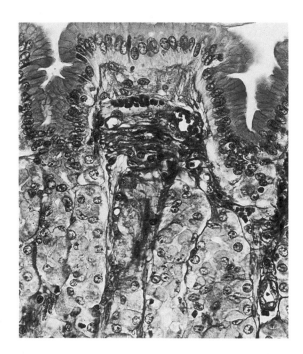

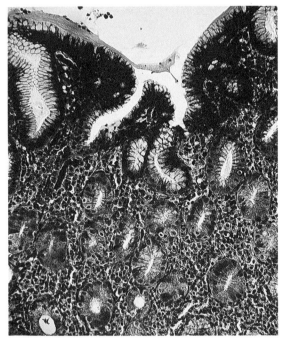

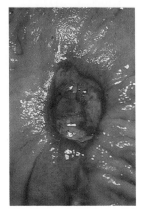

◀ ▲ *Section through the lining of a healthy stomach (top) and a stomach ulcer (above and left). The epithelium layer, here stained blue, becomes thin and broken, allowing the digestive enzymes and acid to attack the body's own tissues. Most ulcers, though not all, are the result of excess acid in the stomach; they may be a side-effect of the body's "Generalized Adaptation Syndrome" to stress (◆ page 88).*

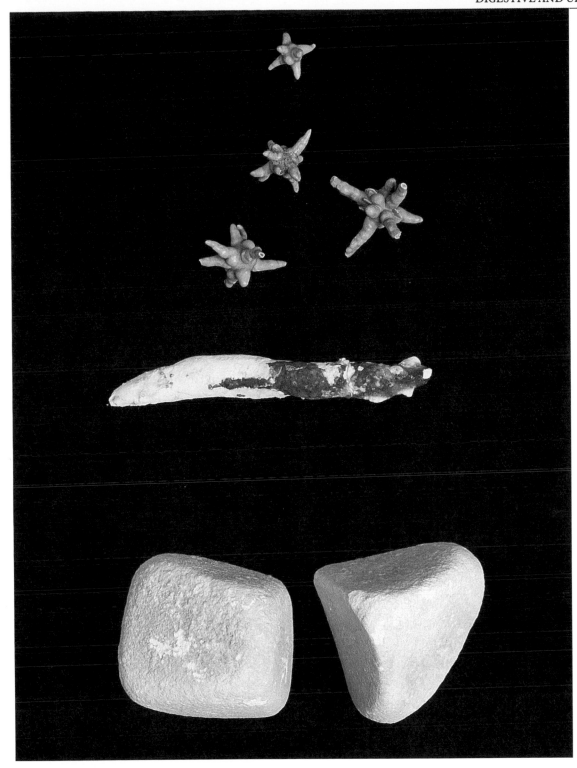

◄ *Stones from the urinary tract, including the knobbly "staghorn" stones from the kidney.*

Ultrasonic probe

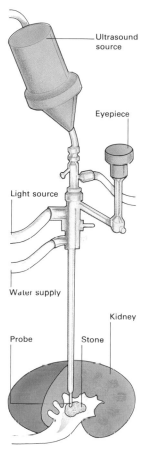

Ultrasound source

Eyepiece

Light source

Water supply

Kidney

Probe   Stone

▲ *Kidney stones can be destroyed using an ultrasound probe inserted into the kidney, allowing the surgeon to view the stone optically, aim the ultrasound source and flush away stone fragments with water.*

► *Lithotripsy is another new technique for destroying kidney stones. The patient is placed in a bath, above a high-energy sound source contained in an ellipse that focuses the sound-waves on the kidney. These waves destroy the stone and the fragments are excreted. Recovery rates are much faster than with conventional surgery.*

◄ *Kidney stones may virtually fill the calyx, or urine-gathering space in the kidney.*

Lithotripsy

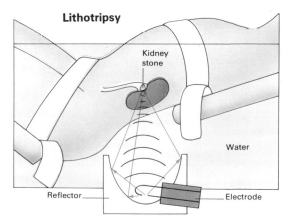

Kidney stone

Water

Reflector   Electrode

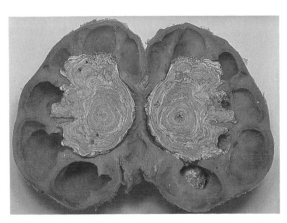

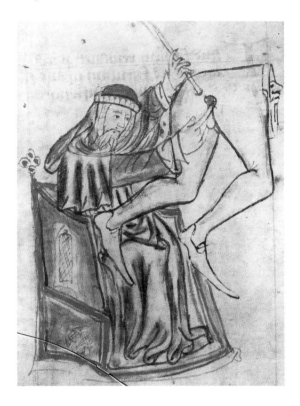

▲ *A medieval operation on piles. These are benign swellings in blood vessels inside or outside the anus which can cause discomfort and pain. Hemorrhoids rarely have a single cause, though constipation and straining to pass feces may often bring them on. Surgery is sometimes necessary in the most severe cases.*

Colostomy – bypassing the intestines

A colostomy is an artificial anus, which a surgeon can arrange by cutting across the colon and diverting it towards a newly-created opening in the wall of the abdomen.

There are two reasons for carrying out a short-circuiting operation of this sort. Intestinal contents may have to be voided before they pass through a portion of the colon which needs to be allowed to heal after disease and/or surgery. Gunshot injuries and the tearing wounds sometimes received in road accidents are other grounds for adopting this measure. A colostomy done for such reasons is temporary, normal function being resumed and the abdominal hole being closed several weeks or months later. Alternatively, when a large section of the bowel has to be removed because of disease (usually cancer), a permanent colostomy is then created. In either case, the patient uses a colostomy bag, which covers the artificial opening and receives the excreta.

Some intestinal operations are conducted in two parts. The surgeon may arrange a temporary colostomy as the first stage in dealing with a tumor that is blocking the colon. He can then remove the tumor, before closing the colostomy and restoring the normal function of the intestine and rectum. Modern appliances and techniques make it possible for an individual to live both comfortably and hygienically with a colostomy, and to conceal its existence from other people.

Whether or not stone disease needs surgical treatment depends on the nature of the obstruction rather than the size of the stone. The aim of conservative (non-surgical) treatment is to get the patient to pass the stone spontaneously. This can be encouraged by a high fluid intake, sometimes coupled with brief diuretic treatment.

Stones can also develop in the gall bladder, where they cause abdominal pain, often accompanied by nausea and vomiting. Gallstones may affect as many as one in five people worldwide. Again, there is a difference in composition between developed and underdeveloped countries. Cholesterol is a major component of western gallstones, while stones containing calcium ions and bile pigments are more frequent in underdeveloped areas. If the stones are wholly organic, they can be dissolved by chenodeoxycholic acid, but calcified (calcium-containing) stones resist this treatment and usually have to be removed surgically. Both gall and urinary stones have high rates of recurrence.

Urinary tract infections

Although the prostate gland is not directly involved in excretion, its position in the body means that its enlargement may cause excretory disorders. When male hormone production ceases, the prostate gland (which produces a secretion that forms part of semen) degenerates and after the age of 60 enlargement of the fibrous residue is common. This can cause pressure on the urethra, which is surrounded by the prostate, so that the bladder does not empty properly. Stones may precipitate in the stagnant urine remaining and infections or cancer may develop. The condition is alleviated by surgery. The prostate may also become infected (prostatitis) causing gut and back pain.

Urinary tract infection may also be a symptom of polycystic kidney disease, which can cause severe abdominal pain and high blood pressure and eventual deterioration of kidney function. It is an inherited disease in which both kidneys are covered with multiple cysts. A cyst is an abnormal piece of tissue which encloses liquid or semisolid material or gases and can occur in or on many parts of the body, notably the liver. Choledocal cysts are cysts of the bile duct which can contain up to eight liters of material. They also cause abdominal pain and if removed surgically can cause biliary cirrhosis.

Swollen prostate gland

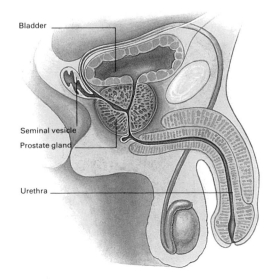

Bladder

Seminal vesicle

Prostate gland

Urethra

◄ *The prostate gland, which provides part of the seminal fluid, tends to become enlarged. This is very common in older men. Since it is situated at the base of the bladder and around the urethra, this swelling can cause disruption to the normal processes of urination. This may result in a sudden inability to urinate, or a gradual failure of the bladder to empty, which may eventually cause kidney problems. In these circumstances it is necessary to remove the prostate.*

Intestinal infection and sanitation...Malnutrition and diarrhea...Cholera, an ancient scourge...Salmonella food poisoning and typhoid fever...Amebic dysentery... Intestinal worms...PERSPECTIVE...The spread of cholera...The agents of gastroenteritis...Recent typhoid fever outbreaks...Food preparation and infection... Modern drugs

The digestive system

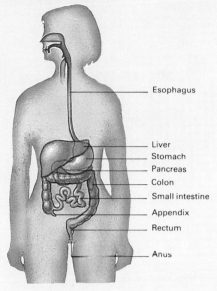

- Esophagus
- Liver
- Stomach
- Pancreas
- Colon
- Small intestine
- Appendix
- Rectum
- Anus

Although we cannot see individual microbes, astronomical numbers surround us from cradle to grave. The vast majority are beneficial, in helping plants to assimilate nitrogen from the air, breaking down dead plant and animal tissues, and recycling elements which are central to the planet's ecology. Many microbes are relatively self-sufficient, finding energy and materials for continued growth in the environment. But some microbes have evolved a parasitic way of life as an easier method of securing the nutrients they require. Known as pathogens, these are recognized by the infectious diseases they cause (◆ page 174). Like other animals, humans acquire such micro-organisms in several different ways – through food and water, by inhalation, sexual intercourse, contamination of a wound, or the attentions of insect "vectors". A few can invade the body by more than one route, but most gain entry through a particular channel and cause their principal damage there.

Diarrheal disease

Intestinal infections comprise one such group. They are caused by microbes ingested with food or water which then proliferate in the gut. The infections are characterized by diarrhea and/or vomiting, perhaps accompanied by abdominal cramps and raised temperature. Eighty percent of all illness in developing countries is linked to water and for this reason the World Health Organization has adopted a target of clean water for all by 1990. Although that percentage includes conditions such as malaria, spread by insects breeding in lakes and streams, it mainly relates to conditions known collectively as "diarrheal disease".

In some regions diarrheal disease is responsible for as much as 40 percent of mortality among infants and young children of up to five years of age. In 1980, intestinal infections alone caused five million deaths – ten every minute of every day – and 750 million disease episodes in Africa, Latin America and Asia (excluding China). Most of the pathogens concerned would seem little more than transient nuisances in the West.

Continual diarrhea promotes malnutrition and impairs defense mechanisms, contributing to a vicious circle in which malnourished children are 50 percent more likely than well-fed ones to succumb to diarrheal disease. Measles in particular forms a horrendous combination with diarrhea, each condition being a common and potentially fatal complication of the other. In 1984 researchers at Moorfields Eye Hospital, London, and Chattisgarh Eye Hospital in India reported a previously unknown link between severe dehydration caused by diarrhea and the development of eye cataracts (◆ page 50). This discovery may account for the puzzlingly high incidence of cataract in a number of developing countries.

Polluted water supplies
In 1854 an English anesthetist John Snow (1813-1858) demanded that the handle be removed from the public water pump in Broad Street, London. A cholera outbreak then raging had caused 500 deaths in ten days in one small area alone. Making house-to-house enquiries, Snow realized that all the victims had collected their drinking water from the same pump. So the handle was disconnected – and a few days later the epidemic abated. Something similar, though on a larger scale, happened in 1971, when cholera swept through West Africa. Although the outbreak seemed indiscriminate, researchers at the Zaria University Hospital, Nigeria, found that the victims' addresses were not randomly distributed throughout the city. Most of the patients came from the old city and the majority of those had been using well rather than tap water. The authorities chlorinated the infected wells, and immediately the epidemic declined.

A cup of cholera
The importance of factors other than specific microbes in causing disease was demonstrated dramatically by the German epidemiologist Max von Pettenkofer (1818-1901) and the Russian pathologist Elie Metchnikoff (1845-1916). Both were unconvinced by claims from the pioneer German bacteriologist Robert Koch (1843-1910) that Vibrio cholerae was the confirmed agent of cholera (◆ page 142). So they drank cultures teeming with this organism, taken from patients with the disease. They developed mild diarrhea and had enormous numbers of the bacteria in their feces – but did not succumb to cholera. Chance probably played a part in the outcome – few if any pathogens cause disease in 100 percent of infected individuals. Nutrition was certainly important – well-fed middle-class doctors are far less vulnerable to a disease such as cholera than are malnourished Asians. Individuals may also have enjoyed inbuilt resistance, of the sort associated with HLA antigens (◆ page 32).

Oral rehydration therapy, developed in the 1970s, has reduced cholera mortality to 1 percent

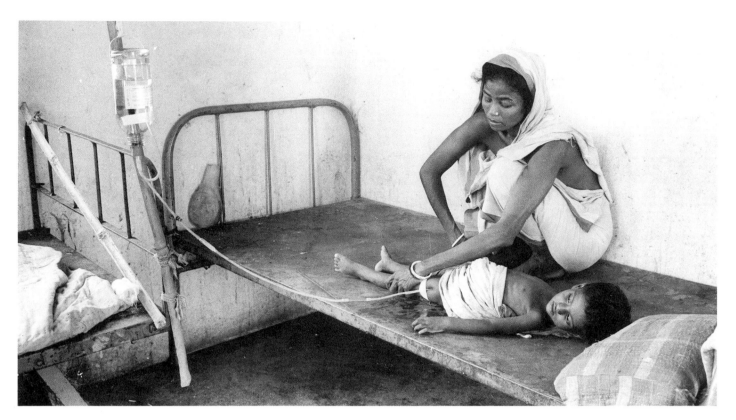

Cholera and its treatment

Pathogens responsible for diarrheal disease include *Vibrio cholerae*, the agent of cholera, plus a wide range of other bacteria and viruses. All are transmitted via food and water contaminated by feces from individuals suffering from the condition, by those of animals, and also by fecal organisms carried by flies. This explains why the problem is so much greater in the Third World than in developed countries with safe water, sewage disposal and food hygiene. The organisms provoke diarrhea by producing toxins (poisons). These make the intestinal tract excrete huge quantities of fluid carrying vital salts.

Dehydration, potentially fatal within a few hours, used to be treated with antibiotics and liquids infused into a vein. But the 1970s saw the advent of oral rehydration therapy (ORT). First employed on a large scale among refugees during the 1971 India-Pakistani war, it reduced mortality from 30 to 1 percent. It is simple to use and (in principle at least) widely available. Patients drink water containing sodium and potassium chloride plus glucose (to help the sick intestine absorb the salts) and sodium bicarbonate (baking soda) to combat acidosis.

Cholera has a very short incubation period between infection and the onset of symptoms – sometimes only a few hours. A comparatively mild illness may ensue, but many victims develop a devastating illness, becoming rapidly dehydrated by vomiting and passing profuse "rice water stools". The bacteria adhere to the microvilli in the intestine. There they generate a toxin which also attaches to cells lining the intestinal wall, activating an enzyme that causes them to excrete water and salts. Losing 15-20 liters of fluid per day, victims develop shrivelled skin and sunken eyes. In addition to ORT, tetracycline reduces fluid loss by reducing the number of infecting organisms. Immunization is short-lived and incomplete, though new, genetically-engineered vaccines promise to give far greater protection. The primary defense will remain good sanitation and hygiene.

▲ *A child with cholera used to be treated by intravenous drip; in poor regions such treatment was prohibitively expensive, and the discovery in 1971 of oral rehydration therapy (ORT) greatly simplified treatment for the disease.*

▼ *Clean water and adequate sanitation is essential to reduce the incidence of intestinal infections in the world.*

Clean Water

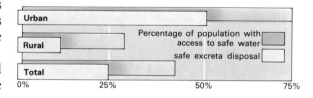

Urban

Rural

Total

Percentage of population with access to safe water

safe excreta disposal

0% 25% 50% 75%

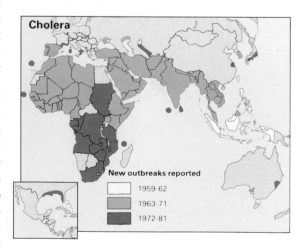

Cholera

New outbreaks reported

1959-62
1963-71
1972-81

▲ *The modern El Tor cholera epidemic originated in South-East Asia in the early 1960s and spread quickly through South Asia and North Africa by 1971. Since 1978 its progress seems to have been halted.*

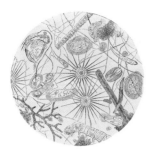

▲ *A 19th-century illustration of the micro-organisms living in drinking water. The discovery that cholera was a disease contracted from micro-organisms in the water rather than from fumes made possible effective preventive action.*

▼ *"The Grim Reaper rowing his boat down the River Thames", a comment from "Punch" magazine on the cholera epidemic in London in 1858. The epidemic of the 1840s and 1850s led to a wholesale reorganization of the capital's water and sewerage systems.*

The ebbs and flows of cholera

Historically, cholera has occurred as a succession of great global waves. The seventh, most recent, pandemic (worldwide epidemic) began during 1961 in Indonesia. It has since spread to Southeast and Southern Asia, the Middle East, west and east Africa, southern Europe, the Far East and western Pacific, and the USA. Caused by the El Tor strain of "Vibrio cholerae" (after El Tor Quarantine Camp in the Sinai where the strain was first isolated), it has largely displaced the previous, classical cholera in India, where the disease has long been endemic (permanently established). Throughout the world there are now some 80,000 new cases of cholera a year.

Man is the only host for the comma-shaped bacterium. Given that the bacterium can survive in water for long periods, even shellfish can be a source of infection. Sporadic incidents also show that, contrary to expectations, the organism is able to establish itself in developed countries and that outbreaks can occur there, given a relaxation in sanitation. Cholera occurs occasionally along the Texas Gulf coast, for example. In 1981 there were 14 cases on an oil rig there among men who had eaten rice rinsed in canal water containing sewage. In 1973 there were 278 cases and 25 deaths in Naples, thought to be the result of contaminated mussels.

Food preparation and infection

Preventive measures can eliminate dangerous organisms, or prevent them growing, in food and water, and adequate cooking kills those in foodstuffs that may be contaminated. Chlorination destroys residual bacteria, already reduced to low levels by filtration, before water is put into the supply system. Milk is pasteurized by being held at 63°C for half an hour, or "flash" treated at a higher temperature for a shorter time. As with boiling to cleanse polluted water, this obliterates intestinal pathogens but not all bacteria.

Techniques which prevent microbes from proliferating, rather than destroy them, include freezing and refrigeration, pickling, smoking, drying, salting and the inclusion of artificial preservatives. Canned food is sterilized to kill all organisms except the most rugged spore-formers. Tomatoes, rhubarb and other acid-containing foods become sterile when heated to lower temperatures for shorter times than, for example, meat or beans. Meat is invariably slightly contaminated at the slaughter-house and must be kept chilled before being cooked for long enough to destroy any pathogens. Particular care is necessary with poultry, which may carry salmonellae. Shellfish are often heavily infected, although oysters offered for sale raw are usually cleansed in clean chlorinated water for some days beforehand.

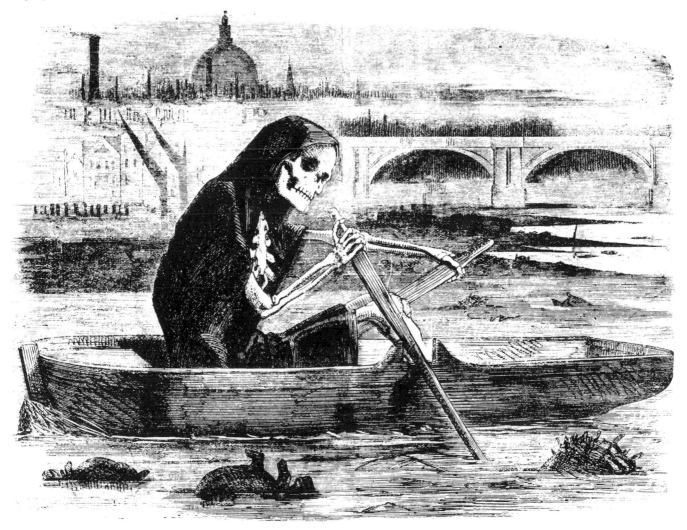

Modern Drugs

BODY SYSTEM	MAIN USES	DRUG GROUPS	TYPICAL DRUG	MODE OF ACTION	
Central nervous system	Pain	Salicylates	Aspirin	Blocks prostaglandins which cause pain, fever and inflammation	
	Severe pain	Opiates	Morphine	Blocks pain receptors in brain	
	Anxiety and insomnia	Benzodiapazepines	Diazepam	Blocks brain receptors	
	Depression	Monoamine oxidase inhibitors	Isocarboxazid	Blocks mood enzymes	
		Tricyclics	Amitriptyline	Uncertain; boosts mood chemicals	
	Epilepsy	Barbiturates	Phenobarbitone	Blocks convulsions via brain neurons	
		Hydantoins	Phenytoin	As above	
	Parkinsonism	Dopaminergic	Levodopa	Affects nerve transmission	
Endocrine	Diabetes	Hormone	Insulin	Reduces blood sugar	
	Growth failure	Hormone	Growth hormone	Replaces deficient hormone	
	Hypothyroidism	Hormone	Thyroxine	Replaces missing hormone	
	Hyperthyroidism	Hormone	Radioactive iodine	Destroys part of thyroid	
	Contraception	Hormone	Estrogen/progesterone	Prevents ovulation	
			Progesterone only	Thickens cervical mucus to prevent sperm reaching egg; may also prevent ovulation	
	Menopause	Hormone	Estrogen/progesterone	Restores female hormone balance	
Joints	Arthritis	Non-steroidal anti-inflammatory drugs	Many	Reduces pain and inflammation	
		Steroids	Prednisolone	As above	
			Gold, penicillamine	Tries to halt disease	
Skin	Acne	Antiseptics	Many	Helps to clean skin	
		Antibiotics	Many	Kills bacteria	
		Keratolytics	Many	Peels off skin	
		Hormones	Cyproterone acetate		
		Steroids	Methylprednisolone	Reduces inflammation	
	Psoriasis	As above	Dithranol		
Digestive tract	Indigestion	Antacids	Many	Neutralizes excess acid production	
	Ulcers	H2 receptor blockers	Cimetidine	Prevents excess acid production	
	Constipation	Laxatives	Methylcellulose	Increases fecal bulk	
			Senna	Stimulates bowel movement	
			Liquid paraffin	Softens feces	
Cardiovascular	Hypertension	Beta blockers	Propranolol	Blocks heart receptors	
		Diuretics	Thiazides	Reduces blood volume and dilates arteries	
		ACE inhibitors	Captopril	Blocks kidney enzyme which affects blood pressure	
		Calcium blockers	Nifedipine	Blocks calcium movement across arterial wall	
Immune system	Allergies	Mast cell stabilizers	Sodium cromoglycate	Prevents overactivity of immune cells to outside allergens	
		Bronchodilators	Salbutamol	Relaxes lung passages in asthma	
		Corticosteroids	Prednisolone	Suppresses immune cells	
	Infections	Antibiotics	Ampicillin, Tetracycline, Sulfonamide, Cephalosporins	Attacks bacteria; drug used depends on causative organism	
		Anti-virals	Amantidine, Acyclovir. Idoxuridine	Attacks viruses; drug used depends on virus type	
		Vaccines	Many	Protects against infection by boosting immunity	
Cells	Cancer	Alkylating agents	Cyclophosphamide	Interferes with cell division	
		Anti-metabolites	Methotrexate	Interferes with cell chemical function	
		Cytotoxic antibiotics	Doxorubicin	Interferes with cell replication and protein synthesis	
		Alkaloids	Vincristine	Halts cell division	
General	Colds	Antipyretics	Aspirin	Reduce temperature	
		Decongestants	Phenylephrine	Unblocks sinuses	
	Coughs	Suppressants	Codeine	Suppresses cough	
		Expectorants	Ipecacuanha	No scientific evidence that they work	
	Vitamins	Single groups of A,B,C, D and E, or combined		Correct deficiencies where diet is poor, or for young children, pregnant women or elderly	

SIDE EFFECTS *	OTHER USES	MARKET SIZE	FUTURE	MISCELLANEOUS
Stomach irritant	Arthritis	Enormous	Stomach problems may reduce use	Better to use soluble aspirin or paracetamol if stomach problems occur
Addiction, constipation, nausea		Stable; only for specific uses	Stable unless non-addictive drugs of same potency developed	
Tolerance, addiction	Epilepsy, major psychotic illness	Enormous	Market likely to decline because of side-effects	Patients should always withdraw slowly from these drugs
Interacts with some foods		Stable		
Dry mouth, sedation		Stable	Use likely to continue unless alternative drugs with fewer side effects developed	
Addiction	Severe insomnia	Decreasing	Declining because of addiction	
Nausea, vomiting		Stable	Stable	Dose has to be tailored carefully to patients
Nausea, insomnia		Stable	May be superseded by more specific drugs	Drug effectiveness decreases with time
Local skin reactions and hypersensitivity		Increasing	Greater use of human insulin to avoid hypersensitivity to animal insulins	
As above		Small	Severe shortages likely to be overcome by use of genetic engineering	
As above		Small		
As above		Small		
Circulatory problems, nausea, weight gain		Large	Stable until safer methods such as vaccines developed	
As above		Smaller		More risk of failure than combined pills but useful for breast feeding women
As above		Growing	Likely to increase	
Indigestion, stomach irritation	Pain	Enormous	Stable until more effective drugs found	
Various, including reduced immunity	Allergies, suppression of transplant rejection	Large		Should be avoided in children because growth is stunted
Severe blood disorders		Small	As above	
		Large		
Overuse of steroids can lead to scarring of the skin				
		Large	Decreasing as some antacids are unnecessary	
Rashes		Enormous	Growing as more cimetidine-like drugs are developed	
Wind, diarrhea		Large	May decrease as people increase their dietary fiber intake	
Nausea, tiredness, vivid dreams, slow heart beat, hypotension	Angina, abnormal heart beat, migraine, acute anxiety	Enormous	May be superseded by ACE inhibitors and calcium blockers	Should never be taken by asthmatics; may have value in preventing heart attacks
Lowers potassium	Reduces edema	Very large	As above	
Nausea, rash, blood disorders	Heart failure	Potentially large	Could take over market if side effects kept down	
Nausea, vomiting, slow heart beat	Heart beat abnormalities, angina	Potentially large	Could have important future role; full potential unknown	
Throat irritation	Rhinitis	Large	Enormous potential with discovery of related chemicals, leukotrienes	
Tremor		Large	Likely to decrease if leukotrienes successful	
Various, including reduced immunity		Large	Likely to decrease for treatment of allergies	
Sensitivity reactions to penicillins		Enormous	Antibiotics becoming increasingly specific but resistance problems mean need for continuing development	
Various		Growing	Enormous potential if more effective drugs developed	
Hypersensitivity		Large	Huge potential if new vaccines can be developed	
Various, from nausea and vomiting to hair loss and major blood disorders		Growing	Enormous potential markets for anti-cancer drugs but unlikely to be a single "cure-all"	
Stomach irritation		Enormous	Continuing large as people seek symptoms relief	
Possible toxicity with large doses of Vitamin A		Enormous	Levelling off and possibly declining because of continuing controversy over supplements for people with balanced diet	

*Side effects are not to be expected in all cases.

Salmonella infections

There are many species of *Salmonella* that cause intestinal infections and diarrhea of varying degrees of severity. These infections are increasingly untreatable because they are caused by strains resistant to antibiotics. In London, scientists at the Central Public Health Laboratory monitored the rise in resistance during the 1970s, and in 1980 announced that all strains of the predominant *Salmonella typhimurium*, causing gastroenteritis, had become insensitive to at least one drug. Some were resistant to six or more antibiotics. The picture is similar in the USA and indeed most parts of the world. Particularly high level of resistance are found in countries, such as those of South America, where people can buy antibiotics across the counter without prescription. It is a paradox of modern medicine that the power of these lifesaving drugs is being reduced considerably as a result of excessive, indiscriminate use. That means that correspondingly more emphasis must now be placed on the importance of preventive action via hygiene and adequate cooking – a need underlined by surveys showing that foods such as sausages are often contaminated with salmonellae.

The agent of typhoid fever

Antibiotic resistance is particularly serious in *Salmonella typhi*. This, the most virulent of all species, is the agent of typhoid fever. Historically a scourge of armies, it killed over 8,000 British troops during the Boer War (compared with 7,500 killed in battle). Nowadays, like cholera, typhoid fever occurs mostly in countries with inadequate sanitation. Elsewhere it causes sporadic epidemics, often originating with organisms brought home by holidaymakers. The organism differs from *V. cholerae* in invading cells lining the gut, sometimes migrating further from there. As many as 80 percent of infected people have only mild symptoms, but the rest develop a potentially lethal infection. During the first week, as bacteria penetrate the gut wall and reach the lymphatic vessels, the victim suffers from fever, malaise and general aches and pains. In the second week, there is diarrhea, delerium and a fever of around 40°C as organisms invade the bloodstream and gall bladder. The third week brings either an improvement or complications such as severe bleeding and perforation of the intestine. Although secondary, person-to-person spread is uncommon, about three percent of those who recover become "healthy carriers", harboring the bacteria in their gall bladder and being capable of transmitting them to others. "Typhoid Mary", a cook in the New York area, caused at least six outbreaks between 1901 and 1907 – one of which may have affected 1,300 people.

Before antibiotics were available, typhoid fever killed about 10 percent of patients. The death rate among those given chloramphenicol is now one percent or less. This is why the emergence of chloramphenicol-resistant strains of the typhoid bacillus in Mexico during the early 1970s greatly alarmed bacteriologists. Around 1974, they infected some 100,000 individuals, killing 14,000 of them. Typhoid fever could again be a major danger if such strains were to proliferate around the world. The possibility of *S. typhi* and other salmonellae becoming insensitive to more drugs is increased by the fact that resistance can be transferred between such species, and even between them and both harmful and harmless strains of *E. coli*. As with cholera, vaccines against typhoid fever and the associated paratyphoid fever afford only limited protection and may well be supplanted by more effective versions made by genetic engineering.

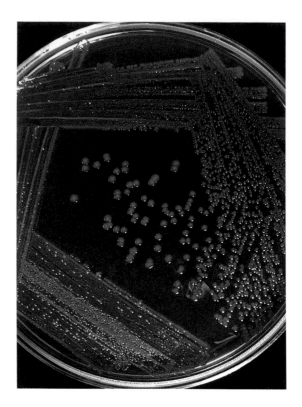

▲ *Salmonella typhi, the agent of typhoid fever, is shown here growing in a laboratory culture. Resistance to the disease may be raised somewhat by vaccination with dead typhoid bacilli. Paratyphoid fever is an infectious diarrheal disease caused by related bacteria, found in temperate and tropical regions. Its symptoms are similar to, though less virulent than, those of typhoid fever.*

Typhoid fever in Aberdeen

Beginning on 12 May 1964, an increasing number of people in Aberdeen, Scotland, went down with what seemed to be gastroenteritis. Four days later one of them was sufficiently ill to be admitted to hospital, where tests revealed Salmonella typhi as the culprit. All the victims were then promptly isolated in hospital and treated for typhoid fever, while public health staff began to seek the source of the outbreak. Enquiries about foods the patients had eaten soon cast suspicions on a dairy, an ice-cream shop and a supermarket. Further cross-comparisons eliminated the first two, and led to the cold meat department of the supermarket, from which three-quarters of the individuals had purchased corned beef. Bacteriologists from the Central Public Health Laboratory in London then confirmed that a six-pound can of this meat, sold in the store, contained S. typhi – and that it was a strain virtually unknown in Great Britain. By tracing the can to its origin, they deduced that the bacterium had entered through a faulty seal while the can was being cooled with sewage-containing water at the manufacturing plant in Argentina. The final toll in the Aberdeen epidemic was 507 cases, and three elderly patients died. Chloramphenicol treatment, seizure of the suspect food, a vigorous campaign to promote public hygiene and the speedy tracing and testing of 4,200 contacts of affected persons, together ensured that those figures were not considerably higher.

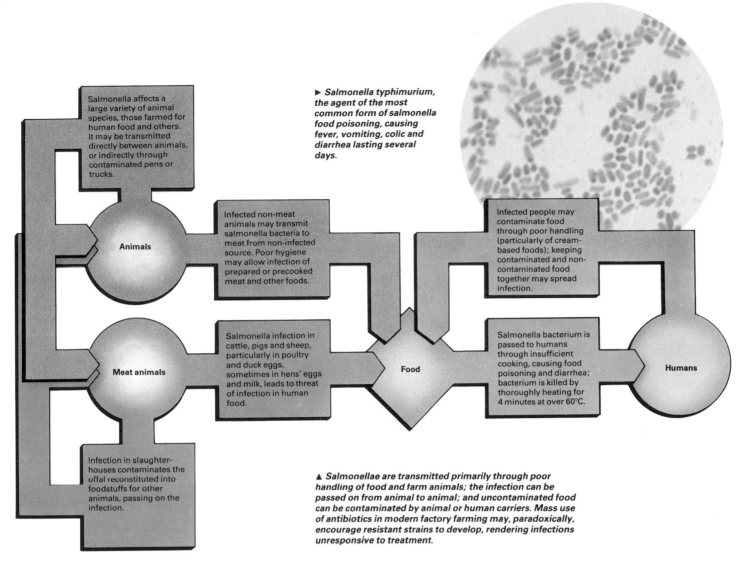

Salmonella affects a large variety of animal species, those farmed for human food and others. It may be transmitted directly between animals, or indirectly through contaminated pens or trucks.

▶ *Salmonella typhimurium, the agent of the most common form of salmonella food poisoning, causing fever, vomiting, colic and diarrhea lasting several days.*

Animals

Infected non-meat animals may transmit salmonella bacteria to meat from non-infected source. Poor hygiene may allow infection of prepared or precooked meat and other foods.

Infected people may contaminate food through poor handling (particularly of cream-based foods); keeping contaminated and non-contaminated food together may spread infection.

Meat animals

Salmonella infection in cattle, pigs and sheep, particularly in poultry and duck eggs, sometimes in hens' eggs and milk, leads to threat of infection in human food.

Food

Salmonella bacterium is passed to humans through insufficient cooking, causing food poisoning and diarrhea; bacterium is killed by thoroughly heating for 4 minutes at over 60°C.

Humans

Infection in slaughter-houses contaminates the offal reconstituted into foodstuffs for other animals, passing on the infection.

▲ *Salmonellae are transmitted primarily through poor handling of food and farm animals; the infection can be passed on from animal to animal; and uncontaminated food can be contaminated by animal or human carriers. Mass use of antibiotics in modern factory farming may, paradoxically, encourage resistant strains to develop, rendering infections unresponsive to treatment.*

Gastroenteritis

In addition to V. cholerae, closely related bacteria such as V. parahaemolyticus, and unrelated ones such as Campylobacter jejeuni also cause considerable amounts of diarrheal disease in the Third World. Other causes are certain strains of Escherichia coli, that usually live without harm in the intestine. Such "wolves in sheeps' clothing" can produce toxins similar to, but milder than, those of cholera. Along with various species of Shigella (responsible for different versions of dysentery) and of Salmonella, these micro-organisms also cause "traveler's diarrhea" and a variety of food poisoning found in developed countries.

Unlike bacteria which produce conditions like botulism (♦ page 238) by making poisons in food before it is eaten, these organisms cause gastroenteritis by colonizing the intestinal tract. The damage they do there is associated with two types of poison. Endotoxins are parts of the bacterial cell wall, which cause fever and shock. Exotoxins, like that of cholera, are excreted by the organisms and provoke diarrhea. Most of these bacteria do not just adhere to the gut wall. They also penetrate the gut lining, particularly in the colon. Salmonellae can invade even deeper tissues.

Rotaviruses, first detected in humans in 1973, are another cause of gastroenteritis in both the developed and developing world, where they are particularly common among young children. They

do not produce toxins, but invade and destroy cells lining the small intestine.

The symptoms of enteritis can be combated by substances ranging from kaolin (which absorbs water) to morphine (which reduces the heightened activity of the lower intestine as it seeks to expel its contents). In severe cases – particularly in the very young and the very old – treatment with antibiotics may be required. But these will be ineffective if the illness is caused by a virus or by one of the increasingly common strains of resistant bacteria.

Various species of Salmonella were once thought to be by far the commonest causes of food poisoning in the USA and Europe. Since the early 1970s, however, they have begun to be rivalled by strains of Campylobacter jejeuni. The disease can be very unpleasant, with explosive diarrhea, offensive watery stools and pain so severe as to suggest appendicitis. Although deaths have occurred in elderly people, the infection usually clears up even before a diagnosis can be made. C. jejeuni occurs commonly in pigs and less often in cattle, dogs and cats, but the sources of human outbreaks are seldom pinpointed. A few incidents have been traced to meat, unpasteurized milk and contaminated water. Campylobacters are destroyed by heat at least as readily as other food-poisoning bacteria. Campylobacters are not yet known to manufacture toxins, but researchers in Australia, Great Britain and Holland suggested in 1984 that they may be responsible for peptic ulcers.

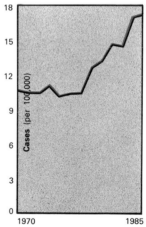

▲ *The cause of the dramatically increased incidence of salmonellosis in the USA is unknown: up to 1977, almost half of those affected were under the age of five, but since that date most sufferers have been in an older age group. Many Salmonella bacteria are now resistant to antibiotics.*

Parasites and the human host

The human intestinal tract is invaded by several organisms larger than bacteria. One is the ameba *Entamoeba histolytica*. Passed in the stools of people with amebiasis, the amebae are ingested in food or water and take up residence in the large intestine. Digesting cells to provide food, they reproduce and sometimes travel to the liver and elsewhere. Symptoms vary from trivial to severe. At its worst there is profuse diarrhea and considerable pain caused by abscesses in the liver. Amebiasis occurs throughout the world but is particularly common in Southeast Asia, Africa and Mexico. Treatment with drugs such as Terramycin is designed to relieve symptoms and to eliminate the parasites – which is less easily achieved than when using antibiotics to destroy bacteria.

Giardia lamblia is a protozoon which, like *Entamoeba*, occurs in developing countries. But it has also caused major outbreaks of giardiasis in the USSR and smaller ones in the USA during recent years. The parasites are transmitted through water (which, because they resist chlorination, must be filtered to remove them). Using two adhesive disks for attachment, they too colonize the small intestine and occasionally the gall bladder. Infected individuals may be virtually free of symptoms, or suffer recurrent pain and diarrhea, which can lead to weight loss and dehydration. Atabrine is an effective cure. *Giardia* is arguably the first pathogen ever seen by man – the Dutch microscopist Anton van Leeuwenhoek (1632-1723) observed it in his own stools.

The largest residents

Worms are the largest creatures to take up residence in the human gut. The World Health Organization estimates that a quarter of the planet's population is infected by the large roundworm *Ascaris lumbricoides*. It lives in the small intestine, laying eggs which are passed out and swallowed in food or water – sometimes after they have survived for several years in moist soil. The infection (which is easily cured by antihelminthic drugs) often causes no symptoms and comes to light only when the worms travel farther afield than the intestine and appear in the lungs, are vomited up from the stomach or pop out of the nose.

Tapeworms inhabit many millions of human bodies as well as using other animals as intermediary hosts. They are composed of head (with suckers to stick to the intestine), neck and a sequence of segments. They have sex organs and simple digestive and nervous systems. Five to ten meters in length and living for several years, discharging eggs continuously, the beef tapeworm (*Taenia saginata*) does much less damage than might be expected, producing only vague symptoms. The larvae of the pork tapeworm *Taenia solium* (which does not occur in the USA) sometimes causes serious injury in the eyes and brain. Tapeworms, which are acquired initially from uncooked meat, can be removed by Atabrine and purgation, usually being expelled intact.

Whipworms (500 million people affected worldwide) and hookworms (900 million people) are the other main groups of intestinal worms. The latter, which can enter through the skin as well as the gut, are now rare in developed countries, though whipworms still occur there among people with poor environmental hygiene. Threadworms are comparatively common in children's colons in Western countries. They seldom cause anything worse than anal irritation, although they may stimulate appendicitis.

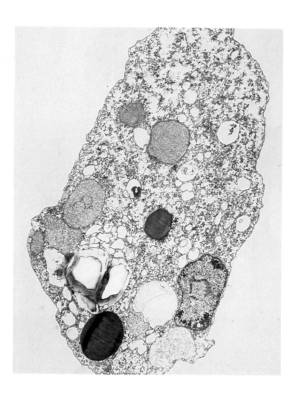

▲ *Entamoeba histolytica causes amebic dysentery when the protozoon penetrates the lining of the colon. In addition to pain and diarrhea, ulcers may develop in the colon, and amebic abcesses occur in the liver. The disease may take months to appear, and people can carry and transmit the disease without showing symptoms themselves. The ameba is destroyed by heat, so boiled water is safe to drink.*

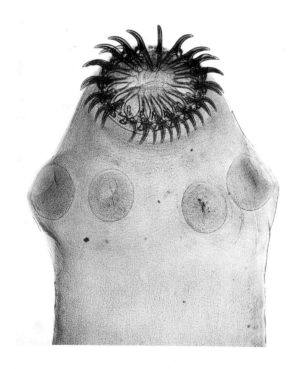

▲ *The head of the pork tapeworm, Taenia solium, carries large suckers as well as rows of hooks to enable it to anchor on the wall of the intestine. Such worms are segmented, and new segments develop continuously near the head. Up to ten segments break away daily, releasing eggs which are discharged in the host's feces, or entering the bloodstream to become established in other tissues.*

*Moving food, gases and nutrients round the body...
The heart, arteries and veins...Blood, its constituents
and functions...The lymphatic system...The lungs and
breathing.. Oxygen and fuel for the tissues...Expelling
gaseous and solid wastes...PERSPECTIVE ...William
Harvey...Early ideas about the circulation of blood...
The composition of blood...Alveoli, interfaces between
air and blood...Studying the structure of hemoglobin*

Transport in the body is almost entirely involuntary – the heart beats, blood vessels contract, we breathe in and out and food moves through the gut without our thinking about these processes.

Pumping blood

The heart is made of involuntary muscle, consisting of single-cell fibers that contract together. However, unlike all other forms of involuntary muscle, heart muscle looks striped under the microscope because the molecules actin and myosin are arranged in groups of sliding filaments like those of voluntary muscle (◀ page 103). The fibers are not parallel with each other, as in both other kinds of muscle, but branching. They form two separate networks – one in the upper heart chambers, the two atria, and the other in the lower two chambers, called ventricles. When a single fiber of either network contracts, all the other fibers in the network do so with it. The heart contracts about 70-75 times a minute. It beats less often in athletes, who have larger hearts as a result of training. Different kinds of nerve stimulation make the heart beat faster or slower (◀ page 55). After each contraction there is a pause, the refractory period, before another can occur.

Adult or child, a person's heart is about the size of their fist and lies at the front of the chest, slightly to the left. It is a blunt cone, with enormous arteries and veins entering and leaving. A surrounding bag containing watery fluid (pericardium) prevents it from rubbing adjacent organs. The atria receive blood and the ventricles pump it out. The atria are separate from each other, as are the ventricles, but each atrium is connected to the ventricle below by a one-way valve. The mitral valve (shaped like a bishop's mitre) is on the left side, and the tricuspid valve (with three cusps) on the right.

The heartbeat is a two-fold sound, lubb-dupp-pause, lubb-dupp-pause, which can be heard by placing your ear against someone's chest. Muscle contraction is silent – the sound is the turbulence in flow caused by the valves closing. The first sound is the valves from the atria slamming shut when the ventricles contract, forcing blood out to the body. Almost immediately comes the second sound, the closing of the outlet valves from the ventricles. When the ventricles have emptied, their pressure is correspondingly low, so blood is drawn passively into them from the atria. Blood leaves the heart through arteries, which have thick, elastic, muscular walls that widen when blood is forced into them and then contract automatically, pushing it onwards. Blood returns to the heart through veins. Because the pressure in veins is lower – the blood has traveled a long way since it left the heart, and its pressure drops progressively – they have thin walls that offer little resistance to the blood entering them. Because returning blood often flows upwards, the main veins of the arms, legs and trunk have valves to prevent backflow caused by gravity.

William Harvey and the circulation of blood

It seems extraordinary that people ever believed that blood did not circulate through the body. However, before the 17th century, doctors imagined that blood was formed in the liver from food and nourished the tissues by absorption like water seeping into earth. Arteries conveyed vital spirits (conveyed with the air from the lungs) which turned blue into red blood, and this animated the tissues. The English physician William Harvey (1578-1657), educated at Cambridge and Padua (Europe's greatest medical school at the time), dissected dead and living animals and found that veins permitted blood to travel only to the heart, and that arteries allowed blood only to leave it. Therefore the blood must circulate, rather than being completely absorbed. He also discovered what the two elements of the heart sound were, and showed that the ventricles refilled passively. Harvey was elected a Fellow of the College of Physicians at the age of 30. Seven years later, when chosen by the College to deliver the Lumleian lectures on anatomy and physiology, he presented his ideas and they found wide favor. Five years later he published his famous treatise on circulation.

In his later years Harvey became physician to Charles I, regularly demonstrating the circulation of the blood to the Court. At the start of the Civil War, when he was traveling with the King, Cromwell's supporters burned his house and destroyed manuscripts.

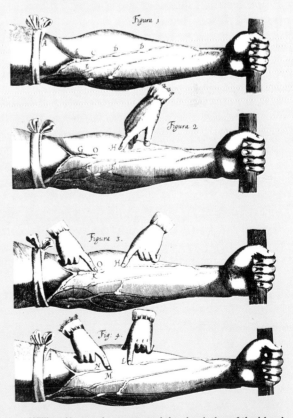

▲ *William Harvey demonstrated the circulation of the blood by showing that an obstruction to a vein in the forearm stopped the flow of blood back towards the elbow and not to the wrist, as had previously been assumed. Galen had taught that venous blood was produced in the liver, and that it nourished the organs and limbs.*

It was not until the 16th century that the passage of blood to the lungs was discovered

The heart

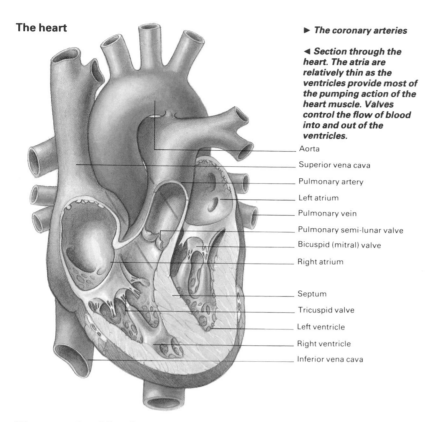

▶ *The coronary arteries*

◀ *Section through the heart. The atria are relatively thin as the ventricles provide most of the pumping action of the heart muscle. Valves control the flow of blood into and out of the ventricles.*

- Aorta
- Superior vena cava
- Pulmonary artery
- Left atrium
- Pulmonary vein
- Pulmonary semi-lunar valve
- Bicuspid (mitral) valve
- Right atrium
- Septum
- Tricuspid valve
- Left ventricle
- Right ventricle
- Inferior vena cava

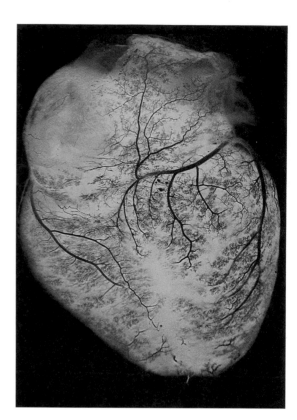

Transporting blood

Blood circulates around the body in a figure-of-eight pattern. Arriving from the lungs with a fresh supply of oxygen, it passes through the heart's left side to the rest of the body. When it returns, carrying carbon dioxide, it goes through the right side of the heart and back to the lungs.

Circulation is different before birth. Because the lungs, kidneys and digestive systems have not started functioning, nutrients and waste products are exchanged through capillaries in the mother's placenta (◆ page 184). Branches from the leg arteries carry waste products (including carbon dioxide) to the placenta, and a vein carries food and oxygen back via the liver to the lower vena cava. The liver also is supplied with blood through a special duct from the aorta, the main vessel from the heart to the body. This means that oxygenated blood from the placenta mingles with deoxygenated blood from the rest of the body before entering the right atrium. Between the two atria is a large opening. Two-thirds of the blood passes through it, going straight to the body instead of the lungs. At birth the vessels connecting the placenta to the baby (and the baby's aorta to its liver) wither. The hole between the atria closes (except in hole-in-the-heart babies, who need an operation to close the orifice).

Arteries leave the heart for the organs, divide into narrower arterioles, and then subdivide into the mesh of tiny capillaries from which oxygen diffuses out, and into which carbon dioxide diffuses in. The capillaries meet up again, forming little veins known as venules which join together to form veins. These leave the organs to return blood to the heart.

Arteries often join with other arteries – and veins with veins – so that some parts of the body receive and send blood along more than one route. Thus, circulation to many tissues continues even if a vessel is blocked by disease or injury.

Early ideas about the circulation of blood
Hippocrates (c. 469-399 BC) and Aristotle (384-322 BC) regarded the heart as the source of blood, blood vessels and an innate heat which caused pulse and heart beat. The physician-anatomist Galen (c. AD 129-199) proved by vivisection that the left ventricle contained blood, but thought that it passed to the right ventricle through invisible pores in the septum. The heart beat propelled blood through the arteries from the left ventricle, while the right allowed waste fumes to leave. The fallacy was first exposed by the Arab physician Ibn an-Nafis (c. 1205-1288), who showed that blood traveled from the right ventricle to the left via the lungs, but his ideas were not assimilated and later were forgotten. Leonardo da Vinci's (1452-1519) anatomical drawings of the heart valves could have helped to dispel the errors of the ancients, but they were privately owned and not widely studied. Andreas Vesalius (1514-1564) noted that the septum between the ventricles appeared impenetrable, but offered no explanation of how blood traveled from the left side of the heart to the right. Michael Servetus (1511-1553) stated that blood coursed from the right of the heart to the left via the lungs, but he was burned for heresy. Later in the same century the tide began to turn: Andreas Cesalpino (1519-1603), who coined the word circulation, stressed the return of venous blood through the veins, and Harvey's teacher at Padua, Fabricius ab Aquapendente (c. 1533-1619) taught that valves in the veins prevented venous blood from rushing downwards. Stephen Hales (1677-1761) measured blood pressure by inserting tubes into the arteries and veins of animals and observed the height to which the blood rose, and its variations with the heartbeat.

Arterio-venous system

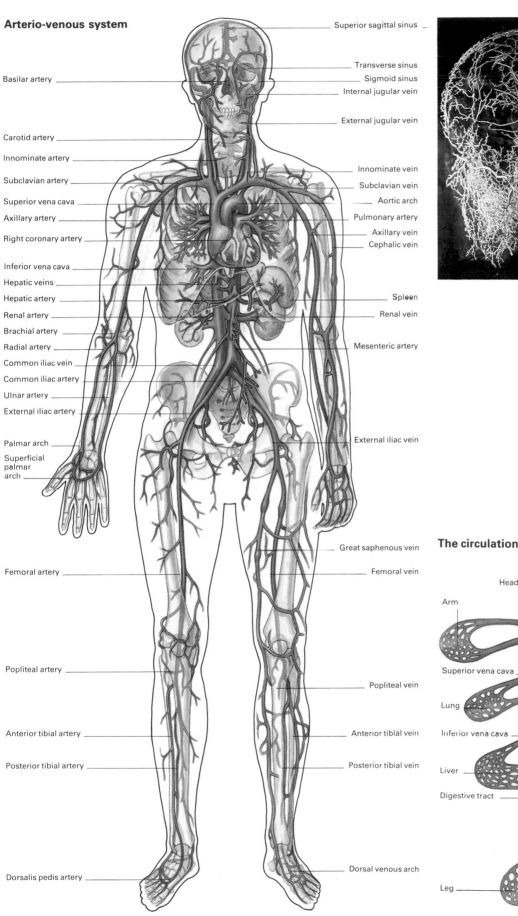

Basilar artery

Carotid artery

Innominate artery

Subclavian artery

Superior vena cava

Axillary artery

Right coronary artery

Inferior vena cava

Hepatic veins

Hepatic artery

Renal artery

Brachial artery

Radial artery

Common iliac vein

Common iliac artery

Ulnar artery

External iliac artery

Palmar arch

Superficial palmar arch

Femoral artery

Popliteal artery

Anterior tibial artery

Posterior tibial artery

Dorsalis pedis artery

Superior sagittal sinus

Transverse sinus

Sigmoid sinus

Internal jugular vein

External jugular vein

Innominate vein

Subclavian vein

Aortic arch

Pulmonary artery

Axillary vein

Cephalic vein

Spleen

Renal vein

Mesenteric artery

External iliac vein

Great saphenous vein

Femoral vein

Popliteal vein

Anterior tibial vein

Posterior tibial vein

Dorsal venous arch

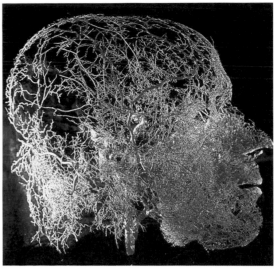

▲ *The face, head and brain have an elaborate and rich supply of blood vessels.*

▼ *The flow of blood around the body. Blood is taken by the pulmonary artery, to the lungs, where it is oxygenated and returned to the left side of the heart to be pumped via arteries to the organs and muscles. There it deposits oxygen and returns via the veins to the right side of the heart. Blood from the gut travels via the liver, where it deposits many of the nutrients it has absorbed.*

The circulation of the blood

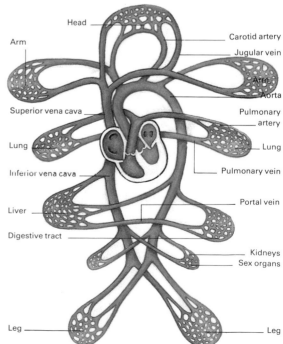

Head

Arm

Superior vena cava

Lung

Inferior vena cava

Liver

Digestive tract

Leg

Carotid artery

Jugular vein

Arm

Aorta

Pulmonary artery

Lung

Pulmonary vein

Portal vein

Kidneys

Sex organs

Leg

All the blood in the body passes through the heart every minute

Blood – quantity and quality

Though blood is a remarkable fluid which carries out many functions of transport in the body, its quantity is even more important than its quality. Even if we bleed heavily, the red blood cells and other cargo (gases, digested food, salts, proteins, hormones and waste products) are all eventually replenished; but a sheer lack of volume of blood can be fatal if it is not treated quickly.

There are four to five liters of blood in a woman and five to six liters in a man, comprising a sixteenth of body weight. More-or-less the total volume leaves the heart every minute during rest. At any moment three of the average five liters are in our veins; one liter is in the lungs, and most of the remaining liter is in the heart, arteries and arterioles – with only a quarter-liter in the capillaries. During exercise, muscles need more oxygen for metabolism, which they get in two ways. The heart's output can increase five-fold by doubling the beat and increasing the volume. (It cannot over-distend because it is enclosed in a fibrous wrapper, the pericardium.) Also, blood is diverted to muscles (including its own muscle, because it is working harder) at the expense of the digestive system and kidneys, which receive only a quarter of their normal quota. The heart supplies blood to itself through two coronary arteries that branch off the aorta.

Blood pressure – measurement and meaning

Blood is pumped out of the heart under sufficient pressure to travel to the organs and back again. Pressure is conventionally measured by the number of millimeters of mercury (mmHg) it would support in a vertical column. In a healthy person's aorta the pressure is about 100mmHg, dropping to 40 in arteries, 25 in arterioles, 12 in capillaries, 8 in venules, and 5 in veins. In the venae cavae (the cavernous veins that return blood to the heart) pressure is 2mmHg, and in the right atrium it is zero. Circulation is helped by exercise, as skeletal muscles contract around the veins, driving blood towards the heart.

Doctors usually measure blood pressure in arm arteries by wrapping an inflatable cuff, attached to a pressure meter, round the upper arm. The cuff is inflated, giving increasing pressure. By listening to the beat through a stethoscope while watching the meter, the operator measures the strength of each beat and the residual pressure (about one-third lower) between beats. The two figures register the person's blood pressure, which in a healthy man aged 20 will be around 120 and 75, usually written as 120/75. Young women are about 115/70. Babies' blood pressure is low; at six months it is 90/60. It increases during growth. In teenagers, blood pressure is related to maturity. Though the figures rise with age, women usually remain lower until the menopause, apart from a rise during pregnancy. Both sexes have an average blood pressure of around 135/85 at 50, rising to 145/80 (men) and 160/85 (women) at 70. The !Kung Bushmen of Botswana do not have this rise, but the reason for this is not known. The reasons may be genetic, dietary, or environmental – they have a tranquil lifestyle. Although difficult to avoid, the rise is undesirable – high blood pressure harms heart, brain and kidneys, and the longest lifespans are found in people whose blood pressure remains below 130/70 between the ages 30-60 (men) and 20-50 (women). Pressure higher than 90, whatever a person's age or sex, needs treatment. The readings are highest in the early evening and lowest during sleep. They can rise temporarily with nervousness (including fear of medical examinations) and during periods of stress (♦ page 166).

Blood cells

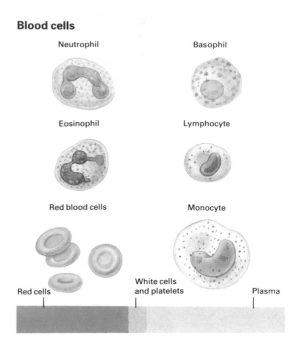

▲ There are five main kinds of white blood cell, which make up 10 percent of the total volume of the blood. Neutrophils and lymphocytes are the most numerous; each has a particular role in the response to infection (♦ page 213). The red blood cells are far more numerous and have the major task of carrying oxygen and carbon dioxide to and from the body tissues. Some 55 percent of the blood volume is plasma, which is mainly water together with proteins and other solutes.

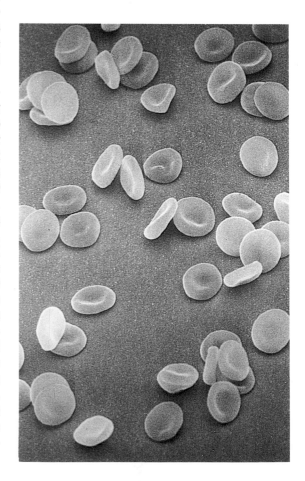

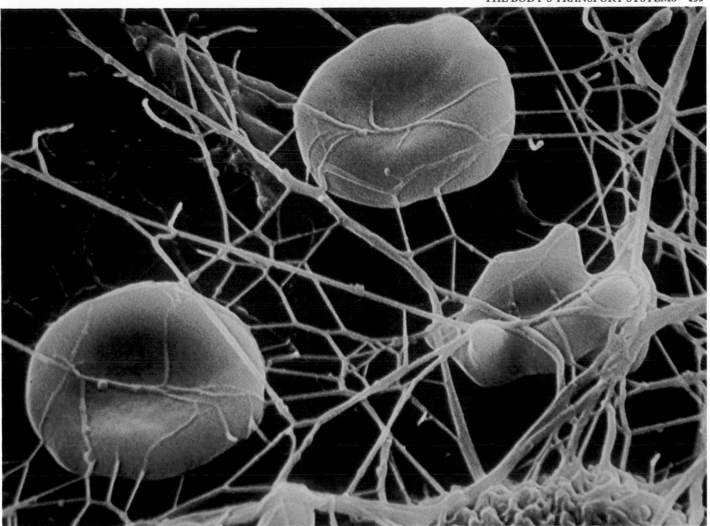

▲ One function of the blood is to clot. This requires fibrinogen, one of the blood's proteins. When a vessel is damaged, platelets collect, stick together and then disintegrate. In doing so they produce thrombin. This converts fibrinogen into fibrin, which is fibrous and holds the red cells into a firm network that obstructs further flow.

◄ The number of red blood cells in the blood can vary: athletes who train at high altitudes develop more than usual. It is possible, as was done by the US cycling team in the 1984 Olympic Games, to have the concentration of red blood cells increased artificially by a blood transfusion.

What blood contains

Blood is three times thicker than water. About half is water containing salts, proteins and cargo, and the rest is red cells, white cells and clotting cells. It ferries oxygen, digested food, hormones and enzymes to cells that need them. It carries unwanted carbon dioxide and other waste products to tissues that dispose of them. It mediates in regulating the acidity and alkalinity of the body. It helps maintain temperature with its water content acting as a heat absorber and cooler. It prevents body-fluid loss through its clotting power. Finally, its white cells attack microbes.

Red cells get their color from the iron in hemoglobin, the chemical that carries oxygen and exchanges it for carbon dioxide (◆ page 158). There are about five million red cells in every microliter of blood. A fall to below four million is usually treated, and women are routinely treated during pregnancy, when the developing baby makes great demands.

Adults' red cells are made in red bone marrow. By the time the cells are mature enough to carry gases and are released into the bloodstream, they have extruded their nuclei, becoming flat disks with thick rims. From the moment they are fully formed, red cells start to die. Their life-span is four months and, to maintain supply, we make two million every second. Old ones are destroyed in the liver and spleen, but hemoglobin molecules are partly reused. In unborn babies the red cells are made in several tissues, including the yolk sac, liver, spleen, and thymus. Fetuses have a different kind of hemoglobin, but switch to making the adult type at birth.

Fighting infection

White cells have nuclei but no hemoglobin. There are five kinds, of two main families, some developing in bone marrow from the same line as red cells, and others from a related line found in marrow and lymph tissue. There are 5,000 per microliter of blood – a thousandth of the number of red cells. Some crawl along the sides of blood vessels by pushing part of themselves forward and then drawing the rest up alongside. Some even creep through the walls of capillaries.

Two of the five kinds of white cells clean up infections, the other three are involved in more specific responses to invasion (◆ page 213). One kind, the basophils, also make an anti-clotting substance, heparin.

Last and smallest of the cells are the platelets, which make blood clot on the surface of a damaged vessel (◆ page 157). Platelets are the shed fragments, wrapped in membrane, of larger parent cells. It may seem odd that in these clotting and anti-clotting agents blood produces substances that oppose each other, but such a balanced system is effective in achieving and maintaining internal stability.

Clotting requires fibrinogen, one of the blood's three main proteins. The other blood proteins are albumin, a substance like thin egg-white, which provides a viscous texture; and the globulins, which include antibodies. When blood clots, a thin straw-colored liquid, serum, eventually separates out. Serum is plasma but without the clotting proteins.

Unlike most bodily functions, breathing can be controlled or can function automatically

The lymphatic system

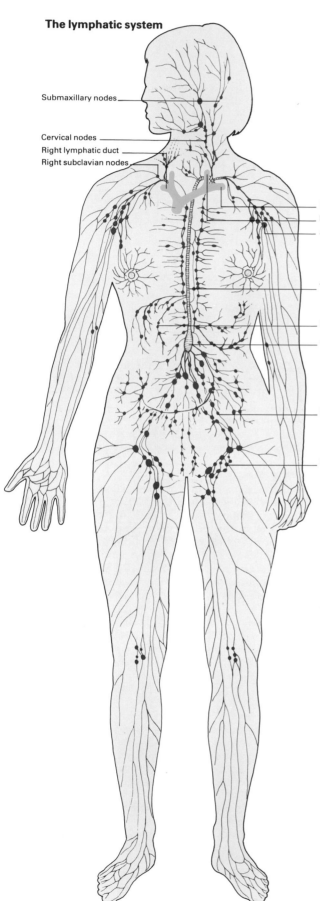

Submaxillary nodes

Cervical nodes
Right lymphatic duct
Right subclavian nodes

Left subclavian vein
Left internal jugular vein
Axillary nodes

Thoracic duct

Intestinal nodes
Cisterna chyli

Iliac nodes

Inguinal nodes

◀ *The lymphatic system drains the entire body, but with particular emphasis on the skin and intestines, where infections could readily enter. The entire system drains into the subclavian veins. Lymph circulation largely depends on activity of the body muscle and skeleton. Many nodes are sited at the knee and elbows, in the groin, along the vertebrae and around the breast.*

Breathing

Diaphragm

▲ *The lungs fill with air when the rib-cage expands and the diaphragm between thorax and abdomen is pulled down. The lungs do not empty completely with an outbreath; the normal flow is known as the tidal volume (often about 500cc); the vital capacity is the amount a person can exhale after taking the deepest breath possible. In a healthy adult this is about 4,500cc.*

Lymph fluid

Plasma and some white cells permeate the spaces between cells over most of the body (the exceptions are brain, spleen and bone marrow). This fluid, lymph, drains into blind-ended lymph vessels, pushed in by the "milking" effect of contracting muscles. It is eventually returned, through a system of lymph vessels, to the vein entering the heart. On the way, lymph passes through solid nodes, which are 1-25mm long (◆ page 215). The nodes in the armpit can be felt and so, sometimes, can those in the groin; other nodes are in the throat – tonsils – and trunk. White cells that live in the nodes remove bacteria, foreign material and cell debris. These white cells are made in the spleen and reach the nodes through special ducts.

Transporting air

Every five seconds we breathe in half a liter of air by moving the voluntary muscles of the diaphragm and ribs. By lowering the diaphragm and expanding certain rib muscles, pressure in the chest is lowered, and air is drawn in through the nose. Here it is filtered by the nostril hairs. The cavity behind the nose, which contains smell receptors at the top, is ridged to give a large surface area. Air is warmed by its plentiful capillary supply (the source of nose-bleeds), and moistened by its mucus. Tears draining from the eye help moisten air and mucus, which covers the ridges and traps fine dust particles that have passed the nostril hairs. The mucus-dust packages are passed down the throat by cilia and coughed out. During speech and when the nose is blocked, air is drawn in through the mouth, and misses this warming, moistening and filtering. Behind the nasal spaces and mouth and linked to both is the pharynx, the passage for air and food which is also a speech resonance chamber (◆ page 68). It houses the tonsils, and leads to the windpipe and gullet.

The windpipe (trachea) lies in front of the gullet. At its top is the larynx (voicebox), covered by the epiglottis, a flap of cartilage that

The respiratory system

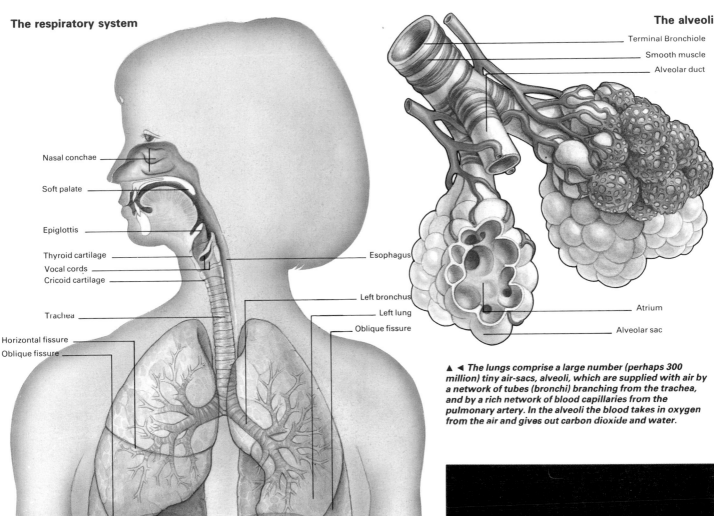

Nasal conchae

Soft palate

Epiglottis

Thyroid cartilage

Vocal cords

Cricoid cartilage

Trachea

Horizontal fissure

Oblique fissure

Esophagus

Left bronchus

Left lung

Oblique fissure

Diaphragm

The alveoli

Terminal Bronchiole

Smooth muscle

Alveolar duct

Atrium

Alveolar sac

▲ ◄ *The lungs comprise a large number (perhaps 300 million) tiny air-sacs, alveoli, which are supplied with air by a network of tubes (bronchi) branching from the trachea, and by a rich network of blood capillaries from the pulmonary artery. In the alveoli the blood takes in oxygen from the air and gives out carbon dioxide and water.*

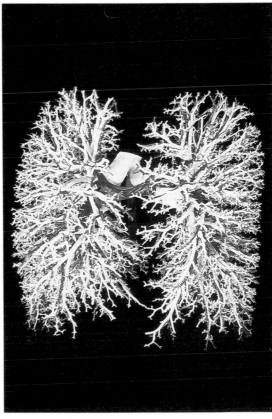

▲ *A resin-cast of the lungs' blood supply.*

closes during swallowing, shutting the windpipe to prevent food going down it. The trachea divides at its base into two bronchi which enter the lungs. These branch into small bronchioles, leading to the chambers (alveoli) where carbon dioxide is added and oxygen removed from the inspired air (♦ page 158). When the lungs are inflated, the expansion triggers stretch receptors that stimulate the muscles used for breathing out.

Breathing is a function we can control when we want to, but which otherwise runs on "automatic pilot" – a decided advantage when we are sleeping. During rest, there is a pause between each breath. When the carbon dioxide in blood exceeds a modest level, it triggers receptors in the brain. These send impulses to the muscles that make us breathe in. If we ignore them, the impulses become stronger, which is why we cannot hold our breath for long under water. (Against this apparent disadvantage, no one can commit suicide by simply stopping breathing.) Breathing is also stimulated by exercise (before carbon dioxide in blood has time to rise), raised blood acidity, lowered blood pressure, overheating and fever, sudden severe pain, stretching the circular muscle of the anus and irritation in the throat.

Although breathing is for the most part a subconscious activity, it has to be regulated. The requisite signals to the brain come chiefly from increased carbon dioxide levels in the bloodstream rather than from depletion of oxygen. Cells in the brainstem respond immediately to even marginal fluctuations in concentrations of the gases, and adjust the lungs' ventilation rate accordingly. Other brainstem cells receive corresponding signals from "chemoreceptors" around the body and react in the same way. The system is exquisitely sensitive: a small increase of carbon dioxide pressure from 40 to 43mmHg triggers a doubling of ventilation in the alveoli.

Internal and external respiration

Although some species of bacteria and other microbes live without it, most living things require continuous supplies of oxygen to break down sugars into carbon dioxide and water, thus releasing energy for upkeep and growth. Simple creatures such as flatworms conduct this process of "respiration" without specialized mechanics. Because none of their cells are far from the surface, they can acquire oxygen and release carbon dioxide by diffusion through the skin.

Larger animals need more efficient machinery for conducting the two gases into, out of and around the body. These include tiny tubes in insects, gills in fish and blood systems of varying sophistication in many different organisms. This has led to the distinction which is sometimes made between external respiration (breathing) and internal respiration (the oxygen use and carbon dioxide release which occurs in the cells).

As with other mammals, the lungs, heart and circulatory system are responsible for respiration in humans. The bloodstream provides all the body's tissues with the glucose they require as fuel. It also makes available oxygen to "burn" this sugar as a source of energy for innumerable activities ranging from muscular contraction and nerve conduction to temperature maintenance and the manufacture of new cell materials. Respiration *is* possible without oxygen. Also known as fermentation, this anaerobic variety of respiration is normal for organisms such as yeast. But it is much less efficient than aerobic respiration and occurs in humans only in certain tissues under conditions of acute oxygen starvation created by prolonged or vigorous exercise. The loss of muscular control observed occasionally in marathon runners is caused by lactic acid released as a consequence of anaerobic respiration.

Converting fuel to energy

Aerobic respiration takes place within mitochondria, tiny energy-generating organelles inside living cells. Each mitochondrion contains over 70 enzymes and other chemicals (including vitamins and minerals) which promote the chemical reactions of respiration. Acting on glucose as their fuel, they break the sugar molecules down step by step, liberating energy at several different stages. This continuous, cyclical series of reactions is called the Krebs cycle, after the German biochemist Hans Krebs (1900-1981) who was largely responsible for discovering it. Energy made available by respiration is stored for immediate or future use in adenosine diphosphate (ADP) and adenosine triphosphate (ATP). These compounds are produced when electrons, released from the Krebs cycle, pass along a sequence of carriers (cytochromes) to oxygen. Called oxidative phosphorylation, this is the key mechanism through which cells obtain their energy.

Breathing in

Breathing out

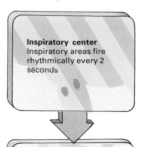
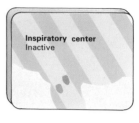

Inspiratory center
Inspiratory areas fire rhythmically every 2 seconds

Inspiratory center
Inactive

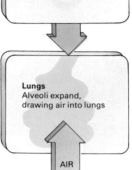
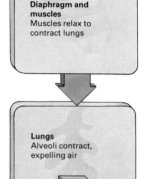

Diaphragm and muscles
Diaphragm and external inter-costal muscles contract to expand lungs

Diaphragm and muscles
Muscles relax to contract lungs

Lungs
Alveoli expand, drawing air into lungs

Lungs
Alveoli contract, expelling air

AIR

AIR

▲ *In normal breathing, the inspiratory area of the brain stem fires automatically and rhythmically in two-second bursts, causing the rib-cage and diaphragm to expand, drawing air into the lungs. When the inspiratory area is not firing, the ribs and diaphragm relax, contracting the lungs and expelling the air.*

▼ *During very vigorous exercise, anaerobic respiration occurs in the muscle tissues. The lactic acid produced from this reaction is mostly taken to the liver, but some collects in muscle tissue, and extra oxygen is required to break it down. Meanwhile the lactic acid and lack of oxygen cause the muscle to feel fatigued.*

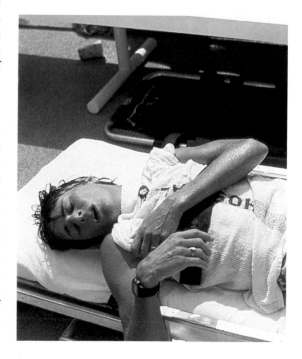

Strenuous breathing

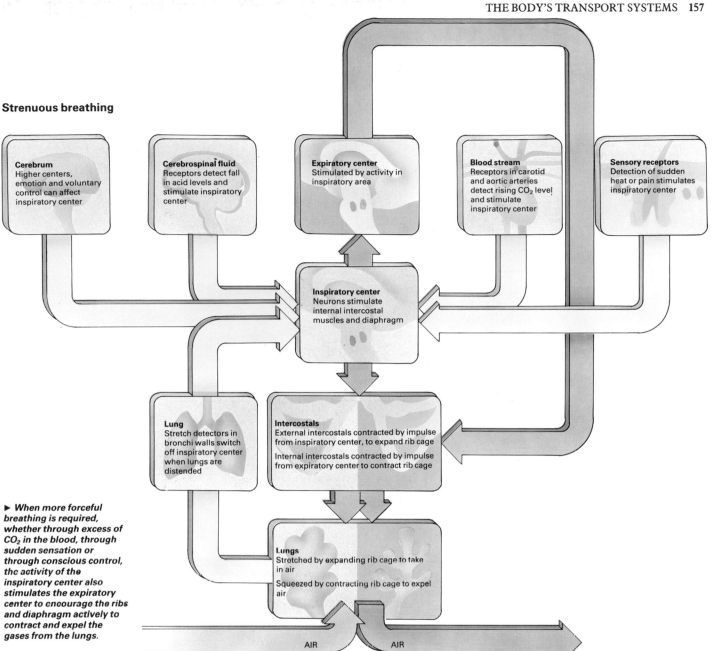

Cerebrum
Higher centers, emotion and voluntary control can affect inspiratory center

Cerebrospinal fluid
Receptors detect fall in acid levels and stimulate inspiratory center

Expiratory center
Stimulated by activity in inspiratory area

Blood stream
Receptors in carotid and aortic arteries detect rising CO_2 level and stimulate inspiratory center

Sensory receptors
Detection of sudden heat or pain stimulates inspiratory center

Inspiratory center
Neurons stimulate internal intercostal muscles and diaphragm

Lung
Stretch detectors in bronchi walls switch off inspiratory center when lungs are distended

Intercostals
External intercostals contracted by impulse from inspiratory center, to expand rib cage

Internal intercostals contracted by impulse from expiratory center to contract rib cage

Lungs
Stretched by expanding rib cage to take in air

Squeezed by contracting rib cage to expel air

AIR   AIR

▶ When more forceful breathing is required, whether through excess of CO_2 in the blood, through sudden sensation or through conscious control, the activity of the inspiratory center also stimulates the expiratory center to encourage the ribs and diaphragm actively to contract and expel the gases from the lungs.

Deep-sea respiration

An outstanding scientific event of recent years was the discovery using the submersible craft "Alvin" of thermal vents in the ocean floor near the Galapagos Islands in the Pacific. First located during the late 1970s, these have proved to be regions where sea water penetrates several kilometers into the Earth's crust at points where two continent-sized plates are moving apart. Plumes of black or blue water up to 350°C in temperature emerge from the vents, which are surrounded by an exotic diversity of living creatures adapted to life under extreme heat and pressure. Mussels, tube worms and microorganisms occur in rich profusion. Particularly remarkable are giant clams, having white shells but with internal tissues colored pink by hemoglobin. Biologists have long recognized that the affinity of different hemoglobins for oxygen varies from one species to another – being greater, for example, in animals living at higher altitudes. So they were interested to find that hemoglobin in the giant clam, occupying a habitat where oxygen is inordinately scarce, had a spectacular avidity for the gases.

When oxygen, carried on the hemoglobin molecules in red blood cells, reaches particular tissues, the amount then released depends upon their requirement at the time. If needs are high (because the tissue is expending large quantities of energy) these are met either by more blood perfusing through the tissue and/or by more oxygen being removed from the hemoglobin. As when oxygen is picked up in the lungs, it passes out of the blood and into the tissues because of the pressure difference in the two domains. Arriving fully loaded with oxygen, hemoglobin has usually given up about a fifth of its load when it leaves the tissues.

Carbon dioxide and water are the waste products of internal respiration. The carbon dioxide is ferried away from tissues in more than one way. Tiny amounts are simply dissolved in the bloodstream or occur as carbonic acid. Most (63 percent) travels in the blood as bicarbonate. A further 30 percent is combined with hemoglobin – the bloodstream's carrier molecule thus plays a dual role. It is adapted for this function, because hemoglobin deficient in oxygen combines more readily with carbon dioxide, and vice versa. The two gases reciprocate in altering the molecule, each fostering the release and transport of the other. When the waste products reach the alveoli, they pass out of the bloodstream into the lungs, and are breathed out.

Scarcity of oxygen at high altitude stimulates the body to produce hemoglobin

Hemoglobin – the blood's transport mechanism

The crucial intermediary role in respiration is played by hemoglobin, of which there are about 280 million molecules in every red corpuscle in the bloodstream. Because it forms an unstable, reversible bond with oxygen, this specialized, iron-containing protein can acquire the vital gas in the lungs and ferry it to tissues throughout the body. When uncombined with oxygen as in venous blood returning to the lungs, hemoglobin is dark blue and known as deoxyhemoglobin. When carrying the gas, as in arterial blood fresh from the lungs, it is bright red and called oxyhemoglobin. Scarcity of oxygen at high altitude stimulates the body to produce more blood cells containing this vital carrier.

The hemoglobin molecule is a huge structure of some 10,000 atoms; each molecule can pick up, transport and deliver four atoms of oxygen. Taking into account the volume of blood passing through the lungs, this means that the human body transports an average of 56 thousand million million million (56×10^{21}) atoms of oxygen per minute. About one-sixtieth of this is simply dissolved in the blood plasma. But if blood cells did not contain hemoglobin, the human body would require some 60 times the volume of blood to accomplish the same task of oxygenation.

At the center of the hemoglobin is globin, a protein consisting of linked pairs of polypeptide chains – two alpha and two beta in adults, two alpha and two gamma in the fetus and newborns (whose hemoglobin is more avid for oxygen than that of adults, so that it is efficient in carrying the gases across the placental barrier). The globin is surrounded by four heme groups, forming a tetrahedral structure. Although heme accounts for only four percent of the weight of the molecule, it contains all of the iron and is responsible for its color.

▲ *liver capillaries.*

▼ ► *After the oxygen-laden blood reaches the body tissues, the oxygen and glucose pass through the cell membrane. A chain of chemical reactions occurs in the cell's mitochondria (right), breaking down the glucose and giving off phosphoryls that convert ADP to ATP. In this way, the cell stores energy for future use. Finally, hydrogen ions combine with the oxygen to form water; this passes into the blood as waste, as does carbon dioxide.*

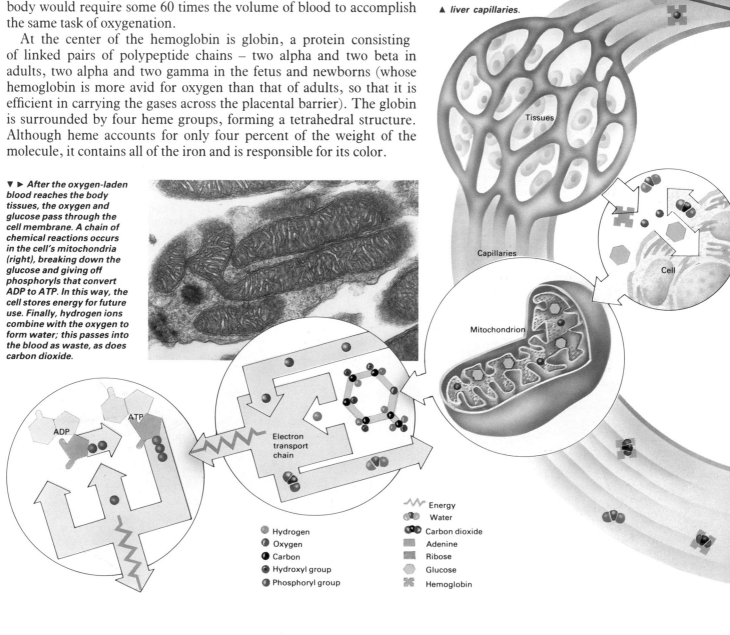

Tissues

Capillaries

Cell

Mitochondrion

Electron transport chain

ADP

ATP

- ⬤ Hydrogen
- ◉ Oxygen
- ◑ Carbon
- ⬤ Hydroxyl group
- ⬤ Phosphoryl group
- 〰 Energy
- ⬤ Water
- ◕ Carbon dioxide
- ▦ Adenine
- ▦ Ribose
- ⬡ Glucose
- ✖ Hemoglobin

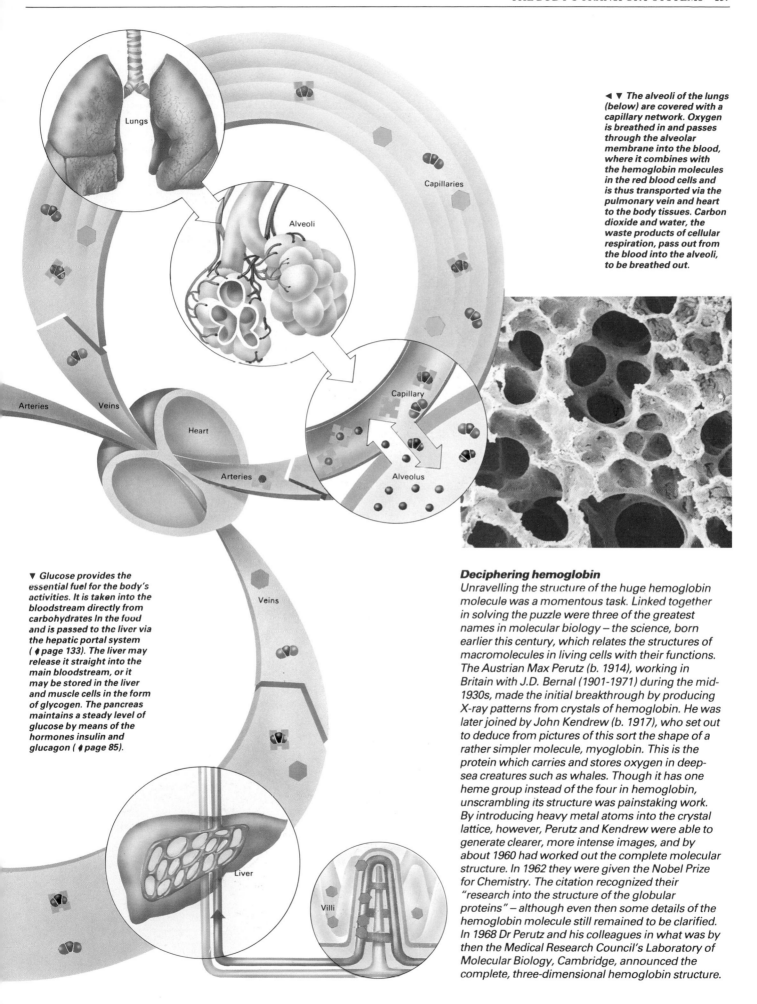

Lungs

Capillaries

Alveoli

◀ ▼ *The alveoli of the lungs (below) are covered with a capillary network. Oxygen is breathed in and passes through the alveolar membrane into the blood, where it combines with the hemoglobin molecules in the red blood cells and is thus transported via the pulmonary vein and heart to the body tissues. Carbon dioxide and water, the waste products of cellular respiration, pass out from the blood into the alveoli, to be breathed out.*

Arteries   Veins

Heart

Arteries

Capillary

Alveolus

▼ *Glucose provides the essential fuel for the body's activities. It is taken into the bloodstream directly from carbohydrates in the food and is passed to the liver via the hepatic portal system (◆ page 133). The liver may release it straight into the main bloodstream, or it may be stored in the liver and muscle cells in the form of glycogen. The pancreas maintains a steady level of glucose by means of the hormones insulin and glucagon (◆ page 85).*

Veins

Liver

Villi

Deciphering hemoglobin

Unravelling the structure of the huge hemoglobin molecule was a momentous task. Linked together in solving the puzzle were three of the greatest names in molecular biology – the science, born earlier this century, which relates the structures of macromolecules in living cells with their functions. The Austrian Max Perutz (b. 1914), working in Britain with J.D. Bernal (1901-1971) during the mid-1930s, made the initial breakthrough by producing X-ray patterns from crystals of hemoglobin. He was later joined by John Kendrew (b. 1917), who set out to deduce from pictures of this sort the shape of a rather simpler molecule, myoglobin. This is the protein which carries and stores oxygen in deep-sea creatures such as whales. Though it has one heme group instead of the four in hemoglobin, unscrambling its structure was painstaking work. By introducing heavy metal atoms into the crystal lattice, however, Perutz and Kendrew were able to generate clearer, more intense images, and by about 1960 had worked out the complete molecular structure. In 1962 they were given the Nobel Prize for Chemistry. The citation recognized their "research into the structure of the globular proteins" – although even then some details of the hemoglobin molecule still remained to be clarified. In 1968 Dr Perutz and his colleagues in what was by then the Medical Research Council's Laboratory of Molecular Biology, Cambridge, announced the complete, three-dimensional hemoglobin structure.

Transporting food

The final transport system of the body involves the automatic movement of food along the gut. Wrapped around the esophagus, stomach and intestines is a tube of smooth muscle that contracts slowly and rhythmically. These contractions are very forceful, although much slower than those of voluntary muscle. Around the gut is a layer of circular fibers and, inside, one of lengthways fibers. Each fiber is a single cell five to ten micrometers wide and 30-200 micrometers long. The fibers are tightly bound together in a continuous mesh. When a nerve cell stimulates one fiber, the impulse travels over the other fibers so contraction occurs in a wave.

The stomach contracts about three times a minute, forcing a ball of food (bolus) into the intestine. (If no food is present, the contractions are felt as hunger pangs.) The bolus is then moved downwards in waves – when circular fibers in one place contract, making the gut narrower, lengthways fibers in the next section relax, making it wider. From mouth to anus the gut is 8m long, and food takes 12-24 hours to travel from beginning to end (◀ page 121).

After food has passed down the gut, the left-overs arrive in the rectum in waves and stay there until their bulk triggers stretch receptors, causing an urge to defecate. The lengthways muscles in the rectum contract, increasing pressure, and voluntary contraction of the abdominal muscles forces the anus open as the feces are expelled. If defecation does not occur, the feces remain until the next consignment arrives from the colon and triggers the receptors again.

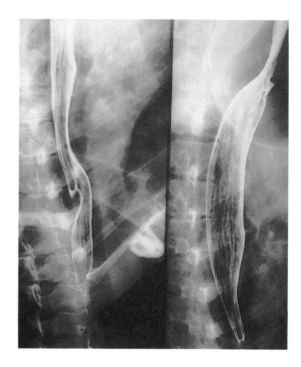

▲ *X-rays of a bolus of food passing down the esophagus After the conscious act of swallowing, the unconscious transport system takes over, relaxing the muscles in front of the bolus and squeezing it along from behind (peristalsis).*

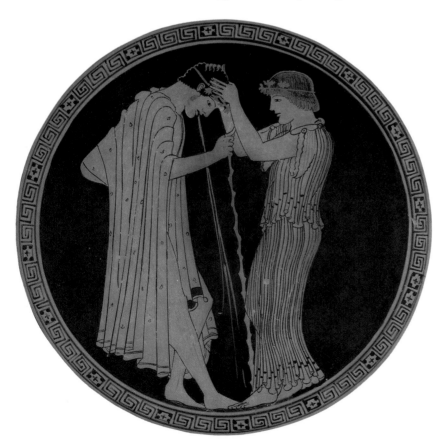

▲ *A Greek vase painting depicting vomiting. Vomiting is the expulsion of stomach contents through the mouth, triggered by poisons in the stomach, stomach distension, unpleasant sights and tastes or dizziness.*

Urinating

Urine is expelled from the bladder by micturition (urination). The maximum capacity of the bladder is 700-800ml, but by the time it has 200-400ml, stretch receptors in its wall send receptors to the spinal cord. This triggers a conscious desire to expel urine and a subconscious reflex (which we can overrule) to the bladder wall and urethra – the canal from the bladder to the outside. In babies under two, the nerve pathways for conscious control are not fully formed. After micturition commences it is almost impossible to stop – a mechanism that prevents urine from going stale and inviting infection.

Coughing, sneezing, laughing, yawning, sighing, hiccuping and vomiting

Coughing occurs when irritation in the throat provokes reflex closure of the glottis (blocking off the gullet), drawing-in of breath, and sudden release of the trapped air at speeds of up to 150 meters a second. Sneezes, triggered by irritation in the nose, are faster still. The tongue rises, closing off the mouth so that the blast exits through the nose, unblocking it and spraying out its contents. In laughter, each deep inspiration is followed by a set of short expirations. Crying is exactly the same, at least as far as breathing goes. Sighing is a single deep expiration with the mouth wide open, and yawning is the opposite – deep inspiration. Hiccups are spasmodic inspirations which end with the abrupt closure of the vocal cords.

In vomiting, the sufferer takes a deep breath, the glottis shuts off the airways, the soft palate rises and closes off the nostrils, the diaphragm and abdominal muscles contract, the gullet opens, and out it comes.

Coronary heart disease...Heart attacks...Heart surgery...Treating heart disease with drugs...Arrhythmias...Valve replacements...High blood pressure...Heart disease in the newborn...Other circulatory diseases...PERSPECTIVE...Heart transplants...Lifestyle and blood pressure

The heart

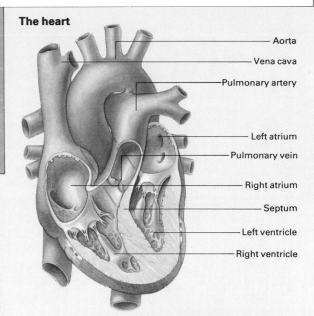

- Aorta
- Vena cava
- Pulmonary artery
- Left atrium
- Pulmonary vein
- Right atrium
- Septum
- Left ventricle
- Right ventricle

The heart is a self-powered pump which drives blood around the body, so that it can oxygenate tissues and carry away waste products such as carbon dioxide (◀ page 150). Heart failure occurs when the heart cannot cope with the body's metabolic needs. If the heart stops pumping so that oxygen no longer reaches the brain, death follows.

Cardiovascular diseases are those in which the heart's performance is impaired. Although the proportion of deaths from such diseases has decreased in the USA, Australia and parts of Europe during the 1970s and 1980s, they still cause about half the deaths in Western countries. In half these deaths coronary or ischemic heart disease is the cause. Hypertension (high blood pressure) is the other main cause.

Ischemic (coronary) heart disease – the sort which leads to "heart attacks" – is caused by narrowing or blockage of the coronary arteries which supply oxygenated blood to heart muscle. In a heart attack, (also known as a myocardial infarction), the interruption of this blood supply leads to the death of part of heart muscle tissue. This can cause the normal heartbeat to be replaced by a rapid, uncoordinated beat (fibrillation), which makes the heart's pumping action ineffective. The brain may be starved of oxygen and death often results soon after the start of the attack. If a heart attack victim is still alive two hours later, the chance of survival thereafter is good.

Heart attacks often strike without warning, although after an attack sufferers may recall that they had felt unusual tiredness for several weeks. The symptoms are severe pain in the chest, which can spread to the arms, neck and teeth, accompanied by breathlessness, sweating, nausea and dizziness.

Though a heart attack may occur unexpectedly, heart disease usually shows symptoms, the severity of which indicate the severity of the disease. The coronary arteries narrow gradually as a result of deposition around the artery walls of atheromatous plaques, mixtures of white blood cells, platelets, fibrin and cholesterol. In males, this atherosclerosis may begin during the teens or early twenties. Females have a low incidence of coronary heart disease until after the menopause, when the incidence gradually rises level to the male incidence for the same age group.

The narrowing of the coronary arteries decreases the oxygen supply to the heart muscles. The heart usually copes with this under normal conditions, but when unusual demands are made on it – as a result of exercise, or even walking upstairs in severe cases – chest pain known as angina results. This is often described as a "crushing" pain. Coupled with the chest pains, there is frequently breathlessness. Because the heart is pumping less efficiently, it may fail to drain the lungs properly. Congestion of the lungs with liquid (pulmonary edema) makes breathing more difficult. Severe angina may also be accompanied by sweating and nausea.

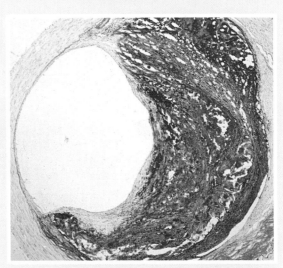

▲ *Section through an artery partly blocked with plaque.*

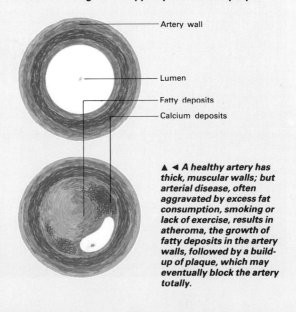

- Artery wall
- Lumen
- Fatty deposits
- Calcium deposits

▲ ◀ *A healthy artery has thick, muscular walls; but arterial disease, often aggravated by excess fat consumption, smoking or lack of exercise, results in atheroma, the growth of fatty deposits in the artery walls, followed by a build-up of plaque, which may eventually block the artery totally.*

Open-heart surgery is one of the great medical achievements of recent decades

If the heart is not working efficiently, one consequence may be swellings in the legs (peripheral edema or dropsy). Liquid passes out of the blood through the capillary walls into the body tissues and accumulates under the influence of gravity; in serious cases, the legs may become swollen up to the thighs. Edema may, however, also have other causes such as kidney or liver disease.

Surgery and coronary heart disease

In extreme circumstances surgery may be needed to treat coronary heart disease. The most common operation is the coronary by-pass. In this operation, pieces of vein from the patient's leg are transplanted into the coronary artery to provide a way around severe constrictions. A person who has suffered a heart attack may have an aneurysm, which can also be removed surgically – often at the same time as a by-pass operation. The aneurysm is a piece of non-functioning ventricle which bulges outward. This can harbor blood clots which may detach and enter the bloodstream. They can then block arteries elsewhere in the body. If this happens in the arteries leading to the brain, the result can be a stroke, which may paralyze large parts of the body by depriving part of the brain of oxygen (◆ page 168), or may even result in death. If such a clot occurs in the pulmonary artery, which takes blood from the heart to the lungs, it is called a pulmonary embolism, and may well threaten the patient's life. An aneurysm may also occur in the aorta, as a result of atheroma. This may swell until it leaks, and immediate surgery is required to strengthen the aorta wall with a woven fabric tube.

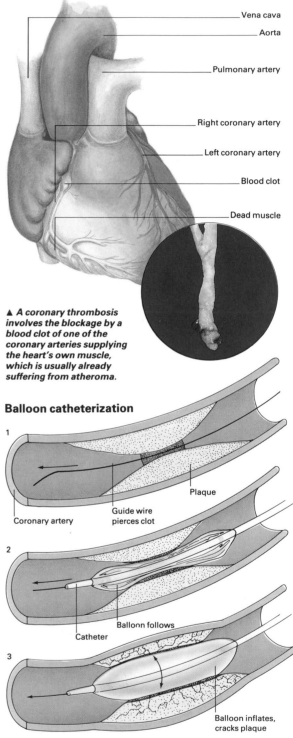

Coronary thrombosis

Vena cava

Aorta

Pulmonary artery

Right coronary artery

Left coronary artery

Blood clot

Dead muscle

▲ *A coronary thrombosis involves the blockage by a blood clot of one of the coronary arteries supplying the heart's own muscle, which is usually already suffering from atheroma.*

Balloon catheterization

1

Plaque

Guide wire pierces clot

Coronary artery

2

Balloon follows

Catheter

3

Balloon inflates, cracks plaque

▲ *A modern technique for unblocking coronary arteries involves the insertion of a balloon catheter in the femoral artery in the thigh. A thread is fed through the arterial system into the coronary artery and through the blockage, allowing a balloon to be passed into it. Inflation of the balloon causes the plaque to crack, reopening the artery, even in cases where it had previously been totally blocked.*

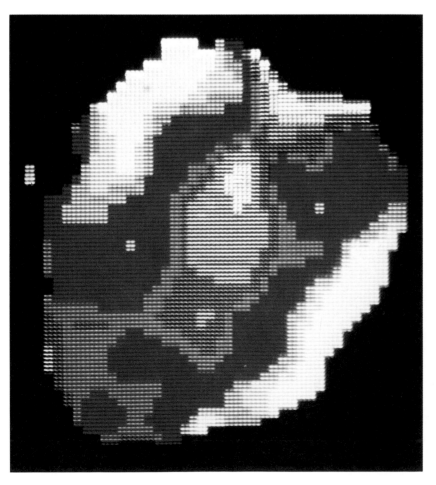

◄ *The condition of the heart can be assessed by computerized scanning after treatment with radio-active isotopes. The image obtained indicates blood flow.*

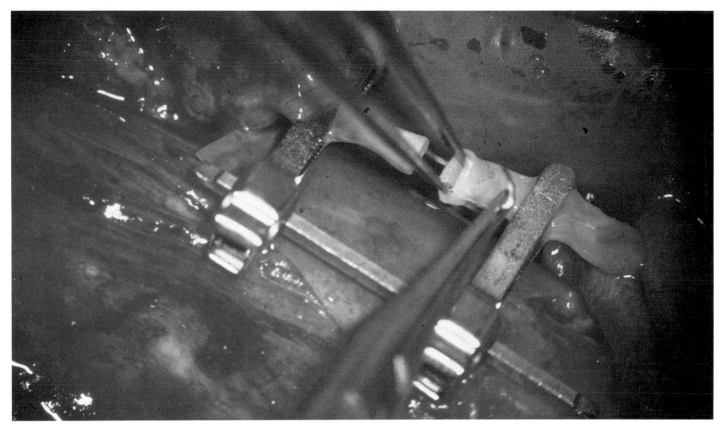

Heart transplants

Although heart disease may be controlled by drugs and changes in lifestyle, surgical treatment is the only hope of survival in some cases. In the past three decades, heart surgery has made major advances. Many operations are now carried out annually that would have been considered impossible before the Second World War. The most remarkable is heart transplantation.

The first human hearts were transplanted in the late 1960s, following many years of experimenting on animals. At first, the survival rate was low. This led to criticism of the surgeons pioneering the technique, Christiaan Barnard (b. 1922) in South Africa and Norman Shumway (b. 1923) at Stanford University, USA. Today the one-year survival rate for patients under 40 is better than 70 percent.

Heart transplantation is performed only on patients suffering from severe heart failure, particularly those under 55 years old. Donors are usually people aged under 35 who are "brain dead" (♦ page 205) as a result of an accident, but whose hearts are still beating when they enter the hospital. Donors and recipients are matched by height and weight (so that the size of the hearts is comparable) and the donors must have shown no evidence of heart disease. In addition, donors and recipients must be of the same ABO blood type and one particular HLA characteristic (♦ page 32) must also be the same. Apart from this, immunological compatibility is not considered important.

When a donor and recipient meet these criteria, the donor's heart is stopped by an overdose of potassium ions. It is then removed, cooled and transported to the recipient. In the Stanford

transplants, which account for nearly half of all those performed, the heart is transplanted within 3·5 hours of removal.

Usually, the recipient is placed on a heart-lung machine and the heart removed by dividing the atria part-way down. The donor heart is attached so that its atria link up with the residual atria of the recipient heart. It is then connected to the arteries.

Heart transplant patients have to take immunosuppressive drugs for the remainder of their lives, to prevent rejection of the new heart. Ninety percent of transplant patients suffer a "rejection episode", a concerted effort by the immune system to destroy the new heart. These episodes are usually overcome by treatment.

Long-term treatment with immunosuppressive drugs can produce side effects. A higher-than-normal incidence of cancers, notably those affecting the lymphatic system, is found in transplant patients. The major effect of such drugs is to reduce the body's ability to deal with infections. More than half the deaths in heart transplant patients are due to infections.

Immune reactions are probably also responsible for accelerated atherosclerosis in heart transplant patients. Attempts by the immune system to reject the foreign heart seem to lead to alterations in the surface of the coronary arteries which help rapid build-up of atheroma. As the new heart is not connected to the nervous system, there is no anginal pain to warn of this. Consequently, heart transplant patients undergo routine checks to assess their cardiac state. If accelerated atherosclerosis is present, the only satisfactory treatment is a further transplant.

▲ **Microscopes are often needed by surgeons when reconnecting tiny blood vessels in heart surgery.**

The artificial heart

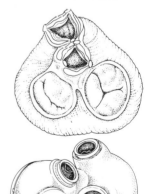

▲ **Artificial hearts (here seen from above, and compared to a normal heart from the same angle) were developed in the 1970s, and the first such heart was implanted into a human in 1982. The use of such hearts is beset with difficulties and is highly controversial among cardiac surgeons.**

Heart stimulants derived from the foxglove plant are among the oldest drugs still in use

Drugs and other treatments for heart disease

Edema and angina can often be treated with drugs. Digitoxin and digoxin, poisons (♦ page 238) derived from the foxglove *Digitalis*, are among the oldest known drugs still in use. They stimulate heart muscle to work more effectively. Many drugs (vasodilators) work by relaxing the veins, so that the back pressure is reduced. Nitroglycerin, better known as an explosive, is a commonly prescribed drug with this effect. Diuretics, drugs which increase urination and so reduce blood volume, can also be used.

More recent are the "beta blockers". The heart beats faster in response to many stimuli such as fear, because of the increase in blood concentration of adrenaline and related substances (♦ page 88). These react with sites on the muscle wall called beta receptors. Some molecules, which are known as beta blockers, can obscure the beta receptors without triggering the normal physiological reaction. These have become a very important class of heart drug. They can, however, induce heart failure in some patients, and sudden withdrawal from beta-blocker treatment may precipitate a heart attack.

Palpitations are a symptom of heart disease, although these may have other causes, such as stress. Occasional palpitations occur in the normal heart, and can be induced by excessive consumption of coffee, tea or alcohol, or by heavy smoking. The most common type is the so-called "missed beat"; the heart does not actually miss a beat. The electrical signal which initiates each contraction fires at the wrong moment, making the beat less effective. As a consequence, the next

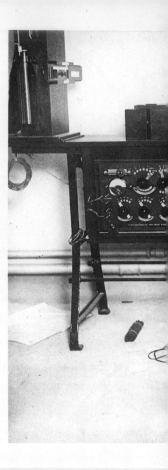

► *Clinical electrocardiography (ECG) was first developed at the turn of the 20th century by the Dutch physicist Willem Einthoven (1860-1927), although earlier studies of the heart's electrical activity had been made by A.D. Waller (1856-1922), seen here. Einthoven recorded ECGs from leads connecting the two arms, and each arm and each leg. He also described the ECG trace and suggested its use as an aid in diagnosing heart disease. Einthoven won the Nobel Prize for Physiology in 1924.*

► ▼ *The ECG trace consists of three main elements, the P-wave, the QRS-complex and the T-wave. Each provides different information about the activity of the heart, as does the interval between the start of the P-wave and the QRS-complex.*

Normal heartbeat

P   R   T

Q   S

Bradycardia

The heart beat

Atrial systole

Ventricular systole

Atrial and ventricular diastole

► *A pacemaker can be inserted to cure bradycardia (slow heart beat). The electronic circuitry is designed to maintain the heart rate at a suitable level. If the heart operates normally, the mechanical pacemaker is inhibited.*

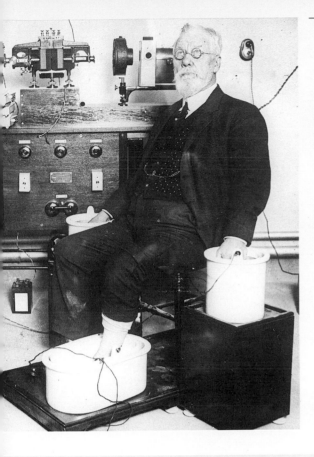

beat has to expel a larger than normal volume of blood from the heart and appears as a prominent or thumping beat. Another type of palpitation causes a fluttering feeling in the chest and may be accompanied by lightheadedness and sweating. Known as tachycardia, this is caused by an abnormally fast heart rate.

Persistent arrhythmias (deviations from the normal pattern of the heart beat) can be controlled by drugs or by surgical treatment. Beta-blocking agents and some anesthetics are useful in treatment. In cases of severe bradycardia (palpitations caused by slow heart beat), insertion of a mechanical pacemaker is often the best treatment.

Inefficient operation of the heart can result from damage to its valves. A common cause of this, particularly in less-developed countries, is rheumatic fever. This can cause scarring of the valve tissue so that it becomes stiff and less efficient at closing. As a result, blood may leak backward through the system. In such conditions, the noise of the heart through a stethoscope changes, to give a "murmur".

In some cases, valve segments become partly fused together, so that it cannot open fully. Stenosis, as this is called, reduces the volume of blood passing through the valve at each stroke. One consequence may be the enlargement of the heart as it tries to compensate for this decline in efficiency. Valvular disease can cause a large number of symptoms, notably angina and palpitations.

Valves can be replaced with either natural or synthetic materials. A new valve may be constructed from tissue taken from another part of the patient, or an intact valve from a cadaver or a pig may be used.

Fibrillation

Mitral stenosis

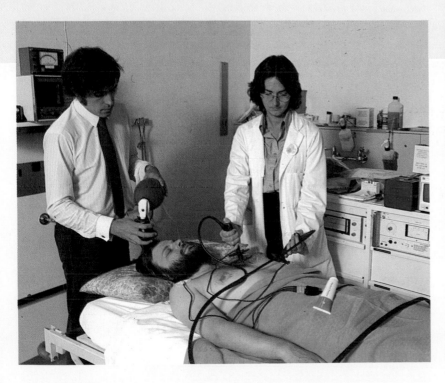

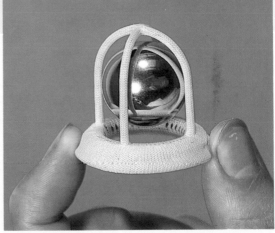

◄ *In ventricular fibrillation, the heart's action is uncoordinated and shows up on an ECG as an irregular wave. Normal action can sometimes be restored by delivering an electric shock from a defibrillator, as shown here.*

▲ *A diseased mitral valve may cause a backflow of blood into the left atrium. It can be replaced by a synthetic substitute of which there are various designs. In the type shown, the base is sewn into the valve position.*

An estimated 10 percent of people in the USA and UK have raised blood pressure

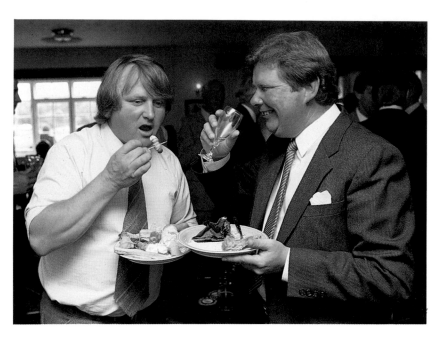

◀ **Overweight, lack of exercise, tension, fatty foods, smoking and the intake of alcohol add up to a recipe for potential hypertension with its associated problems later in life, threatening strokes, kidney failure and hastening the onset of atherosclerosis.**

▶ **The !Kung tribe of Africa do not suffer the usual rise in blood pressure with age. The reasons for this are not clear, but seem to be associated with their low salt intake, the lack of fat on their cattle, their plentiful exercise and, possibly, a lack of mental tension in their way of life.**

Heart disease and lifestyle

Blood pressure increases normally with age (◀ page 152), but when it goes above the norm for the age group, it can be dangerous. The risk of death rises almost proportionally to the increase in pressure. An estimated 10 percent of people in the USA and UK have raised blood pressure, but in only half of them has it been detected.

Although heart attacks may occur without warning, there are factors which predispose people to them. These include raised blood pressure, obesity, smoking and a family history of coronary heart disease. Regular exercise to the point of breathlessness seems to have a protective effect against such attacks.

A number of other correlations have been shown between environmental factors and the incidence of heart disease. Hot climates and hard water are associated with reduced incidences. Alcohol consumption in moderation appears to have a slight protective effect, but alcohol abuse increases the risk. Stressful events, such as a bereavement, seem to increase the likelihood of an attack.

How these factors work and interrelate is not understood. Smoking, for example, appears to predispose people to heart attacks only when other risk factors are present. In Japan the incidence of coronary heart disease is low by Western standards, and smoking behavior seems to have no effect.

Treatment of hypertension improved with the development of new drugs. Special cardiac units in hospitals were introduced, with a view to helping heart attack patients to survive the first few crucial hours after the attack, although the effectiveness of these has been questioned. Finally, developments in cardiac surgery have kept alive people who would undoubtedly have died without the availability of such treatment.

High blood pressure

As many as 20 percent of all deaths in the developed world may be partly attributable to high blood pressure (hypertension). This causes excess wear and tear on the cardiovascular system and can damage the heart, kidneys and brain.

Raised blood pressure can be caused by diseases affecting the endocrine glands or kidneys, and by pre-eclampsia (toxemia) in pregnancy (◀ page 192). The oral contraceptive pill raises blood pressure slightly in most women and seriously so in a few cases. Nevertheless, in 95 percent of cases, high blood pressure is "primary" or "essential" hypertension, the cause of which is unknown. An unidentified hormone which affects the loss of sodium from the body may be a cause. Alternatively, calcium imbalance may be responsible.

Grossly overweight individuals frequently have raised blood pressure. This can be reduced by dieting. For most people, drug treatment is the only option. A wide variety of drugs is used, including the vasodilators and diuretics that are also used to treat angina and heart failure (◀ page 164). More recent drugs given for hypertension are the beta-blockers and ACE-inhibitors – the latter prevent the production of angiotensin II, a hormone involved in the raising of blood pressure.

Coronary heart disease

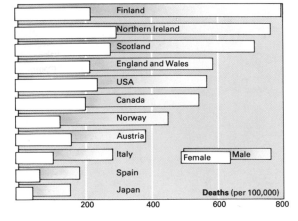

Finland			
Northern Ireland			
Scotland			
England and Wales			
USA			
Canada			
Norway			
Austria			
Italy	Female	Male	
Spain			
Japan	**Deaths** (per 100,000)		

200   400   600   800

◀ **Coronary heart disease mortality rates show surprising variations; Finland has the highest incidence, even though many of its population take regular exercise. It is likely that a higher than average intake of animal fat is to blame.**

▶ **In the USA, about 1 million deaths occur annually from heart disease. About two-thirds of these result from coronary heart disease, but the incidence of death from this cause has been falling since the 1950s. The reason for this fall is not certain.**

US mortality from heart disease

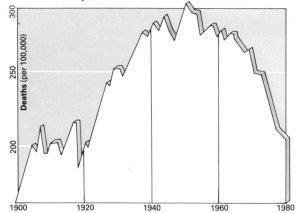

Deaths (per 100,000)

1900   1920   1940   1960   1980

Heart attacks among middle-aged people

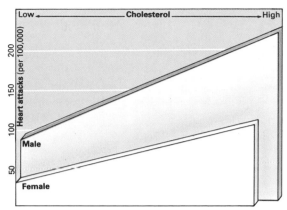

▲ *The amount of cholesterol in the diet has a direct link with the incidence of heart attacks among middle-aged people. Cholesterol is produced by the liver, and plays several metabolic roles including hormone synthesis. If an excess is consumed in the diet, in association with other saturated fats, it seems to promote atherosclerosis.*

Pulse rate when smoking

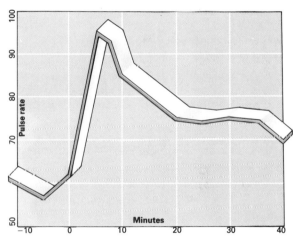

▲ ▼ *Smoking is an important element in hypertension and heart disease. The nicotine from a cigarette remains in the bloodstream for only about half an hour, but in that time stimulates adrenaline production (◊ page 88). Tobacco also stimulates inhibitory cells in the spinal cord, thus lowering muscle tone and causing a feeling of relaxation.*

Stopping smoking and heart attack incidence

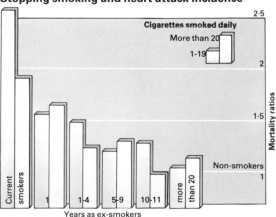

Slightly less than one percent of babies are born with some form of heart disease. In some cases, such as congenital aortic stenosis, the only hope of survival may be surgical operation. In the newly born, the survival rate is often low.

In some babies, the major arteries leading from the heart are transposed. Effectively, this means that the pulmonary circulation which oxygenates the blood is cut off from the circulation around the rest of the system. In the fetus, oxygen is obtained via the placenta and the lungs do not operate. An arterial duct carries oxygenated blood from the pulmonary artery to the pulmonary veins, thus by-passing the lungs. This duct normally closes a few hours after birth, thus establishing the normal circulatory pattern. In a baby with transposition of the great arteries, closure of the duct leads to oxygen starvation. In recent years, there have been developments in surgical treatment of this disability, but mortality is still high.

In some cases, even when the heart is normal, the arterial duct remains open. This can be a symptomless ailment, but needs eventual surgical treatment. Without treatment, pulmonary hypertension (raised blood pressure in the lung system) leads to death in middle age.

Pulmonary hypertension and early death also occur as a result of other types of heart defect, notably those in which the septum – the wall of the tissue separating the left and right chambers of the heart – has a hole in it. This may occur either between the atria or the ventricles. The ventricular septal defect accounts for a quarter of all congenital heart defects. Between a third and a half of such holes close spontaneously during the first year of life; holes in the septum dividing the atria do not close spontaneously. Neither condition threatens life in young children, so operative correction is usually left until later years.

Other circulatory disorders

Apart from the heart, other parts of the cardiovascular system can become diseased. In anemia, the blood is an inefficient carrier of oxygen. To compensate for this deficiency, the heart has to work harder than normal. This may produce the same symptoms as coronary heart disease – breathlessness, peripheral edema and arrhythmias – although usually the patient is at risk only where there is already a history of heart disease.

Reduced oxygen supply is a problem also with emphysema. In this lung disease, which may be caused by heavy smoking, sufferers are unable to breathe out properly (page 172). Consequently, the lungs are never fully emptied and the amount of fresh (oxygen-carrying) air taken in with each new breath is consequently reduced.

Veins can also cause illness. Notably in the legs, veins may become twisted and distended as a result of faulty operation of the valves that should prevent a backflow of blood. Such "varicose veins" cause swellings and a tendency to cramp. In severe cases, ulceration of the legs may occur.

As a result of increased abdominal pressure, in pregnancy for example, swollen blood vessels may appear in the anal region, where they are better known as hemorrhoids or piles (page 140). Testicular varicose veins, or varicoceles, can be a cause of male sterility.

Thrombophlebitis is an inflammatory disease of the veins which can cause blood clots (also known as thrombi or emboli). These may enter the circulation and lead to stroke, heart attack or pulmonary embolism if they then block an artery.

Fetal circulation

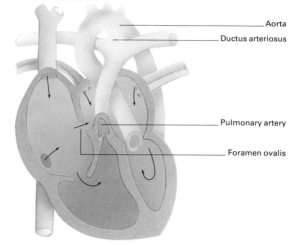

Aorta
Ductus arteriosus
Pulmonary artery
Foramen ovalis

Babies' heart disorders

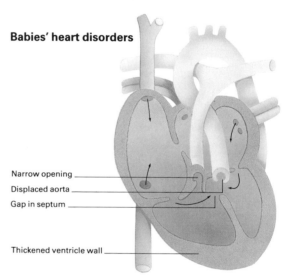

Narrow opening
Displaced aorta
Gap in septum
Thickened ventricle wall

▲ *The fetal heart has a hole (foramen) between the atria, and a ductus arteriosus linking the pulmonary artery and aorta. In some babies these fail to close at birth, and the aorta opening is misplaced. Corrective surgery may be required.*

Stroke

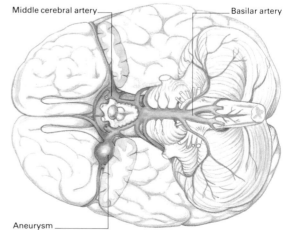

Middle cerebral artery
Basilar artery
Aneurysm

▲ *A "stroke" involves a thrombosis or embolism in cerebral arteries supplying the brain; an aneurysm or weak point in the artery may also cause a hemorrhage in the brain. Both may cause damage to areas of the brain.*

*The threat of respiratory disease...Colds and flu...
Mutating viruses...Bronchitis...Pneumonia...The
appearance of Legionnaires' disease...Tuberculosis,
a disease of the past...Whooping cough and diphtheria...
PERSPECTIVE...Mind over matter...Monitoring
microbes...Vaccination "fever"*

The respiratory tract

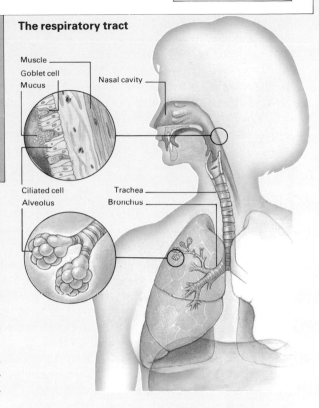

Muscle
Goblet cell
Mucus
Nasal cavity
Ciliated cell
Alveolus
Trachea
Bronchus

Together with diarrheal disease, acute infections of the respiratory tract are the most important causes of preventable deaths in the world. There are no reliable global figures (because some regions do not provide statistics) but the World Health Organization estimates that such maladies are responsible for over 666,000 fatalities each year in 88 countries, representing a quarter of the world's population. Assuming similar mortality rates in areas not reporting figures, this suggests an annual toll of well over two million. Although the microbes concerned are often never identified, viruses seem to be the primary culprits. They attack different parts of the respiratory passages, producing diseases which include the common cold and influenza plus many less well known infections. Bacteria can often appear as secondary invaders, proliferating in tissues which are already ravaged by viruses.

As with intestinal conditions, the effects are far worse in undernourished people. Respiratory infections kill more that 1,500 babies per 100,000 live births in some countries, including Egypt and Mexico – about 30 times more than in the USA. But such diseases are by no means negligible in the developed world. One study, of 1,000 families in Newcastle upon Tyne, England, showed that respiratory infection constituted half of all illness in pre-school children. There are also strong suspicions that one of the organisms, respiratory syncytial virus (RSV), helps to precipitate some of the sudden deaths which occur among infants in the Western world.

Categorizing respiratory infections

Although physicians divide the respiratory passages into upper, middle and lower portions, micro-organisms do not respect such demarcation. So the labels attached to different diseases are only approximate. Least serious are infections of the upper tract – typically the streaming or blocked nose of the common cold. Infections in the middle tract are of major concern because they can block the airways completely. Named after the tissues most affected, these include tonsillitis, laryngitis and pharyngitis (usually caused by *Haemophilus* bacteria) and bronchitis – infection of the bronchi leading to the lungs – which is often due to adenoviruses plus a mixed invasion by bacteria. The principal diseases of the lower tract are pneumonia and bronchiolitis (affecting the bronchioles in the lung, and typically caused by RSV). Particular viruses may, however, produce a diversity of conditions, even among members of the same family. Commoner during the winter, all such infections are worsened by smoking and to a lesser degree by air pollution (as the 4,000 deaths during London's smog in 1952 testify). They are acquired not only by breathing in droplets expelled during coughs and sneezes but also by transferring to the nose viruses picked up on the hands.

Vaccination "fever"
Influenza is an acute, highly contagious disease caused by a virus infection. Since a number of different viruses can cause the disease (◆ page 170), immunity to one does not prevent susceptibility to another.

In February 1976, virologists isolated an unusual influenza A virus from the body of an American army recruit at Fort Dix who died after collapsing on a night march. Tests indicated that it might be identical with the strain that caused the 1918-19 pandemic – the most devastating worldwide epidemic ever documented, killing over 20 million people. So the US public health authorities decided to immunize the entire population against a predicted epidemic. Appropriate vaccine was manufactured and given to nearly 46 million people before evidence emerged linking it with side effects known as the Guillain-Bare syndrome.

The campaign was halted in December. But by that time, the program had become hotly controversial, with delays in vaccine production, accusations and counter-accusations about its safety, refusals of manufacturers to accept the responsibility for inadvertent damage, and claims that the entire exercise had been too precipitate. Critics felt themselves justified when the Fort Dix virus proved not to be the 1918 pandemic strain after all. But those responsible for the program defended their actions on the reasonable grounds that, had the original suspicions been correct, the population would have been just as vulnerable as their forebears to an epidemic of horrendous scale. The lethal potential of influenza was confirmed in 1979-80 when an A-type virus killed 20 percent of the harbor seal population along the northeast coast of the USA.

The mere prospect of inoculation against influenza can reduce a person's susceptibility to the disease

The common cold

Despite its apparently specific name, the common cold illustrates the difficulty of categorizing respiratory infections. The universal characteristics of the common cold are that virus multiplication is restricted to the nose, nasopharynx and pharynx, and that the condition is much more frequent in children than adults and in households with children than those without. Although rhinoviruses were proclaimed to be the cause when they were first identified in 1960, it is now known that this one complaint can be produced by over 100 different rhinoviruses and by a range of others, including coronaviruses, enteroviruses, influenza C viruses, parainfluenza viruses, and the agent known as *Mycoplasma pneumoniae*. Once this huge variety of pathogens came to light, microbiologists realized that the purpose of their earlier search for a single agent of the common cold – to develop a vaccine – was unachievable.

Attention has since shifted towards drugs which, paralleling the antibiotics employed against bacteria, act on a range of different viruses. Although for most people colds are a trivial nuisance, methods of treating or preventing them are especially needed for those at greater risk because of chest or heart disease. Moreover, about a third of industrial absenteeism is attributable to respiratory infections. There has been some success in using the synthetic drug enviroxime to prevent colds, but the greatest hope lies with interferon. Produced naturally by cells in response to virus infection and serving to prevent the virus replicating itself, interferon was discovered in 1957, but difficulties in purifying it delayed substantial progress until the early 1980s. Then research at Britain's Common Cold Unit and elsewhere indicated that interferon from white blood cells, sprayed into the nose, inhibited the development of colds in volunteers. Several different interferons are now known.

In 1978, an investigation conducted at the Amundsen-Scott South Pole Station clarified a formerly puzzling feature of colds – their sudden appearance in a community without any evidence of viruses being introduced from outside. There were two separate outbreaks during the winter months when the station was totally isolated. On each occasion, researchers found parainfluenza viruses in the victims' throats, but they also found them throughout the winter in people not suffering from colds. The existing belief that people harbor viruses only when they are shedding them during infection, and for a short time afterwards, was demolished by the South Pole study. It proved that viruses can persist for long periods in healthy individuals. As with typhoid fever, there are carriers of the common cold too.

Influenza

Whereas colds recur because many different micro-organisms cause them (on average each person has two or three colds per year), influenza comes in epidemics because it changes genetically, spawning new varieties to which populations have little or no immunity. Produced by influenza virus A or B, it is the only respiratory virus infection whose constitutional effects (fever, lassitude, malaise, and aching limbs and head) overshadow more localized symptoms in the respiratory passages. Bronchitis can follow (◗ page 172), but the most serious complication is pneumonia (◗ page 172) – an acute infection of the lungs. When it results from bacterial invasion, this can usually be cured by antibiotics. Pneumonia caused by the influenza virus itself is more lethal, with virtually no effective drugs available.

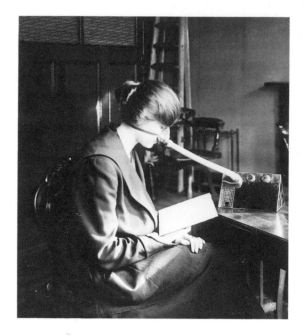

▲ An air-filtering device marketed at the height of the European flu epidemic of 1919, which killed many millions.

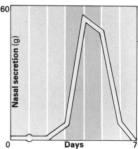

◀ Diagram of the duration of a typical common cold. Nasal secretions, at first containing large amounts of infectious viruses, rise quickly but normally pass after a couple of days.

Mind over matter

Experiments have confirmed that the mind really can affect our receptivity to the common cold. The first was carried out in 1977 at Britain's Common Cold Unit: 48 volunteers were inoculated with rhinoviruses and told they would be expected to develop colds. Half were also warned that after the experiment they would need to have their stomach juices sampled through a tube passed down the nose. Never seriously intended, this was simply a stratagem to make 24 of the volunteers apprehensive about an imminent, possibly unpleasant experience. The outcome was that the colds in this group were significantly more severe, with larger quantities of virus shed in noseblowings, than the colds suffered by the remainder.

Further evidence of the mind's impact on infection came from research into the effect of immunization against influenza among people working in the UK Post Office. Comparisons of the sickness records of 60,000 workers offered vaccine between 1972 and 1977, and those of a matched group not given the opportunity to be vaccinated, revealed two significant differences. As expected, there were signs that immunization, though far from perfect, did protect some people from influenza. But the figures also showed that the mere offer of vaccination, even though not taken up, reduced peoples' chances of developing the infection. The disparity was evident during winters when influenza was prevalent and when it was not.

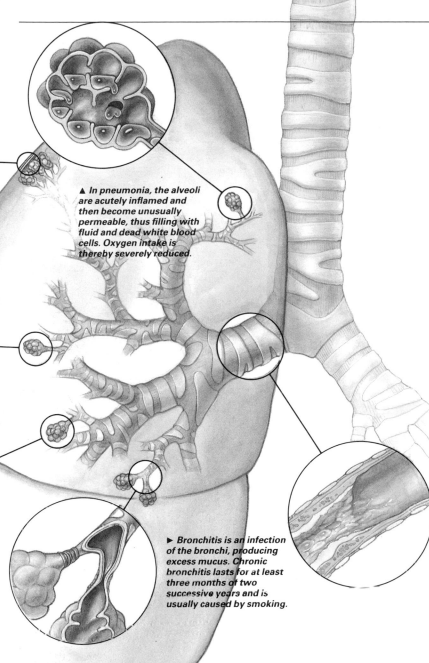

▲ In pneumonia, the alveoli are acutely inflamed and then become unusually permeable, thus filling with fluid and dead white blood cells. Oxygen intake is thereby severely reduced.

▶ Bronchitis is an infection of the bronchi, producing excess mucus. Chronic bronchitis lasts for at least three months of two successive years and is usually caused by smoking.

▲ In asthma (an allergy rather than an infection) the bronchioles go into spasm and give rise to mucus, reducing the passage of air into the lungs and leading to wheezing.

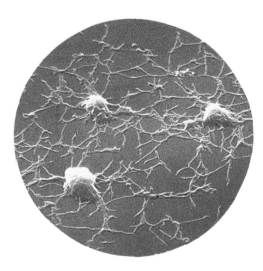

Mycoplasma pneumoniae

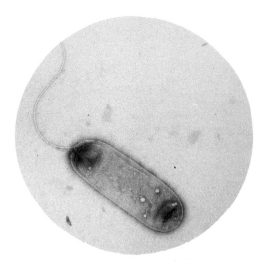

Legionella pneumophila

Whooping cough

Whooping cough (pertussis) persists because the only available vaccine is not fully effective and because some parents fail to have their children immunized through fear of the slight possibility of brain damage caused by the vaccine. By contrast diphtheria has been virtually obliterated by one of the simplest and earliest vaccines ever introduced.

Whooping cough is a highly infectious disease caused by the bacterium Bordetella pertussis. At first, the bacterium multiplies rapidly on the surface of the trachea and bronchi, making the patient highly infectious but not very ill. Then the explosive cough develops. Ten to 15 coughs may follow in rapid succession before a breath is taken, which is the characteristic "whoop". Exhaustion and sometimes vomiting and convulsions often follow.

Whooping cough, which affects mostly the under-fives, occurs in intermittent epidemics and is perhaps the most serious of the acute specific fevers of childhood. Antibiotics diminish its severity, and immunization at an early age (one to two months) prevents or ameliorates the disease. Pertussis vaccine is usually given as part of a triple immunization with tetanus and diphtheria too.

Diphtheria

At one time, one of the most unpleasant and dangerous of all childhood diseases, diphtheria is caused by Corynebacterium diphtheriae. Growing on mucous membranes in the upper respiratory tract, the bacteria produce a toxin which destroys the tissues and provokes such a massive inflammatory response that a grayish "pseudomembrane" forms over the tonsils, larynx and pharynx. The membrane blocks the airways, suffocating the victim if not promptly removed, while the toxin spreads to other parts of the body, damaging the heart, nerves, kidneys and liver. Deaths from diphtheria are often the result of inflammation of the heart.

Even the most powerful antibiotics have little effect on diphtheria. It can, however, be combatted by neutralizing the toxin that is solely responsible for the disease. Antitoxin, an antibody made by injecting small amounts of toxin into horses, is usually given if diphtheria is suspected. But vaccination with a modified version of the toxin known as toxoid is the measure that has made the disease virtually unknown in the developed countries.

Monitoring Microbes

From microfungi to viruses

By definition microbes are living organisms so tiny that they are visible only under a microscope. The vast majority are beneficial. Although pathogenic (disease-causing) microbes are in the minority, techniques of identifying them are important in diagnosing infections, deciding on appropriate treatment, tracing the sources of epidemics, and monitoring the ways in which many strains change their character and behavior over time.

In general, the larger the microbe, the less sophisticated are the methods needed to identify it. At the top of the size scale are the microscopic relatives of fungi such as mushrooms. These microfungi occur as single cells (yeasts) or hyphae, filamentous threads which produce fruiting bodies complex enough for them to be distinguished under a microscope. Athlete's foot is an example of the many infections caused by fungi.

Next in size are protozoa – the agents of such diseases as malaria. Identifying the different species of malarial parasite involves bleeding the patient every six hours and smearing blood across a microscope slide to monitor the changes in the life cycle of the protozoa. Similar methods can identify parasites such as the trypanosomes of sleeping sickness, which may have to be sought in cerebrospinal fluid. Identifying intestinal protozoa, such as Entamoeba histolytica (♦ page 248), requires a fresh specimen of feces.

Although consisting of single cells comparable with those of animals and plants, bacteria are simpler in appearance than most fungi, protozoa and related parasites. They are crudely classifiable under labels such as cocci (spheres) and bacilli (rod-like), but these groups contain many diverse species. Identification is thus more difficult. Technicians apply sophisticated differential stains to search for specific groups of bacteria recovered from specimens such as urine (urinary tract infections), feces (intestinal infections), pus, and swabs from the respiratory tract. Some organisms – such as tubercle bacilli – may be seen at once, using a light microscope. Most become apparent only after the material has been cultured in nutrient medium. Tests of a bacterium's chemical activities aid identification further. Most discriminating are methods of typing bacteria according to their sensitivity bacteriophages (viruses that invade specific bacteria), and of matching them against antibodies.

Viruses are so small that they are visible only under the electron microscope. They are simply fragments of hereditary material (DNA or RNA) wrapped in protein. In order to multiply they have to invade living cells to take advantage of their reproductive machinery. In the laboratory, bottles containing HeLa or other cells (♦ page 211) are used for this purpose, as are fertile hens' eggs in some cases. Inoculated and incubated with material on a swab, such cultures produce plaques – clear patches where influenza virus, for example, has attacked the tissue. Like bacteria, particular virus strains can also be identified by antibody tests.

Magnifications

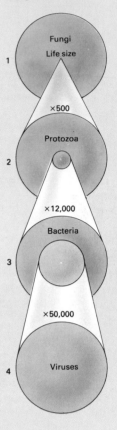

Fungi
Life size
1

×500

Protozoa
2

×12,000

Bacteria
3

×50,000

4 Viruses

1 Athlete's foot occurs when the webs of the toes are invaded by fungi such as species of Trichophyton. Starting with itching and blisters, the skin cracks, making it vunerable to secondary invasion by bacteria. When scrapings from the skin are inoculated onto artificial culture media, the fungus grows profusely, producing a thick felt.

2 Malarial parasites can be seen by smearing a pinprick of blood from the patient on a glass slide, staining it, and examining the smear under a low powered microscope. Repeated samples are needed to identify precise species.

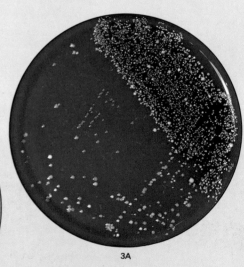

3A

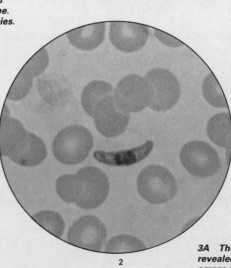

2

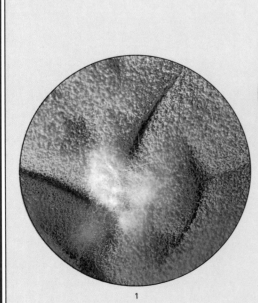

1

3A The skin's normal population of bacteria can be revealed by swabbing the skin and then wiping the swab across a plate containing nutrient medium. After several hours in an incubator at body temperature, colonies of bacteria become apparent. In this plate of blood agar most of the bacteria have proved to be Staphylococcus aureus. Although usually harmless, some strains can cause boils and other infections if they gain access through a skin abrasion.

3B Examined under the electron microscope, S. aureus is a typical spherical coccus, occuring in grape-like bunches.

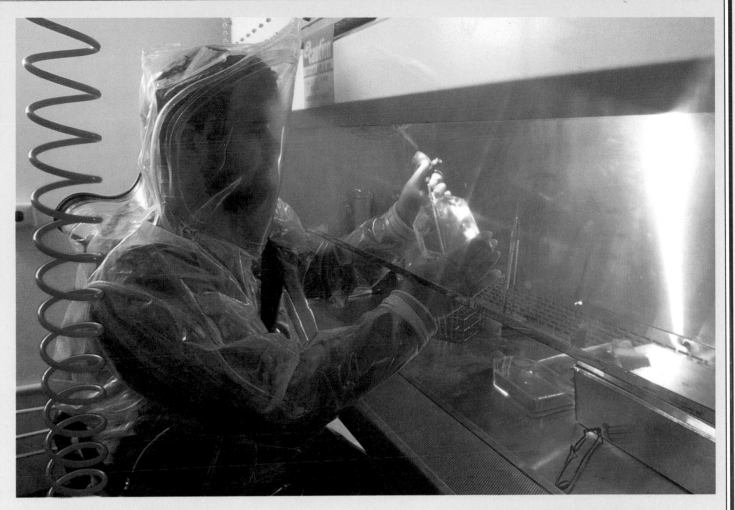

▲ The most difficult task for a microbiology laboratory is to identify a hitherto unknown microbe responsible for an outbreak of an apparently infectious disease, as when Lassa fever occurred in Nigeria in 1969 and Legionnaires' disease came to light in Philadelphia in 1976. It is also a uniquely dangerous task, because technicians may well have little idea of how the suspect and possibly lethal organism is transmitted. They therefore use conventional techniques, such as inoculating swab material into nutrient media and tissue cultures, but do so in high security facilities precluding even accidental contact with the material.

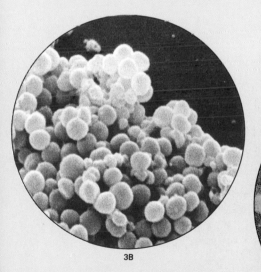

3B

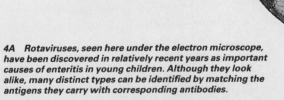

4A

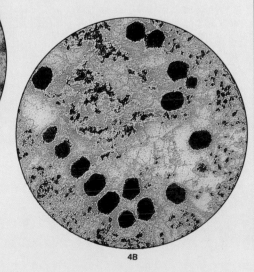

4B

4A   Rotaviruses, seen here under the electron microscope, have been discovered in relatively recent years as important causes of enteritis in young children. Although they look alike, many distinct types can be identified by matching the antigens they carry with corresponding antibodies.

4B   This electron micrograph shows bacteriophages attached to the common bowel bacterium Escherichia coli. Because particular phages attack only particular bacteria, "phage typing" is invaluable as a laboratory tool to identify very precisely bacteria recovered from patients.

Respiratory syncytial virus (RSV)

Not all initially puzzling epidemics turn out to be the work of previously unknown microbes. Thus the outbreak of bronchiolitis, complicated by pneumonia, which killed 121 infants in Naples, Italy, in 1978-9, proved to be a result of RSV infection. RSV is the most important cause of respiratory tract infection among infants and young children. But such was the severity of the Naples outbreak that a novel virus was suspected. In fact, poverty, malnutrition and overcrowding had turned a serious pathogen into a virulent killer.

Pulmonary tuberculosis (TB)

When the pioneer bacteriologist Robert Koch (1843-1910) announced to the Physiological Society of Berlin his discovery of the tubercle bacillus in 1882, there is little doubt that most of his audience had been infected with the organism – yet few if any had developed tuberculosis. *Mycobacterim tuberculosis* is far more likely to cause disease in those debilitated by malnutrition and fatigue. Pulmonary TB, in which the bacteria invade and destroy lung tissue, is the principal type, though TB also attacks bones and other organs. Effective weapons include BCG vaccine and drugs such as streptomycin. Together with improved living conditions, mass radiography to identify early signs, and eradication of the disease in cattle (milk was one source of infection), these have controlled the disease. In the 19th century one person in five died from TB in Britain. Today the death rate is only one per 100,000. But even now tuberculosis kills one person every 30 seconds in the Third World, while elsewhere drug-resistant *M. tuberculosis* persists, particularly among elderly men.

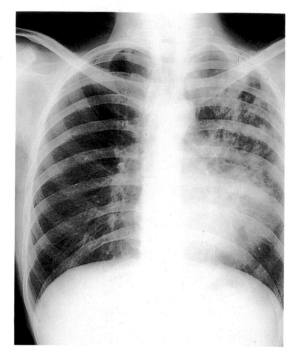

▲ *X-ray of a patient suffering from pulmonary tuberculosis.*

▼ *A tuberculosis sanitorium in England in the 1940s. Such sanitoria were widely built in the late 19th and early 20th centuries. With the advent of mass radiography for early diagnosis and of new drugs, TB became more easily treated and such institutions were no longer needed.*

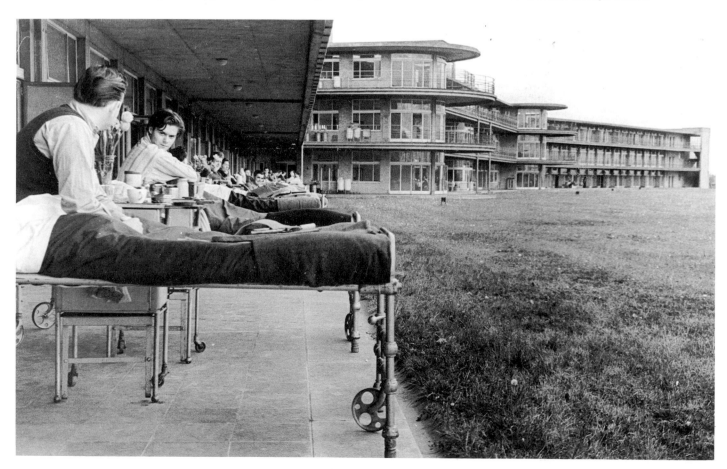

What is sex?...The sexual organs...Intercourse... Fertilization...The developing pregnancy...Giving birth... Breasts and breastfeeding...PERSPECTIVE...Puberty and menstruation...Contraception...Methods of giving birth...Twins

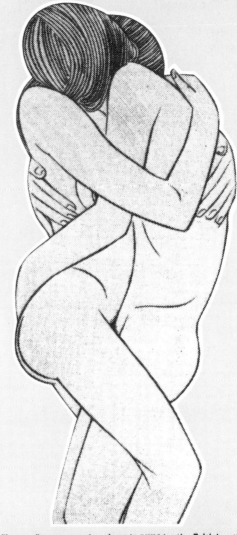

Reproduction does more than sustain the thread of life, ensuring the human species survives. It creates diversity by the mechanism of the two sexes. Although we take it for granted, the difference in form between male and female is the greatest difference in the human race. Women are adapted for child-bearing and men are not, which may allow them to be physically better at other activities. A creature from another planet, unfamiliar with the idea of separate sexes, would think us two different species. Men and women produce different halves of the genetic material needed to make another individual. The process of mixing parental genes in the creation of egg and sperm cells (page 26) ensures that no two children of the same parents are the same, and together they are likely to show more diversity than their parents. Without the existence of sexes, the offspring would have the qualities of only one parent, and perhaps not all of those. This would lead to progressive decline with each generation. In contrast, separate sexes mean diversity, and each generation has a better chance of surviving and thriving.

The male reproductive organs

The fundamental male reproductive organs are the two testicles, which make sperm; the other sex organs merely store and transport sperm. The testicles are oval, 5cm long and half as wide, and contain a fan-like array of tubules. Lining their walls are germinal cells producing sperm, which mature as they move nearer the center. Cells between the germinal cells nourish the developing sperm. Cells between the tubules produce the hormone testosterone (page 90) which is essential for sperm maturation.

▲ *"Lovers", an engraving done in 1924 by the British artist Eric Gill, epitomizing the union of the sexes involved in reproduction of the species. Sexual intercourse is usually preceded by foreplay; stimulation of the erogenous zones stimulates erection of the penis and lubrication of the vagina. Male pleasure derives primarily from ejaculation, female orgasm from stimulation of the clitoris.*

The female genitals

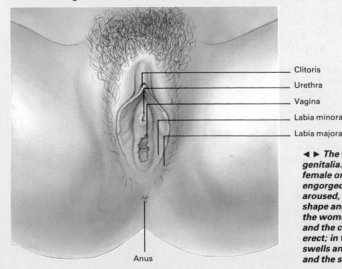

Anus

Clitoris
Urethra
Vagina
Labia minora
Labia majora

The male genitals

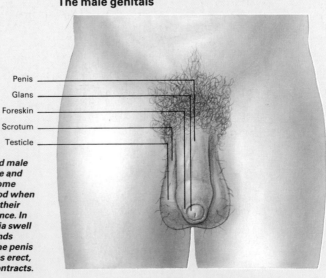

Penis
Glans
Foreskin
Scrotum
Testicle

◀ ▶ *The female and male genitalia. Both male and female organs become engorged with blood when aroused, changing their shape and appearance. In the woman the labia swell and the clitoris stands erect; in the man the penis swells and becomes erect, and the scrotum contracts.*

All the eggs in a woman's ovaries are formed by the time she is born

The male genitals

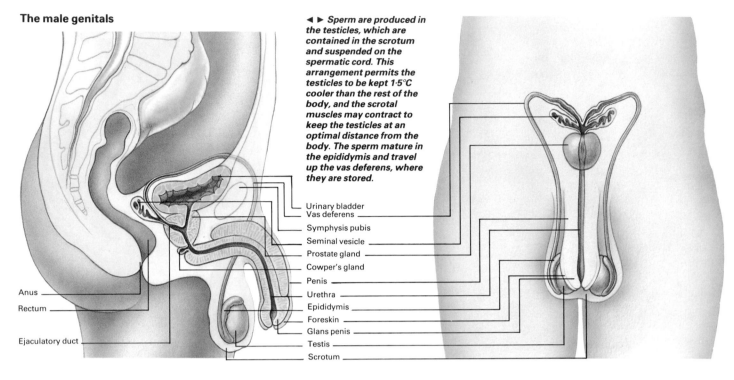

◄ ► *Sperm are produced in the testicles, which are contained in the scrotum and suspended on the spermatic cord. This arrangement permits the testicles to be kept 1·5°C cooler than the rest of the body, and the scrotal muscles may contract to keep the testicles at an optimal distance from the body. The sperm mature in the epididymis and travel up the vas deferens, where they are stored.*

Urinary bladder
Vas deferens
Symphysis pubis
Seminal vesicle
Prostate gland
Cowper's gland
Penis
Urethra
Epididymis
Foreskin
Glans penis
Testis
Scrotum

Anus
Rectum
Ejaculatory duct

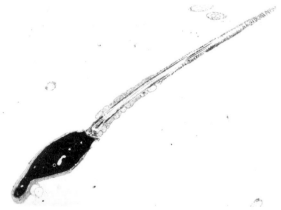

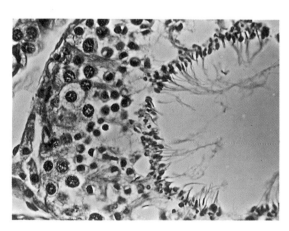

▲ ▲ *A sperm consists of a small head (which contains the nucleus and its genetic information) a body and a long tail. Sperm develop in the germinal cells of the testicles (above), before passing to the epididymis to mature. The coils of the epididymis mean that a sperm may travel some 6m even before ejaculation. It is calculated that a sperm can propel itself at about 20cm an hour.*

Each day an adult male produces three hundred million sperm, which take some six weeks to mature. Only 50µm long and 2.5µm wide (a µm is one thousandth of a millimeter), they are designed to fertilize an egg in a woman's reproductive system, though few succeed. The head bears half the man's chromosomes (◀ page 26), including either his X or his Y chromosome. Behind the head is the midpiece, crammed with mitochondria (◀ page 19) that provide energy for swimming. Beyond is the tail which gyrates to propel the sperm on its lengthy journey to the egg.

Along the side of each testicle is the epididymis, a comma-shaped organ into which the sperm travel, wafted by cilia and maturing as they go. They pass along the 45cm seminal duct (vas deferens), entering the body through the gap in the muscles where the testicles descended before birth. The duct is wide at its far end, and can store sperm for several months. Near the base of the bladder it joins the urethra, the passageway in the penis for sperm and urine.

Three glands mix their secretions with sperm to make semen. The pair of seminal vesicles, 5cm long between bladder and rectum, produce a sugary, viscous, alkaline fluid. This forms 60 percent of the semen and nourishes the sperm. The prostate gland is the size of a chestnut and lies around the bladder's base. It adds a milky alkaline fluid, 30 percent of the semen, that aids sperm motility. The two pea-sized bulbo-urethral glands add mucus for lubrication and a urine-neutralizing substance. Some of its secretion leaves the urethra before the semen. At least 20 million sperm per milliliter are necessary for fertilization, to build up sufficient concentration of enzyme to break down the outer layers of the ovum. From two to six milliliters of semen are issued at a time, either after sexual stimulation or during sleep ("wet dreams"). An emission may contain 50 to 100 million sperm per milliliter.

Masturbation – manual stimulation – is practised by both sexes from infancy, reaching a peak between the ages of three and six, and after puberty. It is harmless.

The female genitals

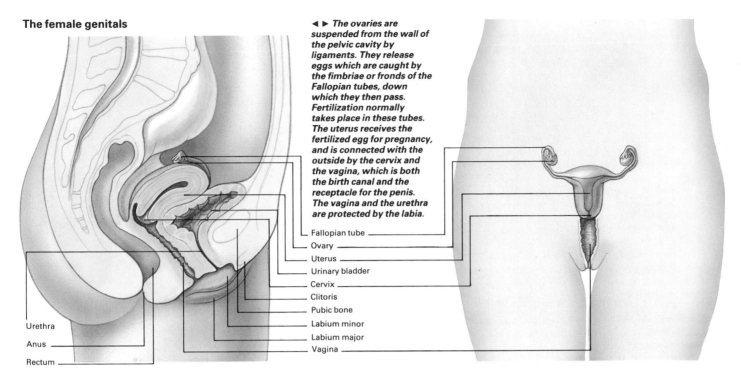

◄ ► *The ovaries are suspended from the wall of the pelvic cavity by ligaments. They release eggs which are caught by the fimbriae or fronds of the Fallopian tubes, down which they then pass. Fertilization normally takes place in these tubes. The uterus receives the fertilized egg for pregnancy, and is connected with the outside by the cervix and the vagina, which is both the birth canal and the receptacle for the penis. The vagina and the urethra are protected by the labia.*

Fallopian tube
Ovary
Uterus
Urinary bladder
Cervix
Clitoris
Pubic bone
Labium minor
Labium major
Vagina

Urethra
Anus
Rectum

At intercourse the penis introduces sperm into the vagina, and must become rigid for this (at other times, rigidity is inconvenient). Inside the penis are three cylinders of tissue, one of which surrounds the urethra. Erection occurs when sexual stimulation enlarges the arteries to the penis, and blood engorges the cylinders to make them swell. Pressure on the veins slows the departure of blood. Erection lasts until sexual excitement stops, when the arteries contract, blood content diminishes and the veins are no longer under pressure. During erection, pressure on the urethra from its surrounding cylinder closes a muscle at the bladder entrance; this stops urine leaving the bladder, and sperm entering it. In addition, the urination reflex is inhibited. The penis is 11-12cm long (along the top) when erect, smaller at other times. Its tip, the sensitive glans (Latin for acorn), is wider than the shaft, and protected by a loose skinfold, the foreskin.

Sex organs in the female

The female reproductive organs are the two ovaries, each the size and shape of an unshelled almond. They are suspended on ligaments about halfway between navel and vagina. They contain undeveloped eggs and, depending on the stage in the menstrual cycle (♦ page 180), a Graafian follicle or corpus luteum. The Graafian follicle consists of a mature egg and its surrounding tissues, and makes estrogen (◀ page 87). After ovulation (release of the egg) the remains of the follicle become enlarged; it is now known as the corpus luteum, secreting three hormones – estrogen, progesterone, and relaxin – to prepare the body for possible fertilization. Ovulation takes place 14-15 days before onset of the next menstruation. All the egg cells in a woman's ovaries – some 200,000 or more – are formed by the time she is born. The number shrinks to about 10,000 at puberty, and only 400 of these are ever matured. Each month, 25 follicles start producing estrogen. One of these (from one or other ovary) matures into a Graafian follicle; the rest dwindle and die. An egg is released into the body cavity at regular intervals of 24-35 days, varying between individuals.

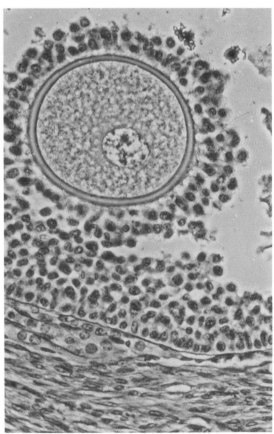

▲ *An egg being shed into the pelvic cavity from the Graafian follicle of the ovary in which it has matured. Several eggs mature in each ovary all the time, but only one is released each month; usually the ovaries produce an egg alternately. The egg is surrounded by other material from the follicle as it is released and passed into the Fallopian tube, along which it is moved by cilia.*

The egg is fertilized not in the womb but high in the Fallopian tubes

Puberty

The age of puberty – sexual maturity and the development of secondary sexual characteristics – varies widely, at different times and places, probably for dietary and social reasons. In girls it generally starts between 9 and 11, when breast buds become noticeable. Pubic hair starts about a year later. Around 13, the nipples darken and armpit hair starts gowing. Menstruation may start at any time during these processes. Ovulation does not occur for the first two years of menstruation, so pregnancy is rare under the age of 15. Puberty in boys occurs slightly later than in girls. The first sign is often testicle growth, generally around the age of 12, followed by pubic hair and penis growth. The first erection may have occurred much earlier, often in infancy. The larynx grows and the voice breaks around 13-14. Mature sperm are not formed until about 16.

The monthly cycle

Menstruation (a "period") is the discharge of 20-100ml of blood, tissue fluid, mucus and surface cells from the uterus. The volume of the discharge often increases with age. Lasting three to six days, it starts 14-15 days after ovulation if a fertilized egg has not implanted. Patches of uterine surface cells are shed gradually – severe bleeding would result if they all went at once. Menstruation is often painful, mainly because the uterus contracts in spasms to expel menstrual fluid.

Ten to twenty days after onset of the last period, depending on cycle length, the ovary releases an egg into the body cavity. Though occasionally lost, this egg is usually drawn into the tentacular, funnel-shaped ends of the Fallopian tubes. Cilia waft it towards the uterus, 10cm away. Fertilization takes place, if at all, in the tube near its junction with the uterus. This muscular organ is an inverted-pear shape, 7·5cm long before the first pregnancy and 10cm afterwards. If not fertilized within 24 hours, the egg decomposes and passes, unnoticed, via the cervix (the neck of the uterus), through the vagina and out. The vagina is about 10cm long when the legs are extended (less when knees are raised). It has three functions – passageway for menstrual flow, receptacle for the penis during sexual intercourse, and birth canal. Its moist lining skin has transverse ridges, and at its lower end is the hymen. This circular membrane varies in size – in many (but not all) women it is torn during the first sexual intercourse.

Outside the vagina are the labia, two pairs of skin flaps. The outer pair are fleshy, with hair outside and oil and sweat glands inside. The inner flaps are thin, with few sweat glands but many oil glands. The inner labia meet in front near the clitoris, a tiny penis-like structure that enlarges during sexual excitement. The urethra, the tube from the bladder, reaches the outside halfway between clitoris and vagina. At each side of the urethra are glands equivalent to the prostate gland of men; at each side of the vagina are glands equivalent to the bulbo-urethral glands. Both pairs of glands secrete mucus for sexual lubrication. The labia and other external sex organs are collectively known as the vulva.

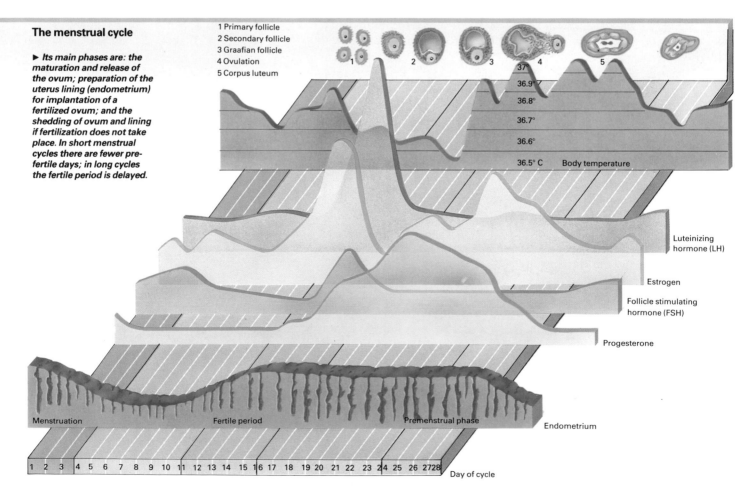

The menstrual cycle

▶ *Its main phases are: the maturation and release of the ovum; preparation of the uterus lining (endometrium) for implantation of a fertilized ovum; and the shedding of ovum and lining if fertilization does not take place. In short menstrual cycles there are fewer pre-fertile days; in long cycles the fertile period is delayed.*

1 Primary follicle
2 Secondary follicle
3 Graafian follicle
4 Ovulation
5 Corpus luteum

37°
36.9°
36.8°
36.7°
36.6°
36.5° C   Body temperature

Luteinizing hormone (LH)

Estrogen

Follicle stimulating hormone (FSH)

Progesterone

Endometrium

Menstruation   Fertile period   Premenstrual phase

1 2 3 4 5 6 7 8 9 10 11 12 13 14 15 16 17 18 19 20 21 22 23 24 25 26 2728   Day of cycle

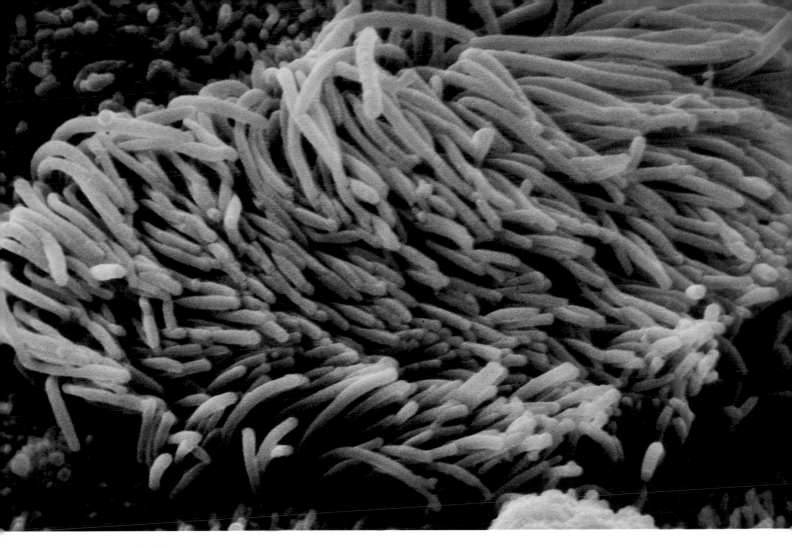

Intercourse and fertilization

The meeting of egg and sperm is made possible by sexual intercourse. The act would never occur without the desire to initiate it (probably stronger in men, especially when young) and its pleasure and satisfaction inviting repeat activity (possibly stronger in women, and increasing with experience). The genital organs become engorged with blood, particularly in men, and glands produce lubricating fluid, more so in women. These reactions can be triggered in two ways – via the brain, through psychological factors, or as a reflex from touch receptors in several places. The woman is receptive as the man eases his erect penis into her vagina. Both contribute to increasing excitement and pleasure with the rhythmic moving that thrusts the penis to and fro. In men, orgasm (climax) and emission of semen occur when stimulation reaches maximum intensity. Reflexes from the spinal cord make the sperm ducts and fluid-producing glands contract, so that semen collects in the urethra. Further reflexes send rhythmic impulses to muscles at the base of the penis, which ejaculates semen in several thrusts. In women, similar reflexes induce rhythmic contractions of the vaginal muscles, inducing a climax which may be less obvious than in men. In both sexes, heart rate and blood pressure increase during intercourse. These subside rapidly after orgasm, and are replaced by warm sweating and relaxation.

Sperm need four to six hours in the female body before they can fertilize an egg, high in the Fallopian tube. While they are swimming through the uterus (and swimming against the cilia in the tubes), female body fluids release enzyme from the sperm heads. It takes many sperm to produce enough enzyme to melt the egg's coat, allowing one to penetrate. As soon as it has – leaving its tail behind – minute electrical changes in the egg's coat prevent other sperms entering.

▲ Tentacle-like projections known as the infundibulum pick up the ovum after it has been shed by the ovary and pass it into the Fallopian tube, along which it is moved by cilia towards the uterus.

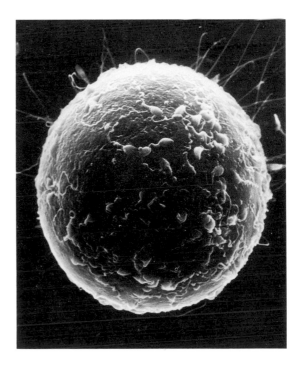

▲ An ovum surrounded by sperm, one of which is piercing the gelatinous covering of the ovum, assisted by chemicals released by all the sperm. An electrical charge is set up which blocks the others from penetrating the ovum as well.

Contraception

Avoiding pregnancy
Conception may be prevented by natural methods, devices and chemicals, hormone pills and injections, or operations. Efficiency differs with the method used and the user's experience, education, age and motivation. Failure rates for experienced and less experienced users, expressed as pregnancies per hundred women per year, are mentioned in the relevant captions.

Natural techniques of contraception
Of the natural methods, the most effective but least enjoyable is abstinence. Coitus interruptus – the withdrawal of the penis before the male partner reaches orgasm – requires self-discipline and a good sense of timing. Some people find it satisfactory; others do not. The safe period (avoiding times when conception is possible) is unreliable, partly because it is poorly understood. Biologists now believe that sperm may be able to fertilize for five days after intercourse, but the egg is fertilizable for no more than 24 hours. Ovulation can be reliably predicted as 14-15 days before the next period is due. A woman should keep note of her cycle length for six months. The first unsafe day in the cycle can then be calculated as the shortest cycle time minus 20. The last is the longest time minus 10. Ovulation is marked by a 0·5°C rise in body temperature, best taken on waking. The Billings (mucus) method relies on examining changes in the mucus on the cervix. This indicates the stage of the cycle. Using the Billings method effectively requires practice.

The diaphragm

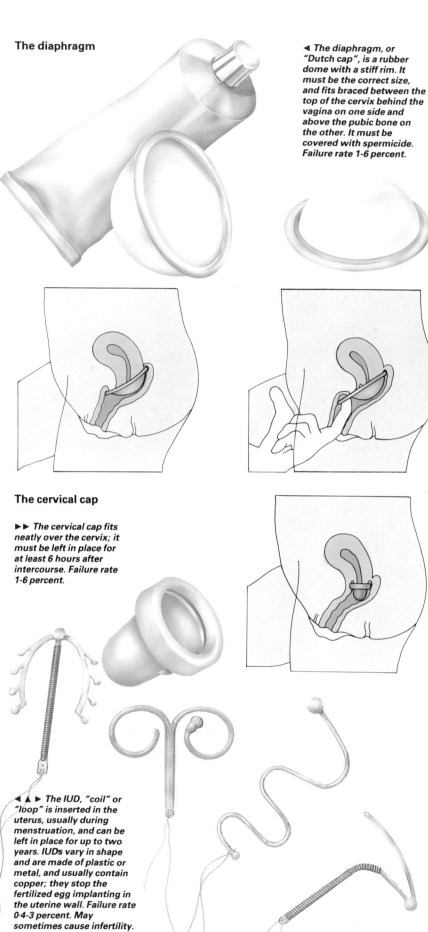

◄ The diaphragm, or "Dutch cap", is a rubber dome with a stiff rim. It must be the correct size, and fits braced between the top of the cervix behind the vagina on one side and above the pubic bone on the other. It must be covered with spermicide. Failure rate 1-6 percent.

The cervical cap

►► The cervical cap fits neatly over the cervix; it must be left in place for at least 6 hours after intercourse. Failure rate 1-6 percent.

The intra-uterine device (IUD)

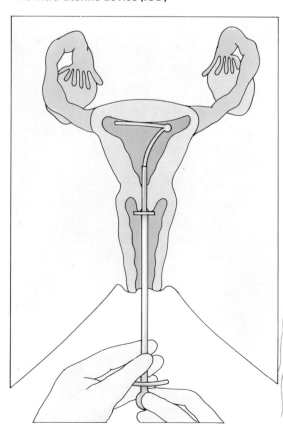

◄ ▲ ► The IUD, "coil" or "loop" is inserted in the uterus, usually during menstruation, and can be left in place for up to two years. IUDs vary in shape and are made of plastic or metal, and usually contain copper; they stop the fertilized egg implanting in the uterine wall. Failure rate 0·4-3 percent. May sometimes cause infertility.

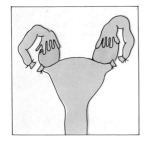

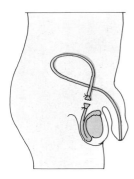

▲ **Sterilization involves removing, severing or placing clips on the Fallopian tubes in women or severing the vas deferens (vasectomy). Female sterilization may occasionally fail in cases where the tube becomes unblocked again. Failure rates 0-0·4 percent.**

The Pill

There are several types of hormonal contraceptive. The ordinary ("combined") Pill, consisting of estrogen and progesterone, prevents ovulation. There are two forms, regular and low-dose. It is taken for 21 days, followed by a seven-day break, during which there is bleeding resembling menstruation, but lighter.

The Pill carries a small risk of cardiovascular disease, low in young women but increasing with age, fatness and tobacco-smoking. Between the ages of 30 and 40 it becomes safer to use a progesterone-only pill. This must be taken, at the same time every day (or within three hours of it), without a break. It obstructs movement of sperm by thickening cervical mucus – ovulation and menstruation take place normally. Its safety does not decrease with age.

Depo-provera is similar, but is injected every three months, though its effect can last twice as long. It is used by people who dislike having (or remembering) to take pills, for women who wish to conceal their use of contraception, for partners of men awaiting clearance after vasectomy, and in remote places where medical care is available infrequently.

The morning-after pill prevents implantation by altering the uterine surface. It consists of four high-dose combined tablets (in Britain, only Ovran or Eugynon 50 are a suitable formula). Two tablets are taken within 72 hours of intercourse, followed exactly 12 hours later by two more. It is 99 percent effective.

A contraceptive pill for men?

Chinese scientists in the 1960s noticed that male infertility was often linked with the use of crude cottonseed oil for cooking. They investigated further and discovered that the active agent was a yellow pigment, gossypol. Since 1972, more than 8,000 volunteers have taken gossypol in clinical trials. A dose of 20mg a day for ten weeks, followed by 50mg once a week, is 99 percent effective at reducing sperm count to a very low level. Ten percent of men remain infertile after treatment stops. Gossypol's adverse effects are fatigue, dizzyness and digestive upsets. Research in the West for an efficient male contraceptive has been unproductive. Based on pituitary hormones, the only effective forms yet developed require twice-daily injections.

Irreversible methods of contraception

Sterilization is done by excising a section of the tubes that carry eggs or sperm. The operation for men, known as vasectomy, takes 30 minutes and is performed under local anesthetic. Even after it has been done, existing sperm are still viable and can fertilize an egg for several weeks, and fertility must be assumed until the sperm count is too low to be effective.

Sterilization in women usually requires a general anesthetic and two to three days in hospital. It is effective immediately. There is no guarantee that either vasectomy or sterilization can be reversed, and neither is recommended for people who may subsequently wish for a family.

The condom

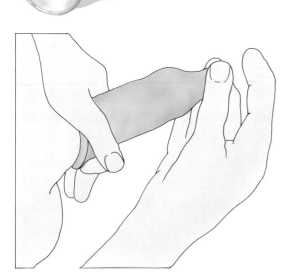

◀ **The condom, or sheath, is the most frequently used mechanical contraceptive. It is a thin latex tube, usually with a teat for the semen. It is placed on the erect penis, and used with care. It must be held in position on withdrawal from the vagina, and must be discarded after use. Failure rate 0·8-5·5 percent.**

▶ **The ordinary Pill consists of estrogen and progesterone, preventing ovulation. It must be taken regularly and without interruption except during periods. The progesterone-only pill prevents the movement of sperm. Failure rates 0-0·5 (standard and low-dose pills); 0·5-2·5 (progesterone only pill).**

The Pill

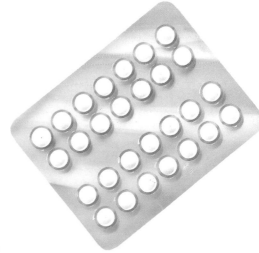

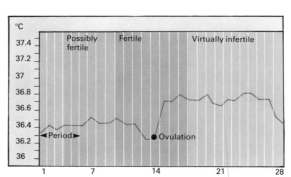

◀ **To follow the rhythm method, a woman keeps a record of her body temperature throughout the month. Since the temperature rises slightly on ovulation, after several months she can predict the date of ovulation, and so calculate the safe periods of the month. This method is often used in conjunction with the Billings method. Failure rate about 15 percent.**

Many of the embryo's internal organs can be distinguished at the age of six weeks

The developing pregnancy

When an egg has been fertilized, it moves towards the uterus, dividing as it goes. At first it stays the same size; its cells get smaller as they increase in number. By the time it is seven or eight days old it consists of two hollow balls of cells, one inside the other. It plants itself in the uterus, the outer cell layer becoming the original placenta. The inner cells form the rest of the placenta and the embryo (developing baby). The placenta immediately starts its two functions – nutrition and excretion for the embryo, and hormone production. These hormones act on the mother's body, maintaining pregnancy and preventing further egg-production (it would be inconvenient to have several overlapping pregnancies of different stages). Initially, only two hormones (◆ page 90) are produced. Human chorionic gonadotropin (HCG) maintains the corpus luteum throughout pregnancy, and human chorionic somatomammotropin (HCS) stimulates milk-producing glands in the breasts. Seven weeks later the placenta starts producing estrogen and progesterone. HCG production falls at the end of the third month, because the placenta's own estrogen and progesterone output is high and the corpus luteum can make less. Towards the end of pregnancy, the placenta and corpus luteum both produce relaxin, which relaxes the ligaments of the pelvic symphysis and helps open the neck of the uterus.

After implantation of the fertilized egg in the uterus wall, cells in the middle of the embryo divide into three layers that will eventually become skin (ectoderm), gut (endoderm), and muscle, bone and blood vessels (mesoderm). The umbilical cord is an outpushing from the embryo, consisting of all three layers. The endodermal and mesodermal layers become the placenta, but the ectodermal layer wraps round the embryo, holding the amniotic fluid ("waters"). By the end of three months the placenta is fully developed, looking like a flat cake of liver, and includes a layer of uterine tissue, shed with it at birth. The tissues of mother and baby meet over a large surface area which is very convoluted. This allows the fetus (as the developing baby is called after ten weeks) to absorb oxygen and nutrients from the mother's blood, and offload waste products including carbon dioxide. Blood sinuses on the maternal side come close to blood vessels from the fetus, but their circulations never mix. The blood sinuses bleed after the placenta is delivered, but this gradually stops as the surge of oxytocin makes the uterus contract.

The first sign of pregnancy is a missed period. Pregnancy tests are usually reliable two weeks later. By this time a woman may "feel" pregnant in an undefinable way. She may experience nausea in the mornings, sleepiness and frequency of urination. After two months, morning sickness has stopped, and weight gain averages 500g. Although very variable, weight gain accelerates, averaging 4kg at 18 weeks, 9kg at 30 weeks and 12-13kg by the full term of 38 weeks. Of this, 3·3kg is baby, 650g placenta, 800g amniotic fluid, 900g increased uterus, 400g increased breasts, 1,250g extra maternal blood and 1,200g extra tissue fluid. The remainder is body fat and milk. Quickening, when the mother can first feel the fetus move, is at 15-18 weeks. A waxy plug forms in the cervix. The breasts enlarge a little at the beginning of pregnancy, stay the same for five or six months, and grow again at the end. The uterus grows so that its top is level with the navel after five months, 5cm above it at seven months, rising another 2cm in the next six weeks. It drops again in the last fortnight of the pregnancy as the baby settles into the birth position.

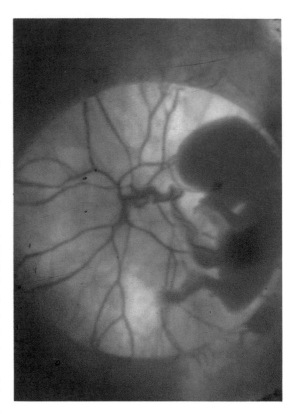

▲ *The fetus at about eight weeks in its amniotic sac, in which it is supported and able to grow without jarring or compression from surrounding organs. The fetus now weighs 1g.*

▼ *The fetus at 12 weeks, by which time all the external appendages are fully formed (including even fingerprints) as are the internal body systems. It moves of its own accord.*

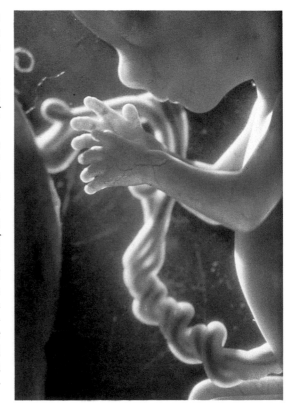

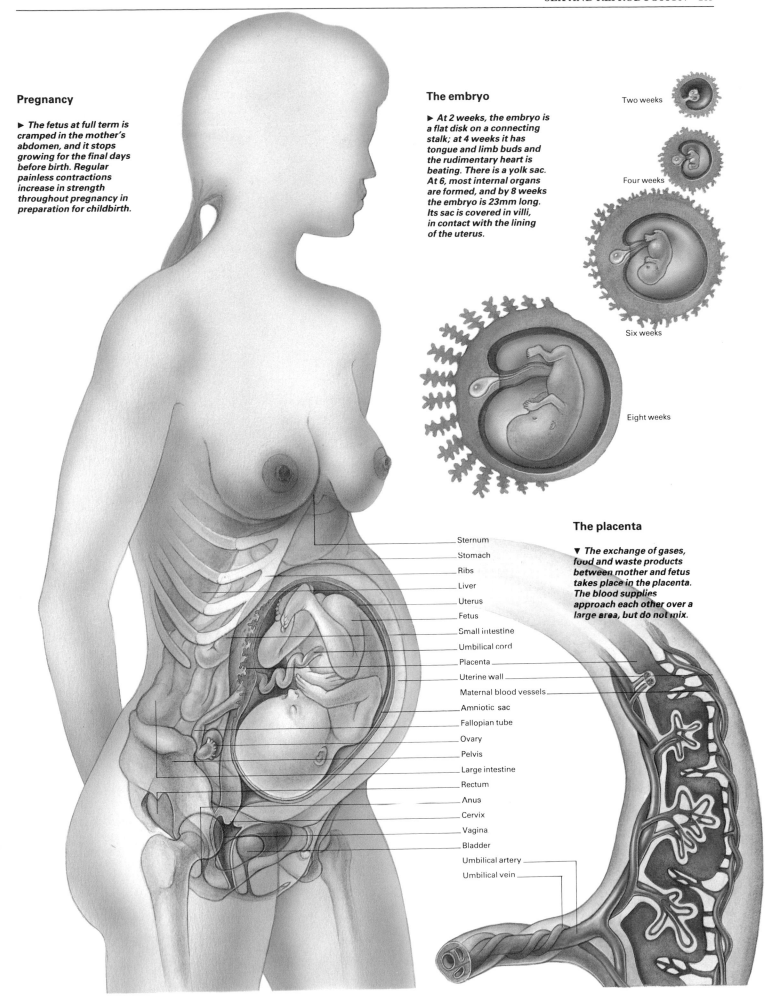

Pregnancy

▶ *The fetus at full term is cramped in the mother's abdomen, and it stops growing for the final days before birth. Regular painless contractions increase in strength throughout pregnancy in preparation for childbirth.*

The embryo

▶ *At 2 weeks, the embryo is a flat disk on a connecting stalk; at 4 weeks it has tongue and limb buds and the rudimentary heart is beating. There is a yolk sac. At 6, most internal organs are formed, and by 8 weeks the embryo is 23mm long. Its sac is covered in villi, in contact with the lining of the uterus.*

Two weeks

Four weeks

Six weeks

Eight weeks

The placenta

▼ *The exchange of gases, food and waste products between mother and fetus takes place in the placenta. The blood supplies approach each other over a large area, but do not mix.*

Sternum
Stomach
Ribs
Liver
Uterus
Fetus
Small intestine
Umbilical cord
Placenta
Uterine wall
Maternal blood vessels
Amniotic sac
Fallopian tube
Ovary
Pelvis
Large intestine
Rectum
Anus
Cervix
Vagina
Bladder
Umbilical artery
Umbilical vein

Most of the effort of labor is devoted to opening the cervix to the diameter of the baby's head

Biologists do not know what triggers the onset of labor, 40 weeks after the last menstrual period and 38 weeks after conception. Progesterone output, which normally inhibits contractions of the uterus, falls. Estrogen levels, which aid labor, rise. The brain produces oxytocin, a hormone that induces contraction, and prolactin, which promotes milk production. Relaxin output rises.

The birth of the child

Labor lasts about 18 hours for the first pregnancy, less on subsequent occasions. It has three stages. The first, lasting 12-14 hours on the first occasion, opens the cervix and pulls it back over the baby's head. It starts with contractions every 20-30 minutes, speeding to every two to three minutes. When the cervix is fully dilated the contractions change, and a feeling of "bearing-down" heralds the second stage. This second stage is the birth, lasting from a few minutes to two hours. The upper part of the uterus contracts and the lower half stretches. The baby's head turns in the basin-shaped hipbone, so that it comes out face-sideways. It then rotates back again (or is helped by the midwife) so that the shoulders emerge horizontally. If the vagina will not stretch sufficiently, doctors make a cut (episiotomy), which is sewn up afterwards. In a breech presentation, the baby's bottom comes out first. Rarely, the feet appear first. In the third stage, lasting twenty minutes, the placenta and cord come away. Although the uterus starts shrinking immediately, about 500ml of blood may be lost.

Most general anesthetics are unsuitable during normal delivery as they can reduce the baby's power to breathe and retard its development in the first weeks of life. Instead, women are usually given a gas/air mixture to reduce perception of pain, or are given an epidural – a continuous injection of anesthetic into the air space around the dura mater (◀ page 56) of the lower spine. This reduces or abolishes sensation in the abdomen and legs. Women may also be given local anesthetics, which do not prevent them pushing.

Normal birth is followed by vaginal bleeding for two weeks while the uterus shrinks. The discharge becomes less bloody and more watery as it dwindles. Most women are briefly depressed about three days after delivery.

The stages of childbirth

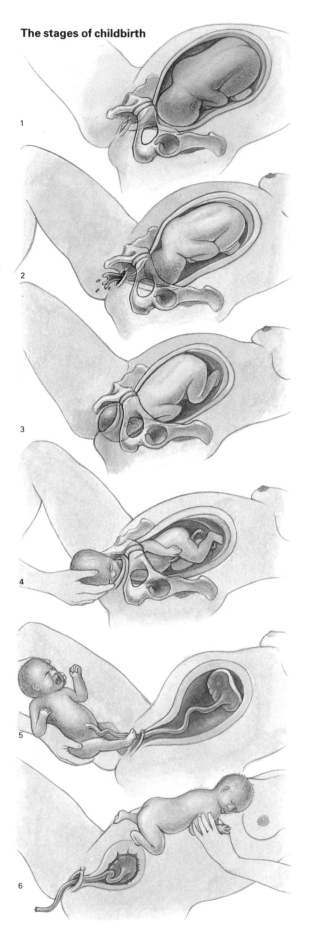

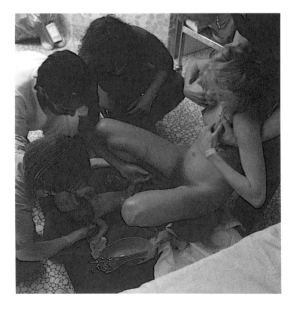

▶ *Childbirth has three major stages. In the first stage, (1) the cervix slowly dilates until it is about 10cm in diameter. At some point the amniotic sac ruptures and the "waters" emerge (2). In the second stage, (3-5) which is much shorter, the contractions bear down on the baby and push it through the pelvic opening. The head is usually born first; its appearance is known as the crowning (3). To squeeze the shoulders through the narrow pelvic outlet the baby rotates through 90°, then emerges completely. In the third stage (6) the placenta is born.*

◀ *Increasingly, doctors are encouraging positions for birth that enable gravity to help the contractions.*

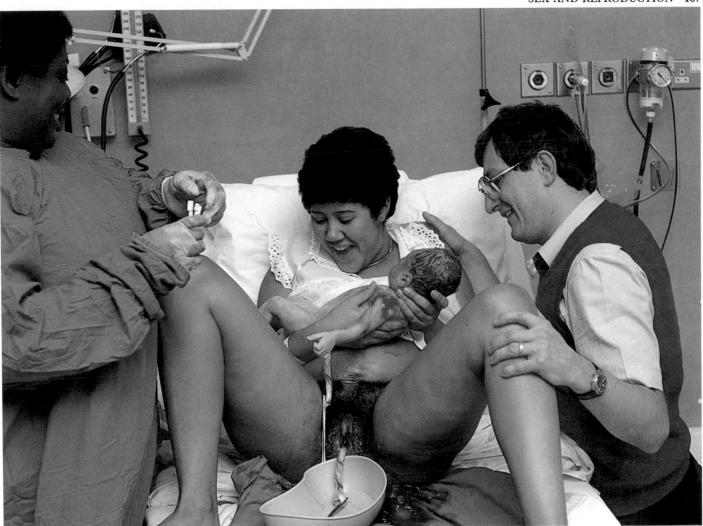

Methods of giving birth

In recent years there has been a move away from the traditional method of giving birth lying in bed (the "stranded beetle" position) in a delivery room resembling an operating theatre. In its place is an attempt to reduce the pain, stress and effort of labor by practising in advance the art of deep breathing and relaxation, which reduces the need for painkilling drugs. Biofeedback (◆page 76) has proved useful help as women relax and participate at the same time, but is surprisingly little used. In 1975 the French gynecologist Frederick Leboyer advocated giving birth in a new setting – sitting upright in a room that is dimly lit and calm, with soft music and attendants who are not wearing operating-theater masks and gloves.

Leboyer's views are echoed by another French gynecologist, Michel Odent. Odent uses a room with no visible medical equipment (it is kept outside the door, available at a moment's notice) and the optional use of a shallow pool so that the baby leaves the waters of the womb to enter a similar pond. In this way, he says, birth is a gentle transition from the womb to the outside world – he has observed that babies seem to find the warm water comforting.

Both Leboyer and Odent originally advocated the presence of the baby's father in the delivery room, but in 1984 Odent changed his view, preferring fathers to stay away. This, he says, is because birth attendants are, by tradition, entirely female – but paradoxically he does not exclude his own presence at the birth.

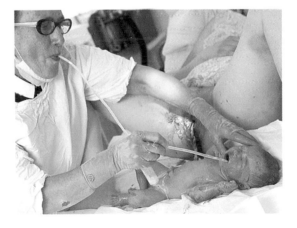

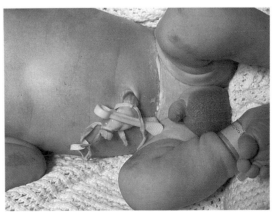

▲ A couple happily meet their new baby. The umbilical cord is usually cut after it stops pulsating, and the baby has begun its independent existence. The third stage, giving birth to the placenta, is still to come.

◄ The new baby may have swallowed some of the amniotic fluid and this is cleared from its lungs. The first breath is usually deep and the baby cries of its own accord. It is checked to ensure its orifices are correctly formed.

◄ After the umbilical cord has been cut, and clamped, the baby's body adjusts. The hole in the heart septum (◆page 168) closes, taking deoxygenated blood to the lungs, and the baby prepares to receive food through its mouth.

Breasts are part of both male and female bodies, but only in women do they they receive the hormones that surround them with fat, mature the milk glands, form milk and eject it. The amount of true breast tissue is much the same in all women, but the quantity of surrounding fat varies. (Breast contours develop in obese men because they make estrogen with their body fat.) Each breast consists of 15-20 lobes of milk-producing cells. Milk reaches the nipple along seven to ten tubes that are wider in one part to allow a certain amount of storage. The nipple is surrounded by a circle of darker skin with fat glands that lubricate sucking and help prevent soreness. The pigmented circle darkens during pregnancy (and stays dark afterwards) as a side effect of pituitary hormone output. Touching the nipples of both men and women triggers a reflex, making them harder.

The presence in the body of estrogen and progesterone from the placenta inhibits milk production before the birth of the baby, but as soon as the placenta is delivered milk production can start.

Prolactin differs from other hormones by, in effect, stimulating its own production. Sucking the nipple sends reflexes to the brain that make more prolactin. It also produces more oxytocin, which makes breast tissue expel the milk it has produced. Thus the more the baby sucks, the more milk is produced. Breast-feeding takes about three days to become established, and requires the participation of a hungry baby. (Many women, not realizing this, give up breastfeeding as they feel they are incompetent and their baby is being undernourished.) It is likely to fail if the infant, given bottled milk, has less incentive to suck hard. The oxytocin produced by sucking has two other effects. It continues making the uterus contract, speeding its return to normal size. It also inhibits LH and FSH (the hormones involved in developing follicles in the ovaries; ◆ page 90), so that the ovaries delay releasing more eggs. This is why breast-feeding is a good contraceptive, though not a completely reliable one.

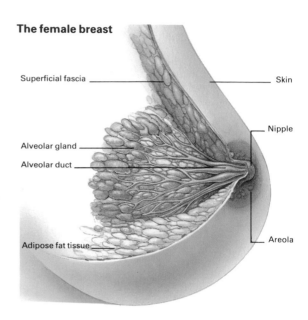

The female breast

Superficial fascia — Skin

Nipple

Alveolar gland

Alveolar duct

Areola

Adipose fat tissue

▲ *The breast consists of fatty tissue and a number of milk-producing alveolar cells. During pregnancy the breasts swell and become capable of producing milk, though the high levels of pregnancy hormones inhibit any actual production. After birth, the breast initially produces colostrum rather than milk. This contains some of the nutrients of milk, but no fat; milk production begins after a few days.*

The breast versus the bottle
Breast milk is the perfect baby food – artificial feeds are merely a good imitation. It is warm, sterile, and carries antibodies against colds and other illnesses. Because it contains no non-human protein it may be good for the developing immune system (◆ page 213). The feeding process strengthens the bond between mother and baby. For the mother, its advantage is its on-line availability. Its disadvantages are often leaking breasts and sore nipples, and it requires her presence every time – which may prove difficult if she is working. Bottle-feeding offers one certain benefit to the baby – it gives the father a chance to do the feeding, and so cements paternal bonding. Weaning usually occurs at six months.

Twins and multiple births
Usually, only one of the 25 follicles that mature each month in the ovaries is allowed to release an egg for possible fertilization. On rare occasions, two or more eggs are produced and fertilized, producing non-identical twins (or triplets, or more). Twins are commonest among Negros and rarest in Eskimos. They are commoner in second and subsequent pregnancies, in older mothers, and in women given fertility drugs (especially by less experienced doctors).

The tendency to have twins can be an inherited characteristic. Very rarely, a single developing egg may split in two producing identical twins. Such twins share a single placenta and have their entire set of genes in common (◆ page 28). Even more rarely the split is incomplete, giving Siamese twins (◆ page 196).

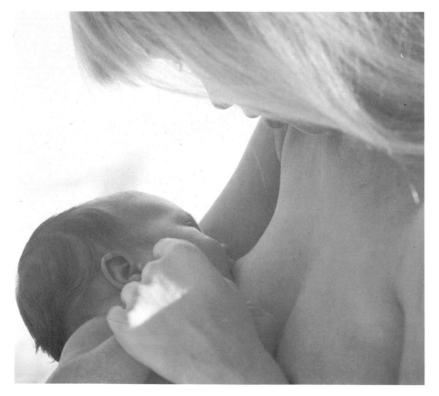

◀ *Breast milk provides nourishment and vital antibodies.*

Reproductive Defects

Mechanical and fundamental infertility...Causes of male infertility...Female fertility problems...Difficulties in pregnancy...Perinatal problems...PERSPECTIVE... Test-tube babies and other new techniques...The rights of the embryo

The male genitals

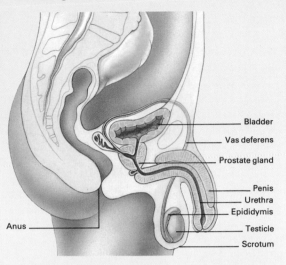

- Bladder
- Vas deferens
- Prostate gland
- Penis
- Urethra
- Epididymis
- Testicle
- Scrotum

Anus

There is no shortage of babies in the world, but infertility can cause considerable anguish to many people. About one couple in six cannot produce children without help. In recent years, better understanding of embryology has led to an expansion of techniques to overcome infertility. This has raised many complex ethical issues concerning the rights of the embryo and the parents.

As suggested by the physiology of reproduction (◀ page 177), the cause of infertility may rest either with the man or the woman. Male malfunctions are responsible in about 40 percent of couples and those of both partners in about 15 percent. As the cause cannot be established in a further 10 percent of cases, infertility may be spread equally between the sexes.

Failure to reproduce may be fundamental or mechanical. In the former case eggs are not produced, and/or sperm are not produced at all, or are produced in insufficient quantity to effect fertilization. A mechanical problem is one in which those elements are produced satisfactorily, but fail to come together, or when the egg is fertilized but does not remain viable. Psychological problems affecting copulation, and more rarely impotence or frigidity of physical origin, can also cause infertility.

Malfunctions of male fertility

Male infertility usually results from a failure to produce sperm (azoospermia), or to produce enough sperm which are normal and sufficiently motile to reach an egg and penetrate it (oligospermia). Infertility of this kind may be caused by hormonal deficiencies, disease, treatment with drugs or the production of antibodies against sperm. These cause the man's defense system to treat his sperm as invaders and destroy them (◀ page 213, 230).

Sperm formation and maturation are assisted by follicle-stimulating hormone (FSH) and luteinizing hormone (LH). These so-called gonadotrophins are released by the pituitary gland, after stimulation by gonadotrophin-releasing hormone, which is manufactured by the hypothalamus region of the brain to control their release (◀ page 86). Consequently, disorders of the pituitary or of the hypothalamus can cause infertility. Such disorders can often be reversed by hormone treatment.

Inflammation of the testes can damage their ability to produce sperm. The common childhood ailment mumps, if caught in adult life, is the best-known example of a disease which can cause such damage. Sperm formation can also be inhibited by some drugs. These include alcohol, barbiturates, cannabis and some antidepressants. Ionizing radiation (radioactivity) and various substances to which industrial workers may be exposed, including some metals and complex organic compounds, may also impair sperm production.

▼ *Seminal fluid can be examined under the microscope to see whether a male is fertile or not. Dilution of the sample, as shown here, enables the technician not only to see whether the sample contains live sperm, but also to assess the number present. Even if live sperm are produced, a man may be effectively sterile if his sperm count is low, since many sperm must be present to allow one to fertilize the ovum.*

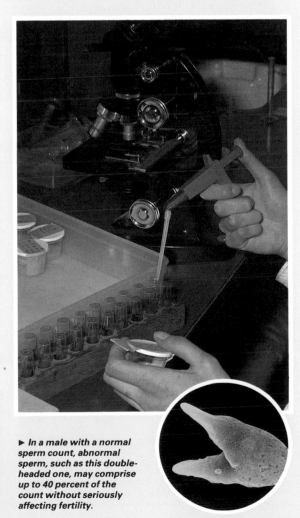

▶ *In a male with a normal sperm count, abnormal sperm, such as this double-headed one, may comprise up to 40 percent of the count without seriously affecting fertility.*

The rights of "test-tube" embryos and babies are still fiercely argued

Drugs may also affect male fertility by reducing the ability of the muscle at the base of the bladder to contract. As a result, sperm are pushed into the bladder instead of being ejaculated. Drugs prescribed for some ailments, including high blood pressure, and some diseases, including diabetes, may also cause impotence, the inability to sustain an erection for long enough to complete intercourse.

Male fertility may also be affected by several other physical conditions. The most common is an enlargement of veins in the spermatic cord (the nerves, arteries, veins, muscle and vas deferens which together form the main supporting structure for the testicles). Such enlarged veins are known as varicoceles, and can be treated surgically. Varicoceles may cause infertility by producing a localized increase in temperature.

Sperm are very sensitive to rises in temperature, and it is known that men whose jobs entail sitting for long periods – truck or taxi drivers for example – tend to have lower sperm counts than average. In some cases relating to the destruction of sperm by heat, male infertility has been cured when the sufferer changed from tight to loose-fitting underpants.

Cryptorchism, in which one or both testicles fail to descend at birth, is a further cause of infertility in which temperature may play a part. This condition usually requires surgical treatment, as does hypospadias, in which the urethra opens on the underside of the penis. This can prevent sperm from being ejaculated sufficiently far into the vagina to achieve fertilization.

The body's immune system sometimes causes infertility by treating the sperm as invading microbes and neutralizing them. This may either happen when the man's own defenses mobilize against his sperm, or when the woman makes antibodies which attack them. Immuno-suppressive drugs are now being used successfully to treat this form of male infertility.

Test-tube babies

In July 1978 the world's first "test-tube baby" was born. She was the result of "in vitro" (literally, in glass) fertilization (IVF), the combining of egg and sperm outside the body. Since that time, many babies have been born to infertile couples as a result of IVF.

IVF involves the removal of a fertile egg from an ovary by laparoscopy (the technique of introducing a fiber-optics tube into the abdomen to enable the surgeon to view the inside of the body without making a large incision). It is then fertilized with sperm obtained by masturbation, and implanted into the mother's womb to develop. This method overcomes infertility only if the partners can both produce viable eggs and sperm.

Fertility drugs may be given to a woman before laparoscopy in order to induce multiple egg production. Then several eggs can be fertilized and placed in the mother, to improve the chances of the pregnancy establishing itself. Or spare eggs may be frozen for use later, if a first attempt fails.

In cases where the male partner is infertile, artificial insemination by donor may be used. If the woman's fertility is unimpaired, sperm donated by a fertile male can be injected into her vagina. If she has fertility problems but produces viable eggs, these may be fertilized in vitro by donor sperm.

If the woman does not ovulate, an egg donated by another woman can be fertilized in vitro by her husband's sperm and then implanted in her. Alternatively, another woman (known as a surrogate mother) can be artificially inseminated and carry the baby. If the woman does ovulate but cannot carry a baby, one of her fertilized eggs may be implanted into another woman's womb (womb-leasing), where it develops normally.

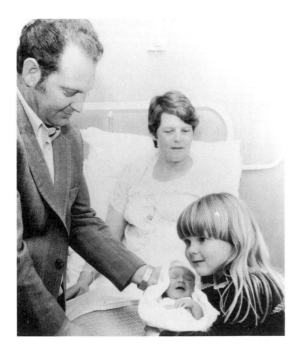

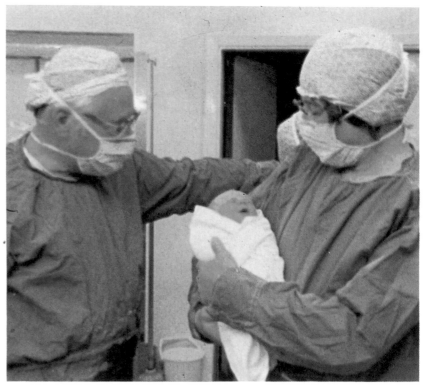

▲ *Louise Brown, the first test-tube baby, with her younger sister, also conceived by IVF.*

▶ *Gynecologist Patrick Steptoe and embryologist Robert Edwards, who did the first successful IVF.*

The debate on the rights of embryos

Unless both sperm and egg are contributed by the couple, the baby is not theirs genetically. This raises questions as to what the baby should be told about its parentage when it grows older. In some countries adopted children have the right to know who their genetic parents were. The rights of babies produced by modern techniques to such knowledge have yet to be established.

The rights of the sponsoring parents, and of the woman who gives birth to their child, are also in dispute. If a surrogate mother proves unwilling to part with the child after its birth, should her contract with the sponsoring parents be binding?

When does the embryo itself have rights? Where more than one egg is fertilized but only one implanted, what should happen to the remainder? Until what time during development should it be permissible to use a "spare" embryo for research?

Some causes of female infertility

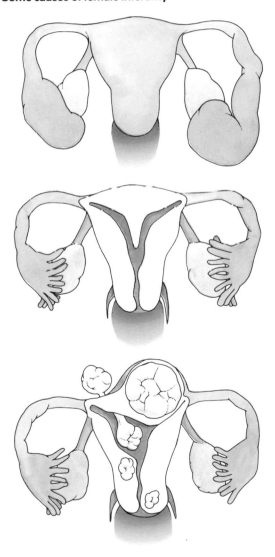

▲ Top, blocked and swollen tubes (salpingitis) may be caused by infection, and may require surgery. Center, a septum may distort the shape of the uterus; below, fibroids, benign tumors of the uterus, may interfere with pregnancy.

Malfunctions of female fertility

Female infertility is generally caused by factors similar to those found in men. Hormonal abnormalities can affect not only ovulation, but also the ability of the uterus to retain a fertilized egg. However, in the female, the mechanics of the system may interfere with reproduction in more ways than in the male. After its release from the ovary, an egg has to travel down the Fallopian tube.

The two Fallopian tubes may be damaged so that the egg's passage is hindered. In some cases, the tubes are blocked (sometimes as a result of damage done by an IUD ◀ page 182). In others, scar tissue formed after inflammation – resulting for example from gonorrhea or acute appendicitis – prevents the egg's passage without there being an actual blockage. Another tubal problem is endometriosis. The endometrium is specialized tissue produced in the uterus into which the fertilized egg can implant. This adherent tissue sometimes forms in the Fallopian tubes and interferes with the passage of eggs.

During the part of the menstrual cycle when an egg is available for fertilization, watery cervical mucus is produced which helps the sperm to swim into the Fallopian tubes. Sometimes infertility is caused by the failure to produce mucus in sufficient quantity or of satisfactory consistency. Blockage of the tubes and disturbance of the cervical mucus can be overcome, in some cases by drug treatment and in others by surgery.

Eventually, all women cease to produce eggs. The menopause (◀ page 95) usually occurs in middle age, but egg production can become increasingly erratic after about 40 years, even though menstruation is regular. Egg production can also fail prematurely. This causes irreversible sterility, usually in the early 30s. Irregular ovulation, which reduces fertility, can be caused by drugs, disease and psychological stress. In some conditions, such as anorexia nervosa, ovulation may stop completely, although not irreversibly.

◀ ▼ *In laparoscopy, a viewing tube is passed into the woman's abdomen through a small incision in her navel; the technique allows microsurgery, sealing tubes or removing ova, often under only a local anesthetic.*

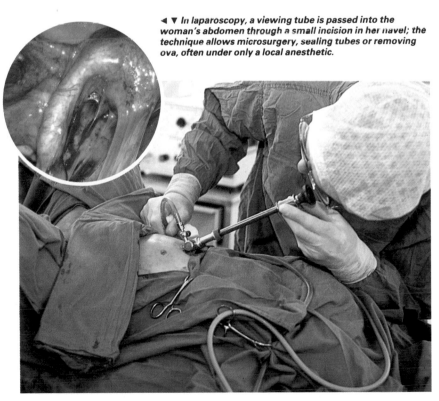

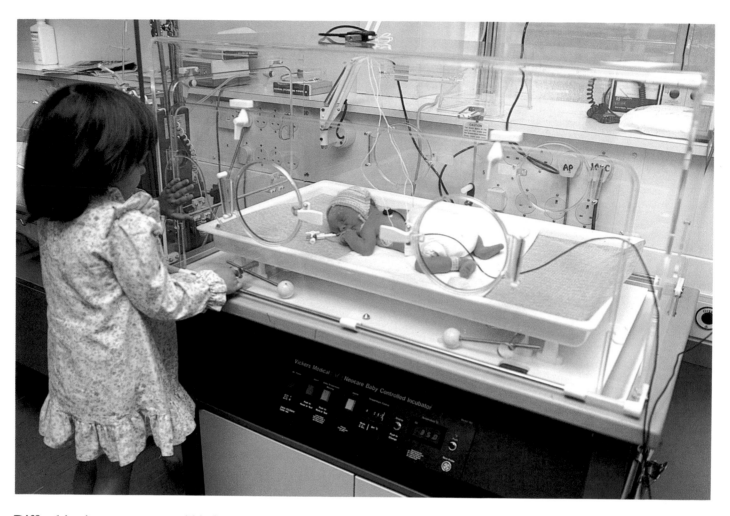

Difficulties in pregnancy and birth

Edema (swelling) during pregnancy, now called pre-eclampsia, occurs in five percent of pregnancies after week 20. Other signs of pre-eclampsia are hypertension and albumin in the urine. If untreated (with bed rest, fluids, intravenous salt solutions and drugs), it leads to eclampsia – fits, and, sometimes, death. It is caused by a partial blockage of arteries feeding the placenta.

Bleeding in the last three months of pregnancy is caused by partial separation of the placenta or implantation of the placenta over or near the cervix. Fetal distress or death may occur if the degree of separation is great. Treatment is bed rest. Birth must be induced – though preferably not before week 35 of pregnancy – if pre-eclampsia or bleeding persist. Labor before week 37 is regarded as premature. If there is bleeding or loss of amniotic fluid the pregnancy cannot last and delivery is necessary; otherwise symptoms can usually be stopped by bed rest and medication, including cortisone to help the baby's lungs mature. Postmaturity – pregnancy lasting more than 42 weeks – is serious because the baby has often defecated and swallowed its own meconium (its first feces). When this happens the uterus shrinks and the fetus is less active.

Premature babies often suffer from respiratory distress syndrome – lack of the chemical released at birth that thins the film of water in the lung alveoli and allows oxygen in and carbon dioxide out. Babies that cannot breathe or have become blue from shortage of oxygen may be given pressurized air from a ventilating machine.

▲ *A premature baby is placed, naked apart from perhaps a bonnet or a diaper, in an incubator, which serves as an artificial womb. It is fed by intravenous infusion or through a nasal tube. The air is kept warm and humid, and the baby may be attached to a ventilator.*

Difficulties in pregnancy

A woman's inability to have a chid may be caused by failure to retain a fetus. There is a 15-20 percent chance of any pregnancy miscarrying. Spontaneous abortion may occur where a fertilized egg has gross genetic abnormalities (♦ page 193). But internal problems in the female can also cause abortion. In the condition known as incompetent cervix, the cervix is insufficiently strong to resist the downwards pressure of the growing fetus and the pregnancy miscarries. As this usually happens without pain to the woman, she may not realize she has been pregnant and may think herself infertile.

A relatively common problem which may interfere with pregnancy is the growth of fibroids, non-cancerous tumors that form in the muscle of the womb. Less common is ectopic pregnancy, in which a fertilized egg embeds outside the uterus, usually staying in the Fallopian tube. Such pregnancies rarely last more than two months, after which time the tube will rupture and death may result without immediate surgery. Such pregnancies are detected after unusual pain and bleeding, and once detected are ended by immediate surgery.

*Hereditary disorders...Imaging the unborn child...
Down's syndrome...Chromosomal disorders...
Anemias...Hemophilia...Genetic engineering...
PERSPECTIVE...Rhesus babies...Abortion...Poisoning
the fetus...Gene therapy*

Pregnancy

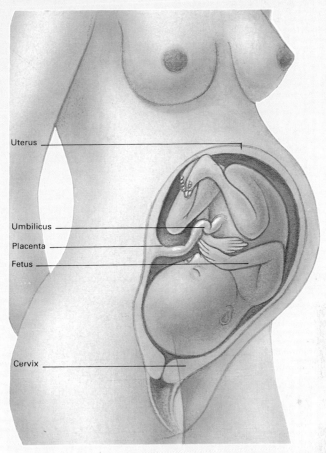

Uterus

Umbilicus

Placenta

Fetus

Cervix

Disease is often seen as an attack on the organism from outside; many diseases, however, are built into us from the moment of conception. When two sex cells combine to create a new organism, the collection of chromosomes which this brings together (◀ page 26) may be faulty in some way.

Assessing the risk

If the embryo's chromosomes are grossly abnormal, it nearly always aborts spontaneously. However, some chromosomal abnormalities, such as Down's syndrome (mongolism), lead to the birth of live but handicapped babies. Increasingly, these problems can be detected before birth. It is also possible to predict that certain people have a higher than average chance of producing an abornomal child before conception. If a couple have already had a child which suffers from a recognized gene-linked abnormality, then "genetic counselling" is advisable to assess the risk of the same abnormality recurring. Similarly, if close relatives have had an abnormal child or suffer from a genetically-linked disease, the risk can also be assessed.

Rhesus babies

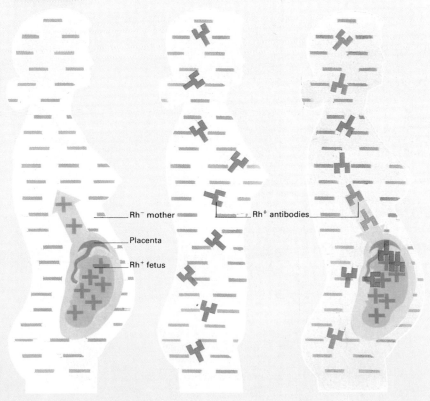

Rh⁻ mother

Rh⁺ antibodies

Placenta

Rh⁺ fetus

Rhesus babies

Blood is characterized by a number of factors (◀ page 30). The rhesus factor is present (Rh⁺) in most of the population, but absent (Rh⁻) in a small percentage.

During birth, there can be interchange of fetal and maternal blood. If an Rh⁻ mother's first baby is Rh+, then the rhesus factor may enter her bloodstream and her immune system (◀ page 213) produces antibodies to it. Circulating antibodies cross the placenta to provide immunity to the newborn against common infections. In a second or subsequent pregnancy, an Rh⁻ mother transfers rhesus-factor antibodies to the fetus. If the fetus is Rh⁺, then these antibodies attack the fetal red blood cells. This may cause only mild anemia, but it can lead to abortion of the fetus.

The problem can be avoided by giving Rh⁻ mothers a large dose of Rh immunoglobulin immediately after the birth of a first Rh⁺ baby. The immunoglobulin reacts with any rhesus factor in the mother's blood before her own immune system has time to respond to it. Using this treatment, it has been possible to reduce sensitization of Rh⁻ mothers more than tenfold. Where sensitization still occurs, the adverse reaction in subsequent Rh⁺ babies is less severe.

◀ So-called Rhesus babies, suffering from erythroblastosis fetalis, occur when a Rh⁻ mother conceives a Rh⁺ child, and her immune system develops antibodies to its blood. Any subsequent Rh⁺ child can be attacked by these antibodies.

Techniques for detecting abnormalities in a fetus are becoming safer and more reliable

Screening techniques

If the risk of having an abnormal baby is above average, screening techniques are used to try to detect abnormalities in the fetus. The most basic is ultrasonography, a study of the developing fetus using ultrasound – electromagnetic waves of a frequency undetectable by the human ear. With this technique, it is possible to tell whether a woman is carrying a single fetus, twins or triplets. It is also possible to detect gross abnormalities such as anencephaly (failure of the brain to develop). Anencephalics mostly die within a few days of birth. Early diagnosis can mean the option of an abortion.

A major advantage of ultrasonography is that it helps to locate the fetus within the amniotic sac and thus makes amniocentesis safer. Amniocentesis is the removal of about 20ml of amniotic fluid by inserting a hypodermic syringe through the mother's abdominal wall. This procedure has immense diagnostic value, mainly because the fluid contains some cells which have been shed by the embryo. As each cell of an individual contains his or her full genetic complement in its nucleus, these can be cultured – much in the way that colonies of micro-organisms are grown – and then examined for genetic abnormalities. In 1968, a case of Down's syndrome in a fetus was diagnosed for the first time in this way.

The fluid itself can also provide useful information. It contains alpha-fetoprotein, the purpose of which is unknown, but which appears to be produced only by fetuses. If the amniotic fluid contains a high amount of this protein, there is a strong likelihood that the fetus suffers a neural tube defect. These defects, including anencephaly and spina bifida, occur when the groove along the back of the embryo, which ultimately becomes the spinal column, fails to close. In some cases, sufficient alpha-fetoprotein escapes from the fetus and crosses the placenta to give detectable levels in the maternal bloodstream. Where it is suspected that a woman may give birth to a baby with a neural tube defect, then her blood is checked for alpha-fetoprotein and she undergoes amniocentesis to confirm the disease.

Amniocentesis usually cannot be carried out before the 16th week of pregnancy because there is insufficient amniotic fluid and free fetal cells before then. The cell culture takes up to four weeks to produce results. Sometimes a second amniocentesis and culturing are necessary to produce a clear result. Consequently, once results are available, there is little time left in which to consider an abortion, as these usually are performed before the 25th week of pregnancy.

A recent advance which may replace amniocentesis is chorion villus biopsy, which can be carried out between 8 and 12 weeks after conception. The chorionic membrane surrounds the amniotic sac and is genetically a part of the fetus. Cells from it can be obtained, either through the mother's abdomen, as with amniocentesis, or via the cervix. Ultrasound is used to guide the instrument to an appropriate point from which to take the cell sample. It is possible to study the genetic makeup of these cells directly, or to culture them. The same types of diagnostic test can be carried out as with amniocentesis. However, there may be a slightly higher risk to the fetus.

Because there is a slight risk with both methods, there is great interest in developing non-invasive techniques. Some fetal cells cross the placenta and enter the maternal bloodstream. If it proves possible to separate these from maternal cells in a blood sample and culture them, even earlier diagnosis of abnormalities may prove possible in the seventh or eighth week of pregnancy.

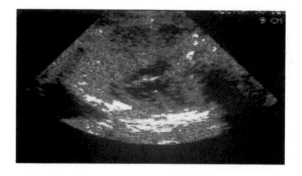

▲ **Echocardiograph of a fetal heart. With this technique, which is a development of ultrasound, it is possible to detect defects in the heart beat and heart structure.**

▼ **Ultrasound scanning of fetuses has become routine in many hospitals. The technique is non-invasive, though some doubts have been raised about the longterm effects.**

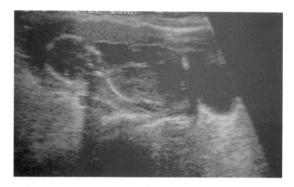

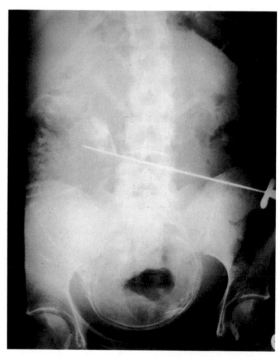

▼ **X-ray of a blood transfusion given to a fetus through the umbilical cord. New imaging techniques have made such operations, and even fetal heart surgery, possible.**

▶ **X-ray of a fetus (colored brown) in its mother's womb, at about eight months, with the head engaged in the pelvic outlet ready for birth, its knees tucked up to its chest.**

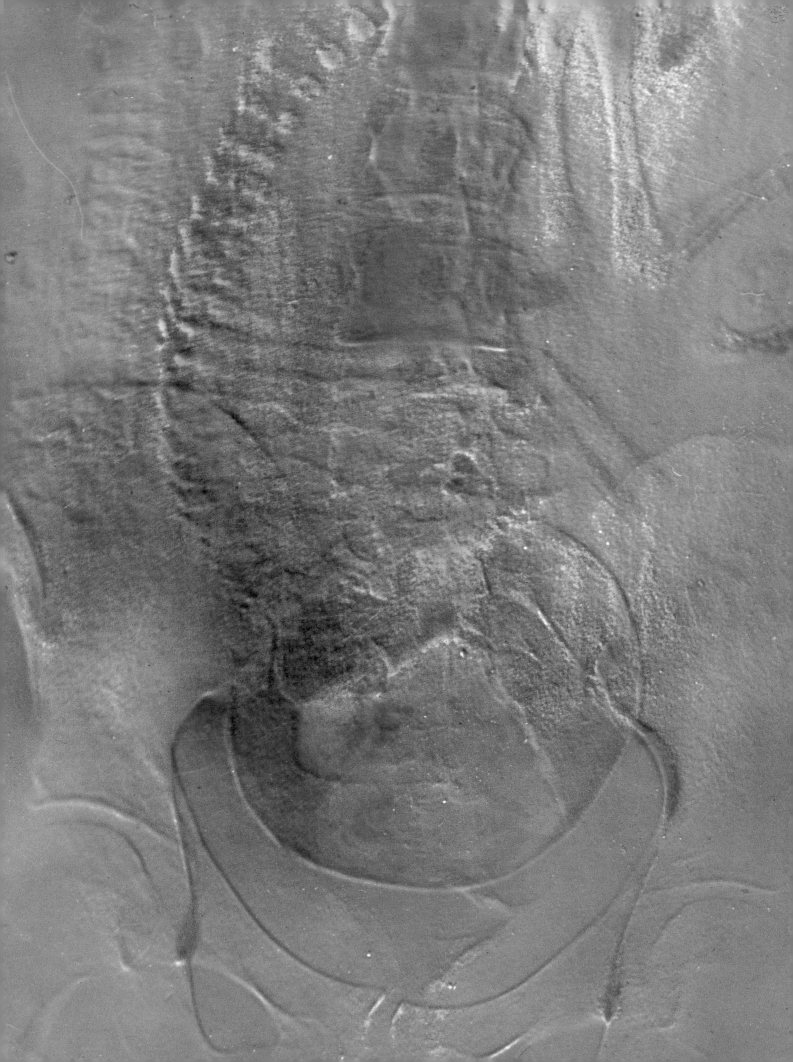

Most inheritable diseases are caused by a missing or defective gene

Inheritable diseases – faulty chromosomes

The most common genetic aberration to produce noticeably abnormal babies is Down's syndrome. Whereas a normal cell carries 46 chromosomes in 23 pairs, in Down's syndrome there are three of chromosome 21, giving a total of 47. The disease is characterized by facial features, which led to the name "mongolism", mental retardation and high incidences of diabetes, heart disease and intestinal disorders.

Of the 23 pairs of chromosomes, one is concerned with sexual characteristics. Several illnesses result from an odd number of sex chromosomes. Klinefelter's syndrome, which occurs with a frequency of one in a 1,000 male live births, is the name given to the condition in which there are two X chromosomes and one Y chromosome. This disease is often not diagnosed until puberty, when male secondary sexual characteristics fail to develop. Sufferers are sterile.

Another triple sex-chromosome disease is XYY syndrome, in which there are two male chromosomes. There has been much controversy about this, because some studies have shown a higher-than-average incidence of antisocial behavior among sufferers. The condition occurs with about the same frequency as Klinefelter's syndrome.

Turner's syndrome is a disease of people who have one X chromosome and no Y chromosome; they are usually physically female. Embryos with this aberration often abort spontaneously and the frequency among live births is between one tenth and one quarter of that of Klinefelter's syndrome. There is little development of the female secondary sexual characteristics and sufferers are usually sterile.

Inheritable diseases – faulty genes

Most of the inheritable diseases are caused by a missing or defective gene rather than a whole chromosome. Because the chromosomes and the genes they carry go in pairs, such diseases may be either dominant or recessive. In the first case, inheritance of the gene from either parent is sufficient to establish the disease. Thus, Huntington's chorea, a degenerative neurological disease, is passed on by sufferers to 50 percent of their children. As the disease does not usually show

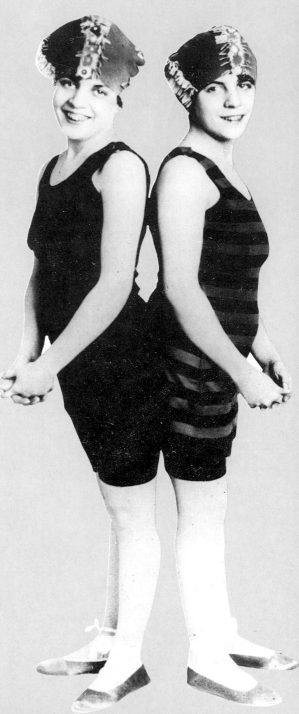

▲ *Twins may result from a single fertilized ovum (identical twins) or from two fertilized ova (dissimilar twins). Exactly how a single egg leads to twins is still not clearly understood. Even less clear is the cause of Siamese twins, identical twins who are partly joined together. The extent of joining differs in this very rare condition. In some cases a vital organ, like the liver, is shared. Where joining is more superficial, Siamese twins can usually be separated surgically. Siamese twins such as Daisy and Violet Hilton, shown here, have lived successfully; Eng and Chang, the "original" Siamese twins from Bangkok, were born in 1811 and lived to the age of 69, having had 21 children.*

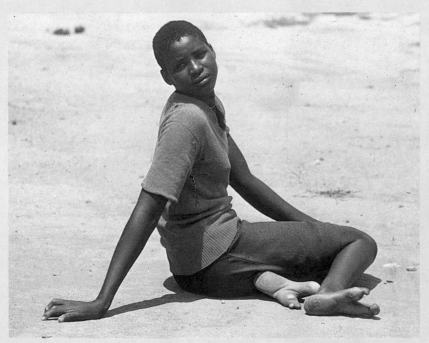

◀ *A girl from the Oysterman tribe of the Botswana-Zimbabwe border, where about 100 people suffer from the lobster-claw syndrome, caused by a faulty gene.*

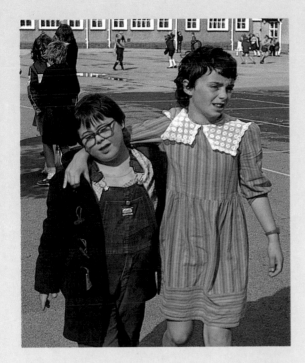

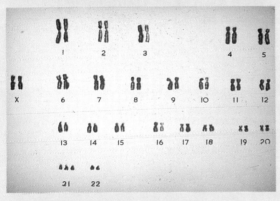

up until middle age, after which it is progressive and incurable, sufferers may have had children before they know they have the disease.

Recessive genetic diseases can be passed on by carriers who have only one affected gene. Hemophilia is caused by a faulty gene which produces an inactive version of a special blood factor (usually Factor VIII) involved in clotting. Sufferers bleed easily and bleeding usually stops only when vessels constrict. Internal hemorrhaging is more common and a major problem, especially in joints such as the knee. The severity of the disease differs between individuals, although sufferers in the same family generally show the same degree of affliction. The faulty gene is located on the X chromosome. A female carrier has one faulty X chromosome and one normal X chromosome and therefore does not suffer from the disease. If she has a male child, then there is a 50 percent chance that it will inherit the faulty X chromosome. As the child inherits a Y chromosome from the father, it has only a faulty X chromosome and therefore is hemophiliac. A female can be a hemophiliac if born to a hemophiliac father and a carrier mother, but this is very rare.

Several other recessive genetic conditions, including Duchenne muscular dystrophy and color blindness (◆ page 29) have been linked to sex chromosome defects. Many other diseases arise through failure of one or more genes on other chromosomes to produce a biologically important substance correctly. In these cases, offspring suffer the disease if they inherit the faulty gene from both parents.

Tay-Sachs disease causes apparently healthy babies to fall ill and die in early childhood. The faulty gene, which fails to produce an enzyme called hexosaminidase A, is found in nearly five percent of Ashkenazic Jews (that is Jews who migrated to Eastern Europe). Carriers can now be detected by a blood test. Cystic fibrosis is another recessive genetic disorder. The frequency of carriers among Caucasions is about the same as Tay-Sachs carriers among Ashkenazic Jews. To date, however, it cannot be detected. Cystic fibrosis is a wasting disease of lungs, sweat glands and digestive organs which usually causes death from infection by the early twenties.

▲ ▲ Down's syndrome is characterized by the moon-shaped face, and is caused by an extra chromosome 21. One child in every 650 live births suffers from Down's syndrome, but the basic incidence is much higher as two-thirds of the embryos abort spontaneously. The likelihood of a mother giving birth to a Down's syndrome baby increases with age, increasing sharply after the age of 35.

Abortion

When a fetus has been diagnosed as abnormal, the parents may be given the choice of an induced abortion. Abortions also may be performed where the mother is unsuited to childbearing. The way in which the fetus is removed depends on its age.

Early abortions, during the first three months of pregnancy, are usually performed either by suction curettage or dilatation and curettage. In both cases, the cervix is dilated, usually under local anesthetic. In suction curettage, a vacuum aspirator is inserted into the uterus and the embryo is sucked out. With dilation and curettage a sharp instrument is used to remove the fetal tissue.

For abortions between 13 and 24 weeks, two methods are most often used. In the first, some amniotic fluid is replaced by a salt solution. In the second, a natural substance called a prostaglandin is injected into the amniotic fluid. Both methods result in expulsion of the fetus through normal labor. The saline method is not recommended for mothers suffering from high blood pressure or heart or kidney ailments, and is usually slower than prostaglandin injection. Both methods usually involve hospitalization.

Intersexes

Intersexes are physically intermediate between a true male and a true female, either as mosaics of sexual parts, or male on one side and female on the other. The condition is either obvious at birth or it becomes apparent at puberty. There are two causes – extra chromosomes or a hormonal abnormality during development of the embryo. True hermaphrodites have both ovarian and testicular tissue, often with ambiguous external genitalia. About three quarters are raised as boys, but develop breasts and begin to menstruate during adolescence. Surgical manipulation can produce normal-looking genitals.

There are a number of diseases producing an intersexual state. Individuals with Turner's syndrome have a female appearance but they do not menstruate and are deficient in the female sex hormone estrogen, which is given as treatment. The inherited testicular feminizing syndrome, produces apparent females who have a male set of sex chromosomes. They synthesize the male sex hormone testosterone, but their cells do not respond to it. The testes tend to form malignant tumors and are removed surgically.

One drug was used for over 20 years on 2 million pregnant women before its abnormal side effects were recognized

Many of the inheritable diseases are caused by the failure of a gene coding for a particular enzyme. As a result, poisonous substances build up in the body which can cause permanent damage. Provided that such deficiencies are diagnosed at birth, they can be controlled, often by diet restriction. Preventive treatment can be carried out from birth on those babies automatically tested for the common forms.

The first such disease for which a test was devised is phenylketonuria. This is caused by failure to metabolize the amino-acid phenylalanine correctly. Toxic products form which can cause severe brain damage. Treatment involves substituting natural proteins in the diet with synthetic protein containing no phenylalanine. This diet needs to be maintained for the first few years of life, while brain development continues, after which it can be relaxed.

By contrast, failure to produce the enzyme adenosine deaminase is almost always fatal. This enzyme is concerned with metabolism of adenosine. If adenosine and the closely related deoxyadenosine reach high levels in blood and tissues, lymphocytes are harmed, leading to severe combined immune deficiency (◗ page 232). The sufferer is particularly liable to severe infections.

Inherited blood disorders

Two blood diseases which affect large numbers in different parts of the world are caused by recessively inherited genes. Sickle-cell anemia, much more frequent among Negros than among Caucasians or Asiatics, is caused by a faulty gene coding for part of the globin protein in hemoglobin (◗ page 158). The difference between the correct and incorrect proteins is only one amino-acid in a protein made up from 140 of them. This single change causes the molecule to deform into a sickle shape that cannot carry oxygen so efficiently. As a result, body tissues receive an inadequate supply of oxygen. Severity of the disease varies greatly. In mild cases, symptoms show up only at high altitude, if the sufferer is flying in an unpressurized aircraft for example. At the other extreme, the disease can be severely debilitating and sufferers may die from a sudden infection which would only rarely prove fatal in a person with normal hemoglobin.

Thalassemia is the name given to a group of recessively inherited blood disorders prevalent in people from countries bordering the Mediterranean; these are also caused by defective globin synthesis. A hemoglobin molecule contains four protein chains in two identical pairs. In the case of sickle-cell anemia, it is the so-called alpha-chains which are affected. The thalassemias are divided into four major types. In two of these, either no alpha globin chains are produced, or only subnormal amounts. In the other two, it is the other – beta globin – chains which are either not produced or produced subnormally. These effects can be produced by many different changes in the structure of the genes which code for these proteins, ranging from point mutations to deletion of part or all of the gene.

The severity of the thalassemias varies, but they are responsible for many infant deaths. In recent years, treatments have been developed based on recurrent blood transfusions. However, these lead to problems, notably the toxic effects of iron, as the iron in the transfused blood accumulates in the body. Sickle-cell anemia and the thalassemias were both originally most common in those parts of the world where Falciparum malaria (the most lethal type) was prevalent. They have probably survived because the genes carrying them offer some immunity to the malarial parasite.

Gene maps

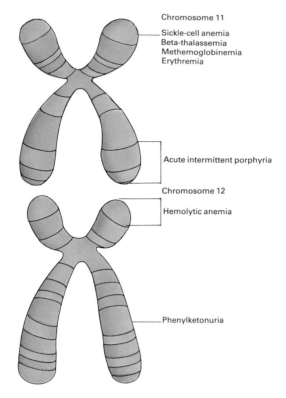

Chromosome 11
Sickle-cell anemia
Beta-thalassemia
Methemoglobinemia
Erythremia

Acute intermittent porphyria

Chromosome 12
Hemolytic anemia

Phenylketonuria

▲ *"Maps" of human chromosomes 11 and 12, showing the locations at which the genetic mutations responsible for various diseases are located.*

▼ *The oxygen-carrying capacity of hemoglobin depends on the shape of the protein (white spheres) around the heme core (red), in turn dependent on its amino-acid composition.*

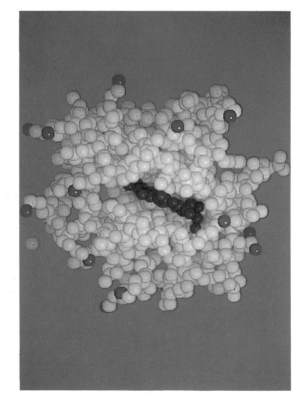

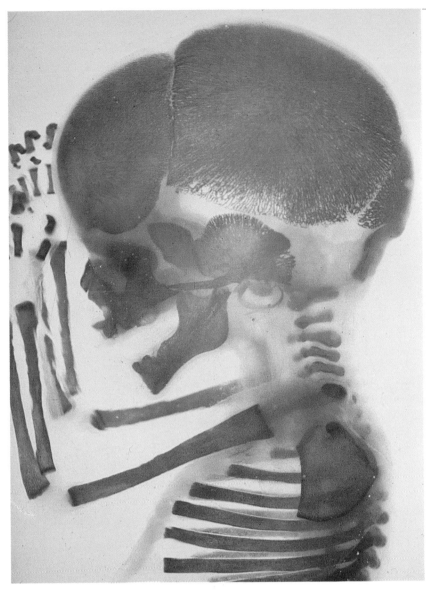

Environmental hazards and abnormal babies

The effect of substances which deform embryos – known as teratogens – is the same for adults, but because embryonic cells are rapidly dividing, poisoning of them may produce very serious consequences.

Substances which interfere specifically with cell division can cause the most severe damage. Thalidomide, a sedative prescribed between 1959 and 1961, is the best known example. Because the generation of particular organs and limbs occurs in a specific sequence, the various types of deformity produced by thalidomide depends on the age of the embryo. The most common affected the arms and legs.

The synthetic hormone diethylstilbestrol (DES) was first used in the late 1940s to help avoid complications in some pregnancies. During the 1970s, genital abnormalities were discovered in a number of children whose mothers had taken DES before the 18th week of pregnancy. Because the abnormalities did not appear until after puberty, the drug was used for 20 years and as many as two million pregnant women may have taken it.

Not all teratogenic effects are produced by man-made poisons. German measles (rubella), if acquired in the first three months of pregnancy, can cause severe fetal abnormalities, as can syphilis, cytomegalovirus infection and toxoplasmosis.

◄ ▼ The side view of the human fetus shows the development of normal arm bones. These are absent in the X-ray of a victim of the drug thalidomide. This drug, when taken by pregnant women, interfered with fetal cell division at the stage when arms and legs were forming. The consequence was a number of live births of children without these limbs.

Embryonic development

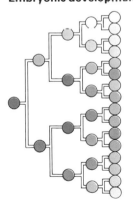

▲ Starting from a single fertilized egg, a fetus develops rapidly via repeated divisions to become a multicelled organism. Between the 3rd and 13th week, cells differentiate to produce different organs of the body. At this stage, the rapidly dividing cells are particularly susceptible to poisoning which can cause a variety of major malformations.

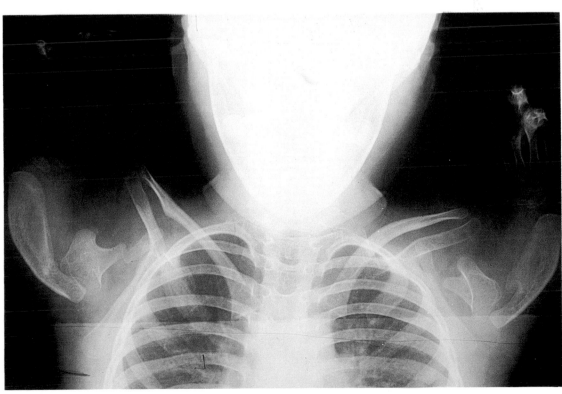

Gene therapy

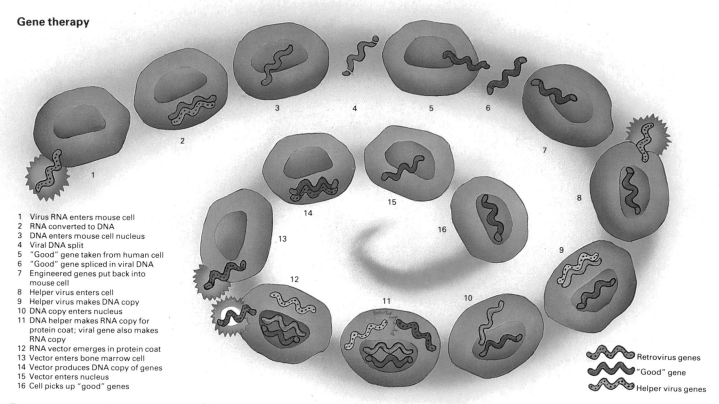

1 Virus RNA enters mouse cell
2 RNA converted to DNA
3 DNA enters mouse cell nucleus
4 Viral DNA split
5 "Good" gene taken from human cell
6 "Good" gene spliced in viral DNA
7 Engineered genes put back into mouse cell
8 Helper virus enters cell
9 Helper virus makes DNA copy
10 DNA copy enters nucleus
11 DNA helper makes RNA copy for protein coat; viral gene also makes RNA copy
12 RNA vector emerges in protein coat
13 Vector enters bone marrow cell
14 Vector produces DNA copy of genes
15 Vector enters nucleus
16 Cell picks up "good" genes

Retrovirus genes
"Good" gene
Helper virus genes

Between one and two percent of babies are born with defects which cannot be attributed to a single faulty gene. These defects often seem to have a genetic component, but the environment is also significant. These multifactorial congenital abnormalities include cleft lip and palate, types of heart disease and neural tube defects. Of the latter, spina bifida has aroused much speculation. At one time, it was thought that a poison associated with blighted potatoes might be exerting a teratogenic effect. Today the high incidence of the condition in manufacturing towns, such as Pittsburgh, USA, and Glasgow, Scotland, makes industrial pollution the possible contributory cause. In addition, the higher risk of a couple with a spina bifida baby having another suggests a genetic link. During 1985 tests based on either DNA "probes" or targeted antibodies were announced for the early detection of conditions such as spina bifida and thalassemia.

The potential of genetic engineering

With the development of genetic engineering techniques, interest has been shown in trying to cure the many kinds of inherited disease by replacing defective genes. Where a single protein is involved, the section of genetic material which codes for it can be isolated relatively easily. The problem is how to insert this material into the cells of sufferers in such a way that it will be reproduced with the cell's own genetic material when the cell divides and, more importantly, will be expressed (will produce protein) at the appropriate time.

Currently, pharmaceutical companies are making some human products, such as insulin, for therapeutic use by culturing bacteria into which the appropriate gene has been engineered. Within the next few years, much of this biotechnological production may be switched into mammalian cell cultures. Developing the technology for that will provide the insights into how similiar insertions might be carried out in living human beings, to overcome their genetic deficiencies.

Gene therapy

In the past, it has been possible to combat damage caused by certain inherited diseases, though without interfering with the defective genes responsible. The ill-effects of phenylketonuria, for example, can be ameliorated by diet, but the gene is still passed on to future generations. In future, however, it may well be feasible to replace certain faulty genes with their normal counterparts. Scientists hope to achieve this feat of genetic engineering by employing a virus to ferry "good" genes into particular body tissues.

As shown in the illustration (above), one chosen vehicle is a retrovirus, so-called because it can make DNA copies of its RNA – the reverse of which occurs in animal cells. Most of the virus genes (including those it requires to make the protein coat which is essential for it to infect another cell) will be removed from such a DNA copy, produced in mouse cells. This will leave room for the "desirable" human gene to be spliced in, yielding a sequence which can then be cloned to generate many copies. These will be added to further mouse cells, together with an RNA "helper" virus which will (again by making DNA copies of its own genes) provide the hybrid sequence with a protein coat. The product should then be a virus which carries the desirable gene and still has the protein coat it must possess if it is to invade human cells – but lacking the protein coat genes it would need to reproduce further. The final projected step is for bone marrow cells to be removed from the patient and be incubated with the tailor-made virus before being reinjected. "Good" genes ferried into these cells by the virus should then enable them to produce the enzyme whose absence caused the disease in the first place.

Sexually transmitted diseases...Changing incidence... The difficulties of diagnosis...Sexual infections and antibiotics...The new threat of genital herpes...Other infections of the sex organs...PERSPECTIVE...The AIDS epidemic...The rise and fall of syphilis

Until the Second World War, "venereal diseases" meant gonorrhea and syphilis. Since that time, a great many more infections have been recognized as being acquired through sexual contact. The entire group now known collectively as sexually transmitted diseases (STD) is attracting growing concern among health authorities throughout the world. Although STDs declined in apparent seriousness when anti-biotics came into widespread use in mid-century, their prevalence has increased dramatically since that time – especially in the 15-19 age group in some countries. Epidemiologists are not sure they know all the reasons, though greater "promiscuity" and the development of international tourism are contributory factors. Transfer of micro-organisms to mucus membranes of the genital tract has also become more likely as the contraceptive pill has replaced barrier techniques such as the sheath.

The incidence of particular STDs has been altering too. Forty years ago most cases of urethritis (infection of the duct leading from the bladder) were diagnosed as being due to gonorrhea, caused by the bacterium *Neisseria gonorrhoeae* invading the urethra and producing a suppurative discharge. In women this can precipitate infection of the Fallopian tubes, blocking them and causing sterility or ectopic pregnancy. In men it can lead to infection of the epididymis, prostate and testes. Arthritis and heart disease may occur in both sexes. Gonorrhea is nearly always acquired during intercourse (the exceptions being eye infection in babies born to affected mothers, and vaginal infection transmitted by towels among infants in institutions).

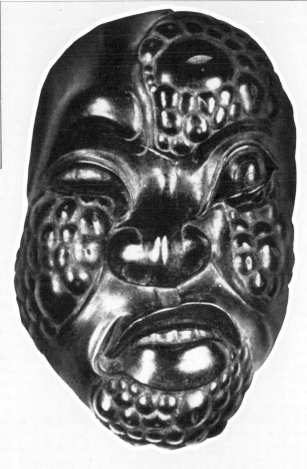

▲ *An Indonesian mask made in the 19th century showing the facial paralysis that can result from advanced syphilis. Western sailors introduced sexually transmitted diseases to the region, where they had previously been unknown.*

▼ *The syphilitic bacterium Treponoma pallidum. It is transmitted either through direct sexual contact or to the fetus via the placenta. Syphilis can be easily detected and is usually treatable by penicillin.*

Female sex organs

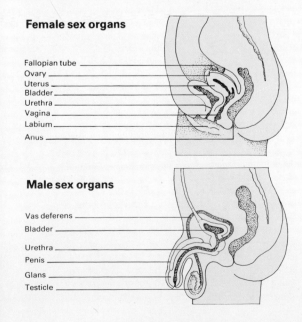

Fallopian tube
Ovary
Uterus
Bladder
Urethra
Vagina
Labium
Anus

Male sex organs

Vas deferens
Bladder
Urethra
Penis
Glans
Testicle

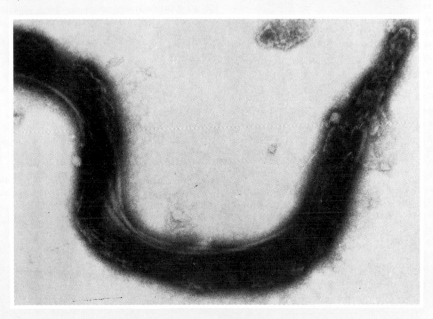

In the 1970s the gonorrhea bacterium became invulnerable to antibiotics

Today, non-specific urethritis (NSU) is as common as that due to gonorrhea worldwide, and twice as common in the West, ranking along with it and syphilis as the trio of most important STDs. About 50 percent of "non-specific" infections are thought to be produced by *Chlamydia trachomatis* – an organism that is related to the trachoma agent (◗ page 241) and is intermediate in size and behavior between bacteria and viruses. The remaining 50 percent are cases in which the cause is uncertain, though *Mycoplasma genitalium*, discovered by David Taylor-Robinson at Britain's Clinical Research Centre in 1983, may play a major role.

The difficulties of diagnosis

Gonorrhea has always proved difficult to control because carriers may show no symptoms but still purvey the disease, and it has become increasingly difficult since the emergence in 1976 of strains of *Neisseria* resistant to penicillin. Common in the Far East and in West Africa, these organisms are being found increasingly in the USA and Europe. The number of patients with such strains doubled each year in Britain between 1977 and 1982, and is still increasing. So, while 150,000 unit shots of penicillin were once considered adequate to obliterate the infection, doses of some 4·8 million units (often accompanied by other drugs) are now necessary. Compounded by a rise in resistance to other antibiotics, the cost of such treatment is growing in parallel. Development of a vaccine has still proved inordinately difficult, but there are hopes for an effective method of immunization in the near future.

NSU due to unknown organisms can also be extremely difficult to treat effectively. But *Chlamydia* (which, like *N. gonorrhoeae*, may also be passed on during birth to infect the baby's eyes) is usually sensitive to tetracyclines. The problem here is identification of the infection. In 1984 one UK specialist estimated that two-thirds of cases were not being diagnosed, leaving thousands of men and women infertile and scores of children with eye disease. There are also strong suspicions that cervicitis (infection of the cervix) often goes undetected. It is hoped that a new spot test for *Chlamydia*, based on highly specific "monoclonal antibodies", will enable all such conditions to be diagnosed and cleared up speedily.

The growing problem of genital herpes

Genital herpes is a major new STD of the past four decades. The characteristic genital sores are caused by a herpes simplex virus (HSV2) related to the one (HSV1) that produces cold sores on the lip (◗ page 244). Although known from much earlier times, the disease increased greatly during the 1970s. So did the frequency with which HSV2 was found in lip sores, and HSV1 in genital sores – a result of more frequent oro-genital contacts. Unlike gonorrhea, NSU and syphilis, genital herpes is incurable. The recurrent and extremely painful blisters can only be relieved by ointments and painkillers before they subside, only to flare up again some time later. As well as interfering with sex life, herpes infection may have very serious complications. At least half the babies born to women with active genital herpes at the time of delivery contract the disease, and half of these will die or suffer permanent neurological damage. There are also suspicions of a link with cervical cancer, though this is not proven. Vaccine trials now under way may provide evidence that the infection is preventable.

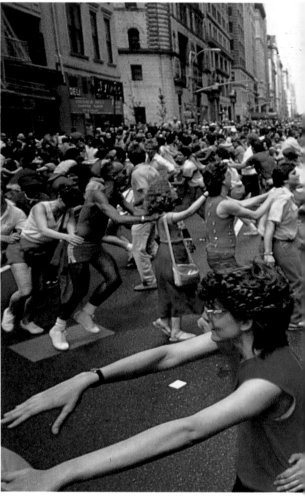

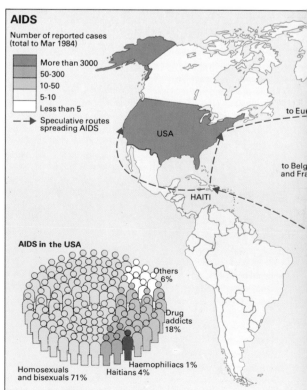

AIDS

Number of reported cases
(total to Mar 1984)

More than 3000
50-300
10-50
5-10
Less than 5

- → Speculative routes
spreading AIDS

USA

to Eu

to Belg
and Fra

HAITI

AIDS in the USA

Others 6%

Drug addicts 18%

Haemophiliacs 1%

Haitians 4%

Homosexuals and bisexuals 71%

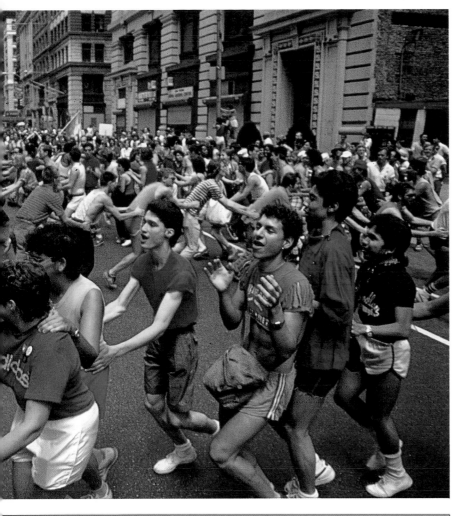

◄ *A demonstration by New York homosexuals demanding action to protect them against AIDS. A great deal of research was quickly begun on the disease, but public awareness often remained at the level of hysteria, with sufferers shunned and some people seeing the epidemic as a "gay plague", even though it is not limited to homosexuals.*

The AIDS epidemic

In June 1981 the US Centers for Disease Control announced that five young homosexual men in Los Angeles had died of pneumonia caused by "Pneumocystis carnii". Shortly afterwards, there were reports that another 26 homosexuals had developed a severe form of Kaposi's sarcoma, a cancer until then extremely uncommon in the USA. Soon it became clear that the two incidents were related. Both groups had been victims of an apparently new condition, acquired immune deficiency syndrome (AIDS), which renders victims vulnerable to a wide range of "opportunisitic infections" and to the onset of Kaposi's sarcoma. Sporadic cases had occurred in the past, but the epidemic which began in 1981 was unprecedented. By April 1984 the disease was claiming 2,000 deaths a year. Four main groups were at risk: homosexual or bisexual men, intravenous drug users, hemophiliacs receiving regular transfusions, and Haitians. But the factor most strongly associated with the illness was the number of sexual partners per year (an average of 60 in one survey). This suggested that AIDS was caused by an agent transmitted during intercourse – probably through the bloodstream. Two groups, one led by Dr Robert Gallo at the US National Cancer Institute and the other by Dr Luc Montagnier at the Pasteur Institute in Paris, have since announced the discovery of the virus which causes the disease (♦ page 232).

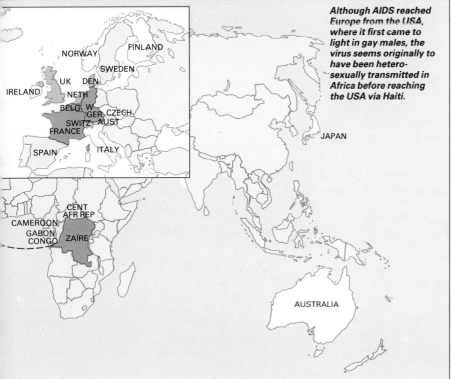

Although AIDS reached Europe from the USA, where it first came to light in gay males, the virus seems originally to have been hetero-sexually transmitted in Africa before reaching the USA via Haiti.

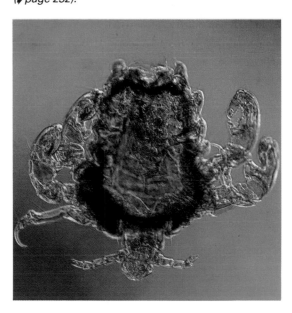

▲ *The crab louse Phthirus pubis is transmitted almost exclusively through intimate physical contact, and not through towels or toilet seats. With front legs capable of grasping just a single hair, it usually resides in the pubic region, but appears occasionally in chest and armpit hair and even eyelashes and thin balding pates. Crab lice are so tiny (1-2 mm long) and well camouflaged that they only reveal themselves after feeding, when they leave bright red feces.*

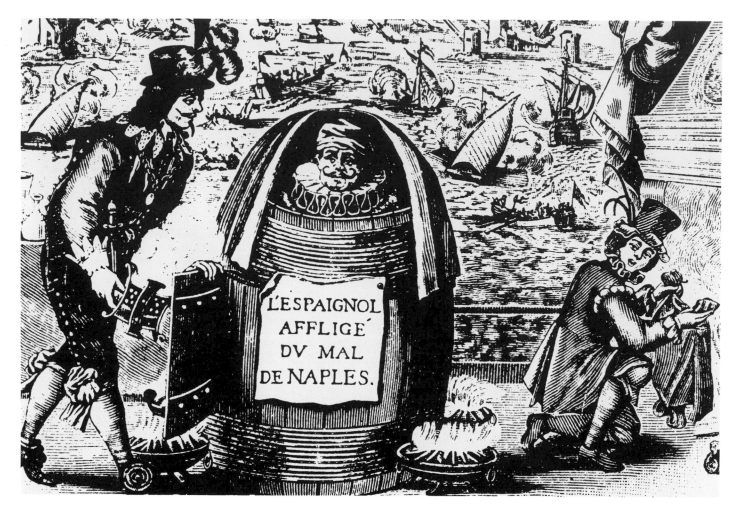

There are 20 or so other STDs. As with gonorrhea, NSU, syphilis and herpes, they are less significant for immediate effects such as urethral discharge than for complications such as infection of the epididymis and Fallopian tubes which can lead to male and female sterility and ectopic pregnancy. Also included in the STD group is trichomoniasis. Caused by the protozoon *Trichomonas vaginalis* living in the vagina and urethra of females, and the urethra and sometimes prostate of males, this generates a watery discharge but is not otherwise harmful. Likewise with the irritating discharge due to vaginal thrush, an infection with *Candida* yeast which is more common than usual among pregnant women, diabetics and women taking certain drugs (including the contraceptive pill). *Gardnerella vaginalis* causes a similarly benign discharge which (despite its odor of rotten fish) often comes to light only during a routine examination.

More than any other group of infectious diseases, STDs act as a monitor of changes in human behavior. So, over the past two decades, microbiologists have found that many bacteria and viruses not previously recognized as being transmitted by sexual activity are being spread in that way. Intestinal pathogens such as salmonellae and giardia are now known to be transmitted among homosexual men by oro-anal contact. Both hepatitis A and B are also particularly common among male homosexuals. They are spread by promiscuous "super-carriers", but there is expert disagreement about the precise routes of transmission. In 1983, the first trials of a hepatitis B vaccine among homosexuals in New York were highly successful.

▲ *Syphilis gave rise to some novel techniques of isolation and disinfection in 17th-century Europe. It spread quickly through Europe from 1500, perhaps brought back from the West Indies by Columbus' sailors.*

The rise and fall of syphilis
Syphilis was unknown to Europe until the end of the 15th century, but quickly reached epidemic proportions. It has declined in comparative importance since the introduction of antibiotics. Like gonorrhea, syphilis is not highly contagious. But untreated, the single chancre which marks the first stage of the disease may be followed within weeks by a secondary stage of fever, rash and possible kidney damage. Years later, after a latent period, some patients develop tertiary syphilis, whose effects range from relatively harmless gummas (lesions of the skin and bones) to paralysis, seizures and other indications of brain infection. Congenital syphilis is a potentially severe, mutilating form of the disease, but infected people can be identified by a simple, routine blood test. One of the bacteria most sensitive to penicillin, T. pallidum has not developed resistance. So the use of this and other antibiotics (plus, as is necessary with all STDs, prompt tracing and treatment of contacts) has made syphilis a less serious danger than before the advent of antibiotics – though there is concern about its global spread among male homosexuals.

*Cell division...Growth from birth to puberty...
Aging...Decline in physical functions...Sleep, a vital
renewal process...Regeneration of the organs...Healing
broken skin and bones...PERSPECTIVE...Taking years
off...Defining death...Hormones for growth...Why do we
age?...Why sleep?*

Growth and degeneration are opposing forces. Growth is necessary to enlarge or repair tissue, and degeneration is inevitable as cells wear out (by use or misuse) or are destroyed (by disease or injury). Growth takes place through the form of cell division known as mitosis. Overall growth slows with age, and stops around the age of 18. Some growth centers disappear completely; the proliferating areas of limb bones vanish at maturity. Very specialized organs, such as the brain and spinal cord, have permanent cells that cannot regenerate. Other less specialized organs, such as the liver, pancreas and thyroid, have stable cells that in adult life divide only after injury or disease – a damaged liver grows until it is big enough, and then stops. Regeneration is best in tissues that are constantly replaced, such as skin, bone marrow, epithelium of lungs, urinary tract and intestine, and the uterus lining.

The growth of the newborn child

Babies grow rapidly. After an initial weight loss of 5 percent in the first week after birth, they gain about 600g by the age of one month and about 1,500g a month thereafter. Some children develop more quickly than others, and these figures (and similar ones throughout this section) can only be rough averages and parents should not be alarmed if their child does not exactly match them. Though babies' heads form a large proportion of their total body size, they grow rapidly to the age of five, and from 10 to 14, then stop around 16. From four onwards, limb bones and muscles grow faster than brain or intestines; the body progresses towards adult proportions.

Taking years off – average longevity

Life expectancy in developed countries is about 73 for men and 77 for women. The gap between the sexes is closing, because treatment of heart disease (the main killer of men) has advanced faster than the treatment of cancer (the main killer of women). The American cardiologist Dr William Castelli believes that, by taking good care of our heart and circulation, most people could live to their late 80s. According to accepted actuarial calculations, heavy smoking (over 40 a day) takes 12 years off this; 20-40 cigarettes, 7 years; under 20, 2 years. Childless women lose 2 months on average, mothers of 7 or more lose 1 year. Sexually active people (at least once weekly) add 2 years to their life expectancy. A thorough annual medical checkup adds 2 years. Occasional drinking adds 1 year, daily light drinking adds 2 years. Heavy drinkers and alcoholics lose 8 years. Overweight – now or in one's past – subtracts 2 years. A diet low in meat, fat and dairy products and high in vegetables adds at least 1 year. Divorce, separation or widowhood loses 4 years for women, 8 for men. Exercise 3 times a week, vigorous enough to cause heavy breathing, adds 3 years.

Defining death

A doctor normally certifies death when the patient stops breathing. However, the development of life-support machines and the need for healthy organs for transplantation has made a definition of death necessary. Scientists have concluded that the most important organ is the brain; death results if it is badly injured or dies when the heart has stopped.

The World Medical Association issued a statement on death in 1968, and amended it in 1983. This points out that death is a gradual process, since tissues differ in their ability to withstand oxygen lack. But death is the fate of a person, not of isolated cells or organs, and the processes must have become irreversible. The entire brain, including the more resistant brainstem, must have ceased functioning.

Mitosis

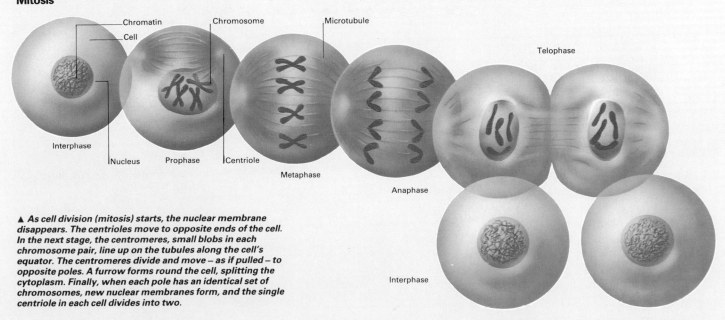

▲ As cell division (mitosis) starts, the nuclear membrane disappears. The centrioles move to opposite ends of the cell. In the next stage, the centromeres, small blobs in each chromosome pair, line up on the tubules along the cell's equator. The centromeres divide and move – as if pulled – to opposite poles. A furrow forms round the cell, splitting the cytoplasm. Finally, when each pole has an identical set of chromosomes, new nuclear membranes form, and the single centriole in each cell divides into two.

Overall body growth in girls ends at about the age of 16, in boys at about 18

Newborns have some inbuilt motor reflexes, notably the ability to hang from their hands, grasp things within reach and "walk" when supported. These are hangovers from our primitive past and disappear within 2 months as the developing motor system overrides them. Motor nerves for coordinated eye movements are formed at 4 to 6 months, and those for bladder control around two years. A baby of 1 month can raise its head slightly and make crawling movements. At about 3 months it holds up its head, and supports itself on its forearms. At 6 months it rolls over, sits well and is able to put its feet in its mouth. At 9 months it crawls, and stands without support. At 12 months it walks, often without help, and cooperates with dressing. At 15 months it may walk well and crawl upstairs, and at 18 months runs and throws things without falling over.

A toddler usually climbs up and down stairs without help at 2 years, and jumps at 2½ years. It climbs stairs with alternate feet and can pedal a tricycle at 3 years, but cannot descend using alternate feet until about 4, when it can also hop and skip. Most children can ride a bicycle by 7 or 8.

Despite their lack of motor skills, newborn babies are far from unaware of their surroundings – they try to defend themselves from approaching objects, imitate adult facial gestures and, by turning their heads, show that they can smell the difference between their own and another mother. From birth, babies hear loud noises and whispers, but do not respond to quieter sounds. From around 6 months they localize sound, and from 12 months onwards ignore repetitive noises that do not interest them.

Newborns make only one sound – crying. At 1 month they utter other sounds and at 6 months they babble, especially when talked to. By 8 months they are forming at least 4 syllables comprehensible to their family, and at 1 year may speak at least 2 or 3 words. Around the age of 18 months they make understandable phrases and babble "sentences"; proper sentences are usually formed by two-year-olds. Three-year-olds can name 16-20 objects and up to 10 actions in pictures. Eye and hand development progresses: most can thread beads at 4 and a needle at 5.

A "cure" for smallness

Normal growth is a complex interaction of growth hormone (GH), nutrition, sleep, and maybe psychological factors; many children are short despite having normal GH output. In 1983 US endocrinologist Selna Kaplan showed that, nevertheless, GH injections could make them taller by doubling their yearly growth to 6cm. In 1984, Britain started a trial of GH injections in children with normal GH but slow growth; it is not given to children with normal growth who are merely small.

Kaplan and colleagues fear their widely-publicised results will lead to indiscriminate treatment of normal short children. The risks are gigantism (◆ page 94), diabetes, and an allergic reaction to GH – their own and injected.

US psychologist Brian Stabler believes that short children who are unhappy are best treated with counselling or family therapy. He fears that ambitious parents will demand treatment for children who may be well-adjusted, and that both child and parents will be dissatisfied by the outcome. Very little is known about the psychology of shortness, its effects on personality, or sex differences in the handicap shortness produces.

Body proportions

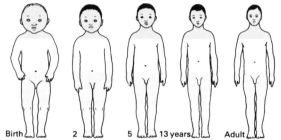

Birth   2   5   13 years   Adult

▲ **As the child grows the proportions of its body change. At birth, the head makes up about 25 percent of the total body length. The brain is 25 percent of its adult weight at birth and 50 percent at the age of only six months.**

The first year of life

▶ *During the first year of life the child gradually acquires motor skills and control over the limbs. At birth, apart from the soon-lost reflex movements, it can do little more than root for the nipple and suck. By about one month, it can lift its head unaided, and begin to focus its eyes. By 3 months it can raise its body on the elbows and turn its head; by 6 months it can sit upright, search out objects with the eyes and reach for them with the hands, though without using the thumb. By 9 months it can crawl and grasp objects firmly. By about the age of one year it can hold objects in the fingertips, and may begin to stand and walk.*

1

2

3

Birth to 1 month

1-2 months

2-4 months

5-7 months

8-10 months

10-15 months

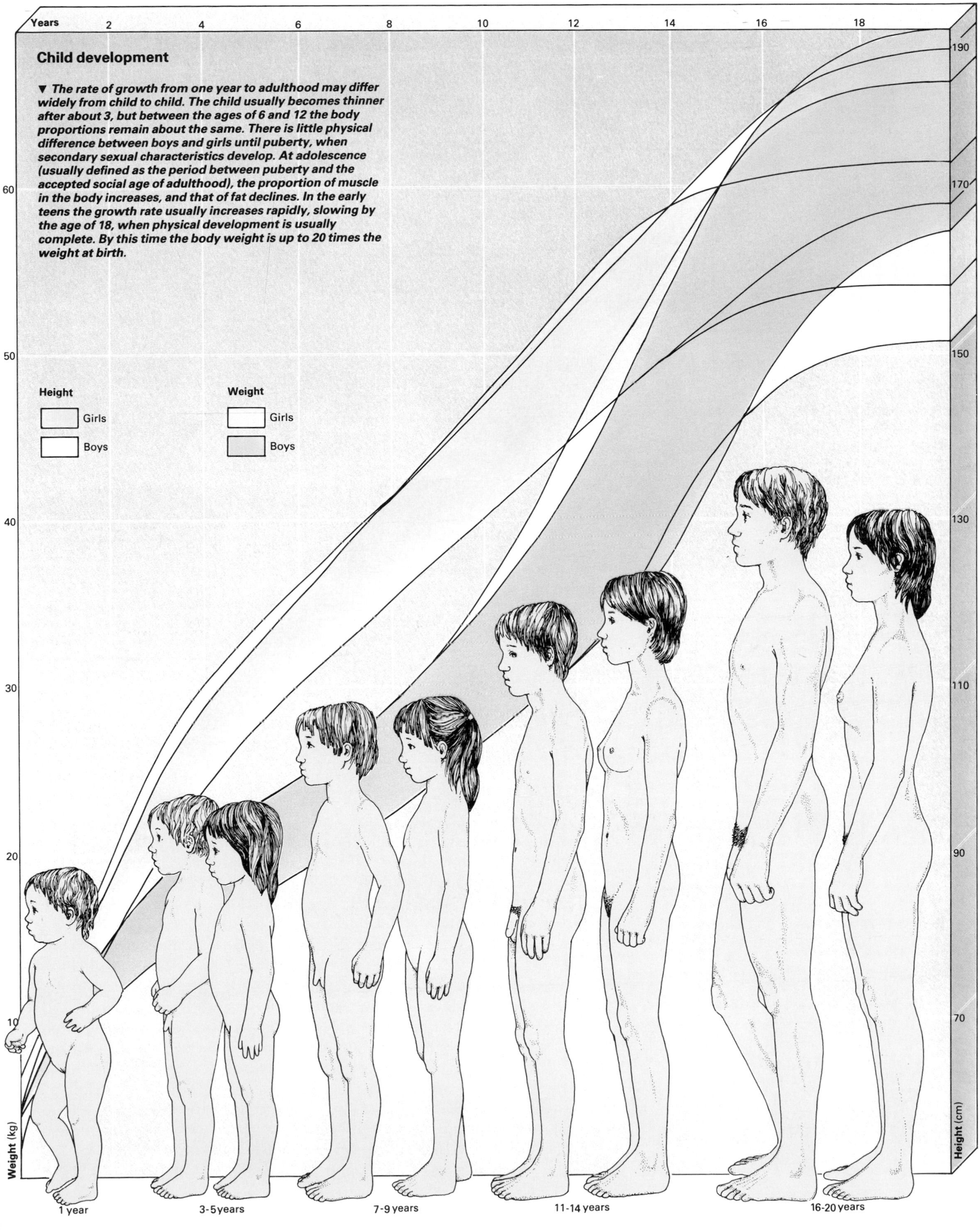

Years
2
4
6
8
10
12
14
16
18
Child development
▼ The rate of growth from one year to adulthood may differ widely from child to child. The child usually becomes thinner after about 3, but between the ages of 6 and 12 the body proportions remain about the same. There is little physical difference between boys and girls until puberty, when secondary sexual characteristics develop. At adolescence (usually defined as the period between puberty and the accepted social age of adulthood), the proportion of muscle in the body increases, and that of fat declines. In the early teens the growth rate usually increases rapidly, slowing by the age of 18, when physical development is usually complete. By this time the body weight is up to 20 times the weight at birth.
Height
Girls
Boys
Weight
Girls
Boys
60
50
40
30
20
10
Weight (kg)
190
170
150
130
110
90
70
Height (cm)
1 year
3-5 years
7-9 years
11-14 years
16-20 years

Many of the effects of aging may only become troublesome in extreme old age

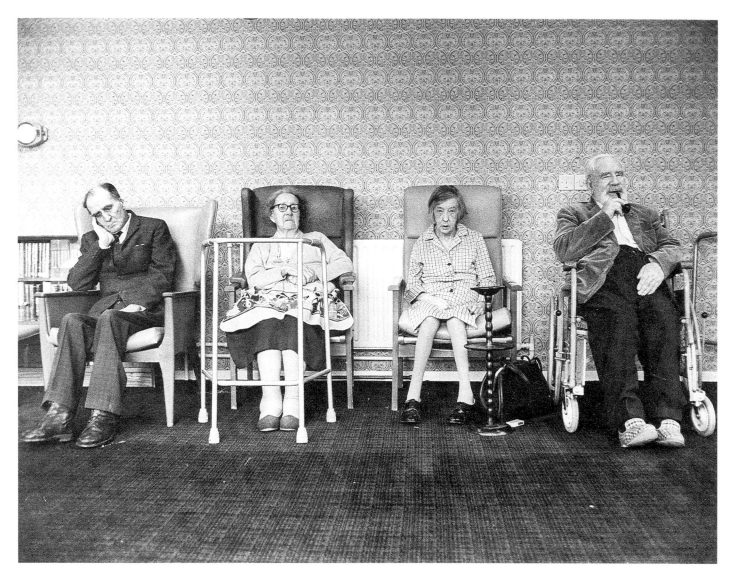

▲ ▼ *Old people may suffer the shock of enforced inactivity at retirement; the difficulties of adjusting to this causes a rise in the death rate in the years immediately after the usual retirement age. Old people may remain integrated in society, or may be institutionalized and hidden away to waste their last years; in Britain in the 1980s, some five per cent of old people live in institutional homes.*

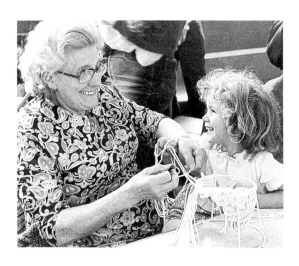

The aging process

Aging is a progressive wearing out or failure of the body's adaptive responses. It consists of loss of cells or changes in them, reducing the efficiency of individual organs and the whole body. These changes occur slowly, and a person is barely aware of them much of the time. Metabolism slows down: body temperature drops 1·1°C between the ages of 20 and 75. Cells consume less oxygen, divide more slowly and less accurately, and perform their functions less efficiently. The personality changes – tolerance of others increases, but so does selfishness, obstinacy and emotionality. One person in ten develops confusion, dementia or depression (◀ page 79). Brain-body coordination deteriorates, so that actions such as crossing the road or mounting steps become difficult. The body deals less well with poisons and harmful metabolic products. The immune system responds less well than before, so infections are more common. Collagen fibers (◀ page 97) become thicker and stronger; skin loses its fat layer and elasticity, becoming thin and wrinkled; artery walls lose their extensibility. Sweat and oil glands wither, making the skin dry and vulnerable to infection. Some pigment cells wither, making the skin paler; others grow into harmless brown "liver spots". Hairs turn white (◀ page 115), and men may develop pattern baldness, inherited via both

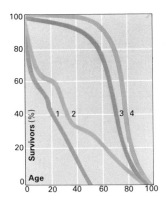

▲ Though Western societies (3) have increased the likelihood of survival to an old age over the rates found in India in 1900 (2) and those of the Stone Age (1), it does not seem possible significantly to increase lifespan on the theoretically optimal life expectancy curve (4).

Theories of aging

Animal research has produced information about aging, not necessarily relevant to humans. Some theories of aging assume the presence of an inbuilt and inherited "clock" that ticks away, but may be speeded or slowed. If several generations of fruit-flies are not allowed to breed until they are old, they produce longer-lived descendants. In contrast, old rotifers (minute freshwater animals) have short-lived offspring, and the foals of old stallions are slightly weaker and shorter-lived than their elder siblings. However, long-lived parents, whether horse or human, have relatively long-lived children. In some animals, the "clock" can be slowed: water fleas (daphnia) live twice as long when the water is 10°C colder. Rats which have been fed a nourishing but low-calorie diet live two to three times as long as normal rats, and look a third of their chronological age. Part of their long life is due to better health – they resist the bronchitis and other respiratory infections that normally kill rats. A similar effect does not occur in humans.

Longevity and genetics

Is lifespan determined by a time-bomb in the genes? The female advantage is probably genetic, but no-one knows how or why. In birds and butterflies the males have two X chromosomes (♦ page 26) but show no "male advantage". Biologists have failed so far to identify genes that are involved in aging. However, they have found that genes become increasingly unable to perform their functions with age, especially in nerve and muscle cells, which lose the power of division early in life. In old age such cells become poorer at making the substances needed for their own special tasks or even for their own maintenance. Genes may be damaged by chance processes: chemicals or radiation may alter or destroy them, cause them to produce faulty enzymes or set off dangerous uncontrolled division. The British biologist John Maynard Smith (b. 1920) has shown that the normal mutation rate of human cells is not fast enough to account for aging, unless the mutant cells also have harmful properties and multiply fast.

The Australian immunologist Sir Macfarlane Burnet (1899-1985), winner of the 1960 Nobel Prize for Medicine, has suggested that if it were true that lymphocytes (white blood cells) mutate, losing their tolerance to a person's own antigens, this would account for the increase of autoimmune diseases with age (♦ page 230). However, lymphocyte abnormalities (there are 4 percent abnormal at the age of 10, and 14 percent at 80) are mainly confined to the sex chromosomes, leaving the others intact.

Is atmospheric radiation to blame for aging? It is pointless comparing populations from countries with high and low radiation because of differences in nutrition, climate and general health. Radiation decreases the lifespan of most animals, moving some causes of death forward more than others. But it prolongs the life of many female insects by causing infertility, so the animal is spared the burden of laying thousands of eggs.

parents, often with increased growth of beard and chest hair.

Bone becomes brittle as it gradually loses its collagen framework and hence its ability to hold calcium. This condition, osteoporosis, occurs in everyone, but produces symptoms in only a few. Caused by loss of sex hormones, it develops faster after the menopause (♦ page 95) in women. It is commonest in thin elderly people; plump people make estrogen in their fat cells. Muscles shrivel and muscle reflexes diminish. Joints wear out as the joint cartilages deteriorate and bony outgrowths form. This condition, called osteoarthrosis or osteoarthritis, is found in most over-50s but only a few have symptoms (♦ page 109). Teeth fall out because the anchoring membrane weakens and is vulnerable to infection (♦ page 112).

A hundred thousand nerve cells die each day, and the brain shrinks by 2-3g a year in middle age, 3-4g in old age. The endocrine and immune systems, which are controlled by the brain, suffer as a result. Nerve cells conduct less quickly, both reflexes and voluntary movement are slower and the sense of balance becomes poor. Hearing becomes dimmer and we lose the power to hear high tones or focus on sounds. Eyes lose their range of focus and may develop cataracts (cloudy lenses ♦ page 51) or glaucoma (excessive pressure in the eyeball). It becomes harder to remember new things, though old memories often become more vivid. Hormone output declines and, in women, the ovaries cease producing sex hormones.

There is a loss of elasticity of the aorta and weakening of heart muscle cells. Reduced heart output may lead to congestive heart failure (♦ page 161). Arteries acquire a hard lining of cholesterol, narrowing vessels, raising blood pressure and reducing the brain's blood supply. The air sacs and tubules of the lungs become less inflatable.

The gut secretes less digestive juices than in youth. Gut movements become slower and weaker, leading to constipation and piles. Swallowing may become difficult. The sphincter (closing) muscles become weaker and food may flow back from stomach to esophagus. The muscles of the urinary system weaken, rendering it liable to infection from microbes in a half-emptied bladder. The bladder stretches less, so urination is more frequent. Men's prostate glands enlarge, impeding urination (♦ page 140).

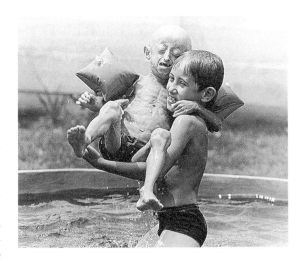

▲ Progeria is a bizarre condition which results in individuals at the end of their first decade developing shrunken skin, cataracts, and other physical signs of aging. Normal growth suddenly decelerates in children as young as eight or nine years of age. As a result of atherosclerosis and high blood pressure, children suffering from progeria usually die of coronary heart trouble.

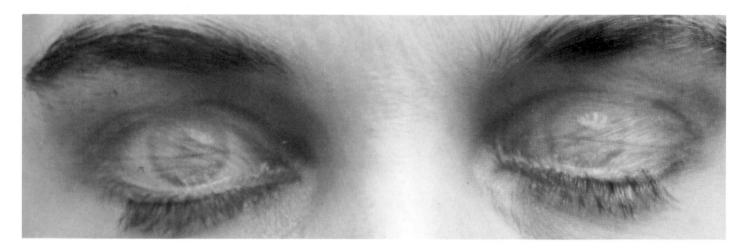

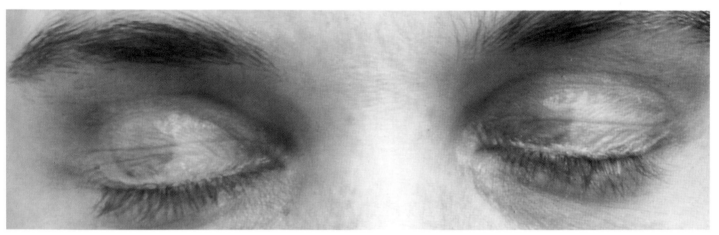

Sleep – the daily renewal

Two kinds of sleep have been discovered by recording the brain's electrical activity. The first stage of the night is "orthodox", and has four progressively deeper stages. Heart rate, blood pressure and metabolic rate fall. In the light stages the sleeper will move, but in deep stages both muscles and brain are at their most inactive, output of growth hormone (◀ page 87) increases, protein production rises and the body repairs itself. Dreams, if any, are matter-of-fact and occur only in the light stages; they may be about the next day's chores. After about 80 minutes, orthodox gives way to "paradoxical" sleep, also known as rapid-eye-movement (REM) sleep, with brainwaves similar to the waking state, increased but erratic heart and respiration rates and sexual arousal. The hands and feet may twitch but the rest of the body is profoundly relaxed. The first REM sleep lasts five to ten minutes and often has a dream about problems left over from the day. Orthodox and REM sleep alternate through the night in 90-minute cycles, the orthodox spell becoming shorter and shallower, and the REM spells longer. The second and third REM sleeps may have dreams comparing the day's problems with similar problems resolved in the past; the fourth is often about life without the problem; the fifth and longest may be a stirring finale incorporating the other four.

Deprivation of either kind of sleep leads to a rebound; we take more of it the next night. Sleep seems essential – deprivation rapidly causes delusions, and kills faster than starvation. REM sleep deprivation makes normal people slightly excitable; it improves depressed people. REM sleep accounts for 20 percent of adult sleep but 40 per-

▲ *The eye movement of REM sleep may stimulate dreams rather than vice versa. Studies of REM and orthodox sleep have produced a very different interpretation of dreams from that proposed by early psychoanalysts (◀ page 77).*

What is sleep?

All mammals have both orthodox and REM sleep, and the REM proportion of sleep is greater in more complex animals, as well as in babies and children. Since sleeping pills reduce or abolish REM sleep without causing apparent harm, what is its function?

Sigmund Freud (1856-1939) suggested that dreams were necessary to express subconscious desires and anxieties; Harvard University scientist Allan Hobson disagrees, saying that dreams are created to accompany the physical activities of REM sleep. He has investigated neuronal activity during sleep and dreaming, and has found that giant cells in the reticular formation of the brainstem are stimulated during REM sleep and dreaming, whereas locus ceruleus (LC) cells, which affect muscle tone, are correspondingly active during orthodox sleep and also during periods of wakefulness.

Other scientists have suggested that sleep is the natural state of the brain (we wake only to eat, mate and make a shelter) or a strategy for conserving energy. None of these ideas explains why we lose consciousness while asleep, rendering us vulnerable to attackers.

Immortal human cells

In February 1951, a 31-year-old Baltimore woman consulted doctors about blood loss between periods. She had a 2·5cm soft purple mass of cells on her cervix that proved malignant. She died eight months later. Cells taken for examination multiplied in tissue culture. They are still continuing to grow and divide over 30 years later.

Little is known about the patient whose tumor cells are now found in laboratories the world over. Called HeLa cells, they are named after her, but no-one knows her real name. She was a Black American, probably called Henrietta Lacks, or perhaps Helen Lane – her hospital record sadly was destroyed. Although she died young, her cells have contributed to advances in the study of viruses, protein synthesis, and the chemistry of cell growth.

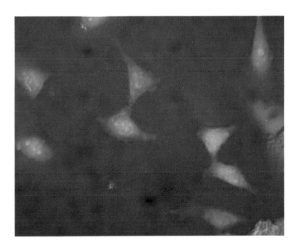

Other theories of sleep

In 1983 Nobel Prizewinner Francis Crick and Graeme Mitchison, suggested that REM sleep is necessary to unlearn or "reverse-learn" certain patterns of thought they regard as parasitic; otherwise, they say, the brain becomes overloaded with memories, causing delusions, obsessions or hallucinations in waking life.

The British computer scientist Chris Evans likened the brain to a computer which, having performed the day's tasks, needs to remain functioning by going "off-line" for reprogramming. He saw the brain as being "on-line" during orthodox, but "off-line" during REM sleep – when woken during REM sleep, the dream we see is the reprogramming taking place. Evans' theory explains why complicated animals sleep more, as do those whose day has been full of stress, change or depression. It fails to explain the beneficial effect of anti-depressant drugs.

British-based US psychiatrist Morton Schatzman thinks that an important function of sleep is problem-solving, and has set problems in magazine articles which readers have subsequently solved during sleep. Otto Loewi discovered the existence of neurotransmitters (♦ page 60) after dreaming about them.

Finally, British sleep researcher Jim Horne has suggested that REM sleep, which begins during the last third of fetal development, starts as a method of relieving the boredom of life in the womb.

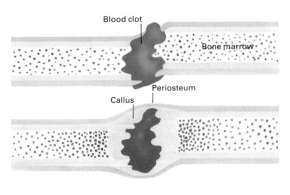

▶ Broken bones heal as osteoblasts or bone-forming cells form a callus that bridges the broken edges and is slowly remodelled. Osteoclasts remove any bony splinters and macrophages clear away the debris. The fracture mends in four to six weeks. If a broken bone cannot be immobilized (as in the case of a rib) or is badly set, the callus forms a lumpy buttress between the broken ends. Otherwise the bone resumes its correct shape.

Bone healing

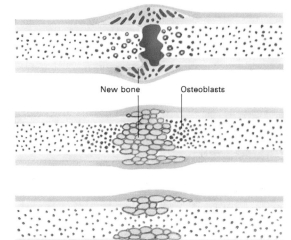

◀ Some of the HeLa cells, obtained by chance from a malignant tumor. They are unique in having survived over 30 years, whereas no culture of normal cells has survived more than a few weeks. There are enough HeLa cells to outweigh a small town, and they are used for medical research throughout the world.

cent of babies', more still in premature babies. Depressed people have increased REM sleep, which is reduced or even abolished by antidepressant drugs; this does no apparent harm.

In 1982 John Pappenheimer and colleagues at Harvard University discovered a sleep-promoting glycopeptide, factor S, in human urine. It increases deep, dreamless sleep by 50 percent, and one day it may prove to be a remedy for insomnia and a research tool for studying the chemistry of sleep and what parts of the brain are involved. Found in the brains of various mammals, its concentration increases after sleep deprivation.

Regenerating organs

Damaged skeletal muscle tissue is regenerated because surviving ends of injured fibers grow about 1mm daily, and parent cells form new fibers. Smooth muscle heals, but biologists do not know whether new fibers form or adjacent ones migrate. Damaged heart muscle (a complication of diphtheria and some other infections, and of heart attacks) is regenerated in children, but in adults a fibrous scar forms.

The moist surface of the lungs, gut and excretory system are constantly renewed, even during health, and therefore heal well. Gut has a wavy surface with proliferating cells in the depressions that constantly divide and migrate upwards. Lung epithelium damaged during infections heals in the same way as skin. Repeated infection such as chronic bronchitis leads to faulty regeneration: the mucus-forming cells have no cilia. Kidneys damaged by infection regenerate only slowly, and the new cells are less efficient.

Skin healing

Making good the damage

The liver suffers little wear and tear; occasional damaged areas are replaced by division of neighboring cells. Divisions may be faulty, producing large cells with two or more nuclei, but this does not seem to matter. Liver damaged by disease (such as hepatitis) or abuse (poisoning or alcohol) regenerates rapidly but irregularly, without its lobular pattern.

Mature brain cells cannot be replaced, though their function is not missed if (as often happens) conduction is diverted along other routes. However, peripheral nerve cells – those outside the brain and spinal cord – often reconnect when cut. The far end degenerates but the Schwann cells (◀ page 60) surrounding it proliferate within their sheath, forming a pathway for the axon which sprouts from the other end. It grows by 3mm daily, fattens, and eventually forms links with motor end plates.

Developing nerves depend on a peptide (small protein), nerve growth factor. Suspected in the 1960s, it was purified in 1979 from the salivary glands of many thousands of male mice. Other growth factors have since been isolated, including factors that sustain sensory nerves, stimulate bone growth, and regulate cell division in skin and connective tissue. All are peptides or glycopeptides (peptides with sugar molecules attached).

How damaged skin heals

If the skin is cut, sooner or later the blood from the broken blood vessels form a clot. The clot has three functions: it fills the gap, protects the wound and bonds the edges together. After the formation of the clot, white polymorph cells arrive at the wound, "eat" bacteria and disintegrate. Macrophages arrive on the third or fourth day and clear up the debris or, if the wound is infected, initiate an immune response to deal with the infection. For 3-4mm around the cut, the convoluted epidermal layer (◀ page 115) flattens and multiplies. Cells around the cut migrate over the wound, sliding over each other as they go. Having formed a continuous layer, they divide. Similar processes occur in the dermis, where new capillary vessels grow at the rate of 2mm daily. Solid at first, these unite with each other or with existing capillaries before hollowing. Some acquire smooth muscle cells and become arterioles or venules. New lymph vessels are formed in the same way.

Fibroblasts (fiber-makers) arrive after four or five days and make a scar of collagen (◀ page 97). Collagen content is highest at three weeks after the injury but maximum strength comes later as the fibers gradually develop molecular bonds with each other. New scars look raised and red because blood vessels and tissue overproliferate; they diminish later. Sensory nerves reach the scar after three weeks but specialized touch receptors, if destroyed, never re-form.

Open wounds start to heal in a similar way to a simple cut. A sheet of epithelial cells advances from the edges of the undamaged skin beneath the blood clot. At first only loosely attached to the dermis, this sheet is easily torn off if bandages are removed roughly. In deep burns the cells have to burrow under a thick layer of dead, burnt collagen. The watery tissue that oozes from many wounds keeps infection away and, when drying, helps to draw the edges together. The tissue below the wound expands upwards. Infected wounds take longer to heal because bacteria have to be destroyed by white cells, which then die and ooze away as pus.

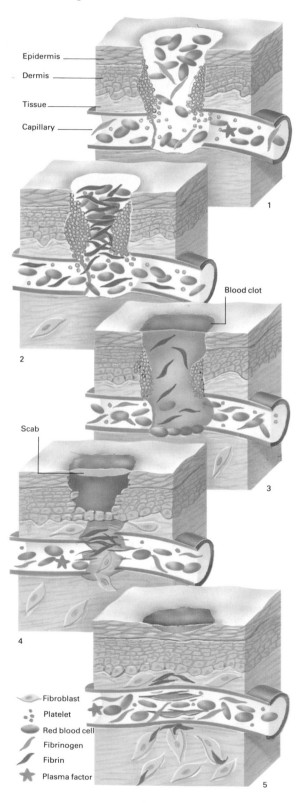

Epidermis
Dermis
Tissue
Capillary

Blood clot

Scab

Fibroblast
Platelet
Red blood cell
Fibrinogen
Fibrin
Plasma factor

▲ **When the skin is cut (1), fibrinogen from the blood plasma combines with platelets to form a fibrin network which enmeshes the red blood cells (2), enabling a clot to form and plug the wound (3). The cells of the epidermis divide and grow back, pushing off the scab (4). Meanwhile fibroblast cells stimulate the regeneration of the underlying connective tissue and blood vessels, healing the wound fully (5).**

The primary defenses against infection...The immune system...The lymphatic system...Macrophages... Lymphocytes, antigens and antibodies...Destroying the infection...Immunity... Vaccination...PERSPECTIVE... Should tonsils be removed?...Interferon, the body's vital poison...The structure of antibodies...Why does the body tolerate itself?

The body is continually liable to attack from infective organisms or to damage from poisons in the environment. Through evolution, protective mechanisms have developed. Some of these are very general, whereas others are much more specific and involve the activation of a highly elaborate defense mechanism. The physical barrier to invasion provided by skin is enhanced by surface secretions containing fatty acids that generally inhibit microbial growth, and the enzyme lysozyme which damages bacterial cell walls. Similarly, the acidity of the stomach helps to protect it from harmful organisms ingested with food. The lungs are protected by nasal mucus, which both traps and destroys foreign bodies, and by cilia which help to expel particulate matter with their beating motion.

If foreign material does enter the body, additional defenses come into play. Inflammation of local tissues may prevent the invaders from spreading through the body. Some viruses are inactivated by slight increases in temperature, so fever can be a defensive response to such invasions. Blood contains substances which are harmful to bacteria. Transferrin, for example, robs them of the iron they need for growth, while white blood cells (leukocytes) digest foreign matter.

There is also a complex system of "specific immunity", the details of which are not yet fully understood. This is characterized by three factors: specificity, memory and self-tolerance. Whereas a nonspecific response does not alter with time or experience of the invader, a specific response allows the body to memorize the structure of a particular foreign body and to react far more quickly and vigorously to any subsequent attack from it.

The body's main defense system

The specific immune system has three major components, comprising two types of lymphocyte and the macrophage. Macrophages are leukocytes; some circulate in the blood, while others reside in tissues throughout the body. They, like granulocytes (◀ page 152), scavenge unwanted material such as old red blood cells. Macrophages also co-operate with the lymphocytes to produce specific immune responses.

The lymphocytes – of which an adult has a trillion (10^{12}), weighing about one kilogram – arise from stem cells in bone marrow. Some are transferred via the bloodstream to the thymus, a gland overlying the heart in the chest. Here they rapidly produce many daughter cells, most of which die. The survivors emerge from the thymus and travel to lymphoid tissue as mature T-lymphocytes (T-cells), able to respond to foreign matter. Lymphocytes of the second kind are produced in the bone marrow and the body's other lymphoid organs, which include the spleen, tonsils, gut lining, appendix and lymph nodes. In birds, this type is produced in an organ called the bursa, from which they were given the name B-lymphocytes.

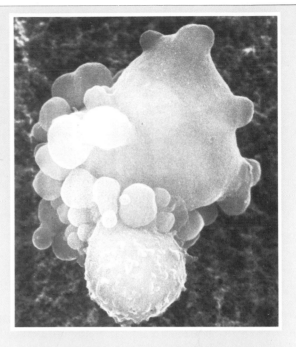

▲ *A cancer cell being attacked and destroyed by lymphocytes, the agents of the body's system of defense against invasion from inside or out. The lymphocytes have caused blisters to grow on the cell before finally killing it.*

Infected wound

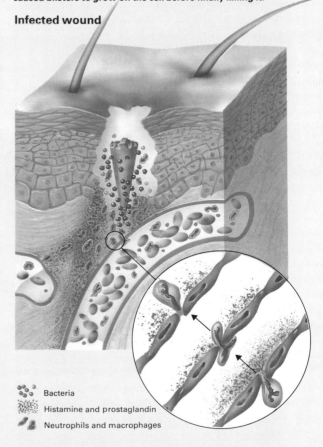

Bacteria

Histamine and prostaglandin

Neutrophils and macrophages

▲ *If body cells become infected, they release histamine and prostaglandins to cause inflammation and trap the infection. Blood vessels dilate and allow neutrophils cells to pass through their walls to the tissues, where they and macrophages attempt to destroy the bacteria. If the infection is too virulent, a specific immune response is invoked.*

Lymphocytes circulate through the lymphatic system (◀ page 154) and the blood. Lymph nodes, capsules of tissue which occur at intervals throughout the lymphatic system, filter the lymph and control the direction of its flow. They are also sites where B- and T-cells mature after challenge by an invader. In some infections, a proliferation of lymphocytes causes enlargement of the nodes, the symptom often described as "swollen glands". The spleen plays a similar role, as filter for microbes that have entered the bloodstream, and stimulates lymphocytes into activity.

The B-cells produce immunoglobulins, complex proteins which cover the cell surface and are also released into the blood. A foreign body that reacts with immunoglobulin is called an antigen. Generally, antigens are large molecules, notably proteins and carbohydrates. Small molecules can be antigenic, but usually only in combination with a large molecule; thus, some reactive chemicals are antigenic because they form complexes with the body's own proteins. Similarly, the allergy shown by some people to penicillin derives from its ability to combine with protein and create a new antigen (◀ page 230).

Immunoglobulins – antibodies as they are also called – combine with antigens like a key fitting a lock. Only a small part of each molecule fits together and a single large antigen molecule may have many such sites – called antigenic determinants – on it. Different ones may react with one or more distinct immunoglobulins. Often, several different immunoglobulins will react with several different antigenic determinants, thus producing a large aggregate which the body can attack more readily.

While the immunoglobulin molecules are much the same general shape, each has variable regions which are the antigen-combining sites, so one type of immunoglobulin usually reacts with only one antigenic determinant. In this variability lies two of the strengths of the immune system, its specificity and its memory.

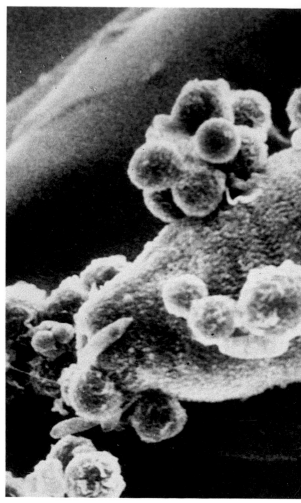

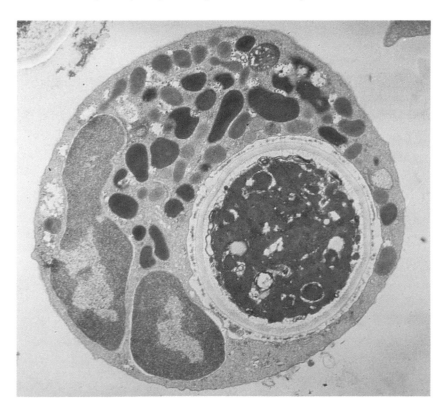

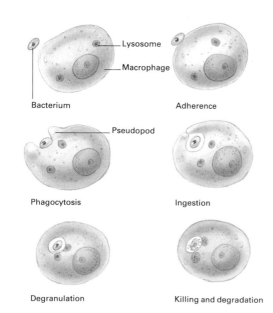

▲ *Macrophages play an important role in the body's defenses, passing through the connective tissue and approaching unwanted tissues or invading organisms. They take the organisms within their cell membranes (phagocytosis) and digest them.*

◀ *A macrophage after ingesting a round yeast molecule.*

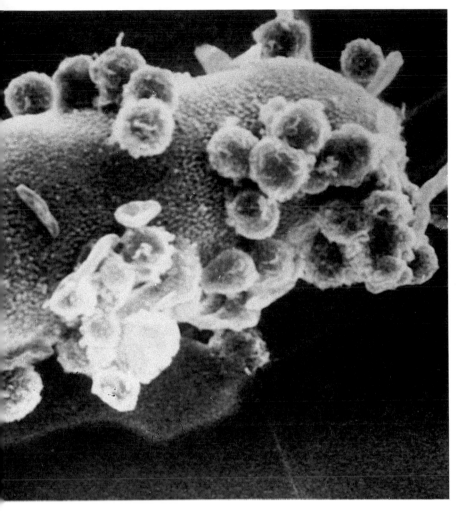

Lymph flow

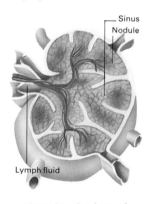

Lymphatic duct

Veins
Arteries
Heart

Blood capillaries

Lymph node

Lymphatic capillaries

◄ Electron micrograph of lymphocytes attacking a schistosomiasis (bilharzia) parasite; once activated, the immune system can launch a powerful attack on invading organisms.

▲ The lymph flows through the lymph vessels by muscular activity, draining and filtering the body tissue fluid and allowing the lymphocytes to reach the site of invasion quickly.

Should tonsils be removed?

Until recently, tonsils were a part of the body often removed during childhood. They were considered to be a nuisance, liable to infection, and serving no useful purpose. In fact, tonsils are a major defense against invasion via the oral cavity. There are three types. The ones which used to be removed commonly were the palatine tonsils. The exposed surface of these in the roof of the mouth is pitted and can accumulate debris. This can be a source of infection, which is known as tonsillitis; the swelling may block the pharynx and interfere with breathing and swallowing.

The pharyngeal tonsils, or adenoids, can also produce harmful effects if they become infected, making nasal breathing difficult. The third set of tonsils, the lingual tonsils, are at the back of the tongue and usually cause no trouble.

If tonsils are not completely removed, they may grow again in young children. However, now that their role as a source of lymphocytes in a vulnerable part of the body is known, tonsillectomy is considered undesirable unless there is persistent infection. It can lead to greater susceptibility to some diseases, notably polio and Hodgkin's disease (♦ page 228).

Lymph organs tend to decrease in size and activity as we get older. Consequently, tonsillitis is generally only a childhood disease.

Immunomodulators

In recent years, it has been shown that the immune system uses a variety of chemical messengers – similar in a way to hormones – to communicate between different parts of itself and to activate specific responses. The exact function of many of these immunomodulators, of which there may be 20-30 major ones, is still unclear.

These molecules, all of which are soluble and can therefore travel freely around the lymphatic system, are called lymphokines. Their roles in modulating the immune system are both activating and passivating. Thus, macrophage migration inhibitory factor will prevent overreaction by part of the immune system, while macrophage activating factor has an opposite effect.

In therapeutic terms, it is the role of some of the less well understood lymphokines, such as the interferons and tumor necrosis factor, which may ultimately be important. Self-generated diseases, such as cancer, frequently arise through the failure of the immune system to destroy material that is or has become "non-self".

Attacking these diseases successfully will probably depend on mimicking accurately the immune system response which has failed. Increasingly, it seems likely that a key part of this effective response is the production of a "cocktail" of appropriate immunomodulators.

Lymph node

Sinus
Nodule

Lymph fluid

▲ Lymph nodes, located on lymphatic pathways, are made up of fibrous connective tissue. T- and B-cells are made and congregate in their nodular compartments, as do other phagocytic cells. Lymph nodes tend to be clustered near parts of the body most susceptible to invasion; they filter the lymph fluid of injurious particles and act as the operations center for the fight against any invading organisms.

The body can remember and recognize 100 million different invading organisms

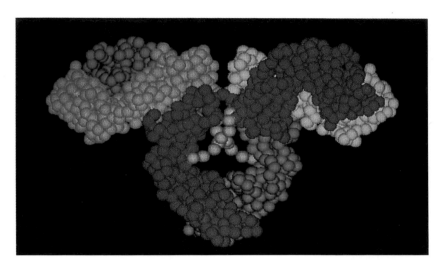

The types of immunoglobulin

*Immunoglobulins – the antibodies released from
the surfaces of B-cells that react to invaders and act
as the crucial memory part of the immune system –
are proteins. Five varieties have been identified.
The most abundant is immunoglobulin G (IgG).
One of its key functions is to pass on immunity
to babies, by crossing the placental barrier.
Macroglobulins (IgM) are aggregates of five
immunoglobulin molecules. Like IgG, IgM can
activate the complement system, but it cannot
cross the placental barrier.*

*A first line of defense is provided by IgA, found
in tears and saliva and released into the gut and
lungs. This helps to inactivate viruses and toxins.
Part of its structure makes it adhere to the lining
of the gut and respiratory tract. It combines with
foreign material and immobilizes it. Bacterial cells
are particularly prone to destruction by lysozyme
after interaction with IgA. This type of immunoglobulin provides resistance in the gut of the
newborn, who obtain it from their mothers' milk.*

*The other two types of immunoglobulin – IgD and
IgE – are less well understood. IgE is implicated in
hypersensitivity and allergy, one of its effects being
the rapid release of inflammatory substances such
as histamine (♦ page 229). It also may have a role in
fighting parasitic infections. The function of IgD is
not clear. Its main role may be as a B-cell surface
receptor, to help to recognize antigens.*

Producing the right antibodies

*Proteins are manufactured in the body from
instructions coded into the genes. The immune
system seems able to produce antibodies specific
to any foreign matter with which it is challenged,
yet it is impracticable to suppose that we have a
gene for every possible antigen sequence that
we might encounter. Different genes each code
for a part of the antibody molecule; these can
combine in different ways, thus creating diversity.
Further diversity arises from the two variable
regions. A third form of diversity is probably
supplied by mutation. While most cells contain
mechanisms to repair genetic material accurately,
lymphocytes may have an error-prone repair
mechanism, increasing the number of changes in
the genes coding for the variable regions.*

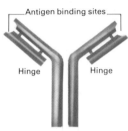

▲ ▲ *An immunoglobulin is
a Y-shaped molecule; the
binding sites, specific to
one antigen, are shaped by
the structure of variable
regions on the arms.*

▶ *After a B-cell has been
matched to the antigen, a
"helper" T-cell with the
same antigen determinants
stimulates the B-cell to
divide (4A), making
memory cells to await
future attacks, and plasma
cells which produce huge
amounts of the right
antibody. This pours into
the bloodstream, binds to
the antigen and neutralizes
it (5A), clumps it to enable
macrophages to attack (5B)
or stimulates the
complement system to kill
its cell membranes (5C).*

The structure of immunoglobulins

*Basically, all immunoglobulins consist of four
protein chains, linked together by disulfide bonds.
There are two identical heavy chains and two
identical light chains. Both types contain regions
which are constant in structure and others which
are variable regions. The constant regions of the
heavy chain define which of the five types a
particular immunoglobulin belongs to, while the
variable regions determine which antigen it will
react with, and therefore these regions give
immunoglobulins their specificity.*

*It is estimated that we have the capacity to
produce 100 million different types of antibody.*

*When the variable part interacts with an antigen,
the shape of the molecule changes. This can help
the antibody-antigen complex to attach to a
phagocyte or, in the case of IgG and IgM, it can
activate the complement system to destroy the
antigen.*

The blood's secret weapon: complement

*The complement system involves eleven different
proteins, some of which are latent forms of the
natural catalyst molecules called enzymes. The
system works in a complex but coordinated
manner called a cascade; it has a variety of effects
all of which help the destruction of the invader.
These include making cells more easily digestible
by macrophages; releasing chemical attractants
which draw leukocytes to the scene; and disrupting
the cell membranes of the foreign organisms,
thereby causing the cell to explode.*

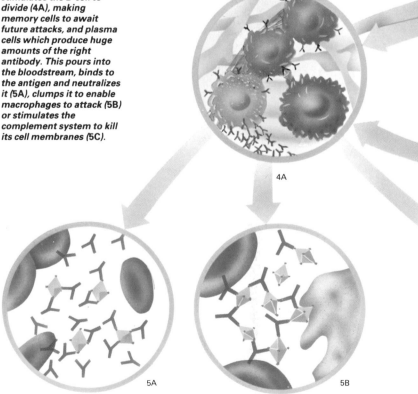

4A

5A

5B

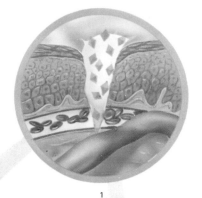

The immune response

▶ *If an invader (antigen) enters (1) the blood stream (2) or body tissues (2A), the first nonspecific response sees it attacked by neutrophils and the complement system. Macrophages may then take it to a lymph node (3), where the antigen is presented to the many T- and B-lymphocytes that are collected there. An appropriate antibody on a B-lymphocyte (or an equivalent site on the T-cell) is matched to the antigen; if none yet exists, a cell with an almost-correct antibody structure is found to mutate and provide an exact fit.*

	Antigen
	Antibodies
	Macrophage
	Neutrophil
	Complement
	B-lymphocyte
	T-lymphocyte

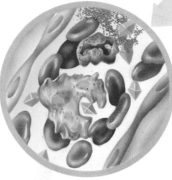

2

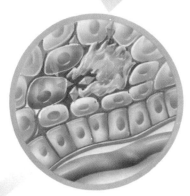

2A

◀ ▼ *After a T-cell in the lymph node has been found with determinants that match the antigen, it then divides and creates four kinds of T-cell (4B). Memory cells await future attacks by the antigen, so that these attacks can be dealt with in a matter of moments rather than days; helper cells assist B-cells to produce antibodies against the antigen; and killer cells pass to the body tissues invaded by the antigen, where they release cytotoxic substances that kill any infected cell and the invader in it (5D). They also release factors which stimulate other lymphocytes (5E) and macrophages (5F) to the site. Finally, suppressor T-cells are produced which also travel to the infected area to suppress the activities of the killer cells and macrophages when the danger is over.*

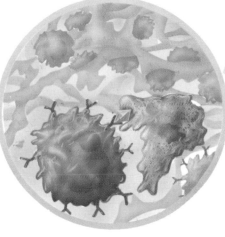

3

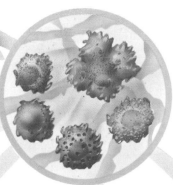

4B

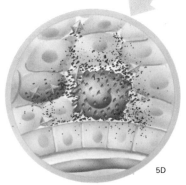

5C

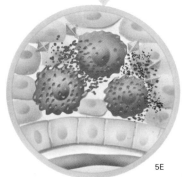

5D

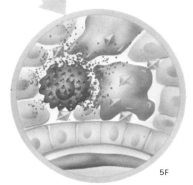

5E

5F

Memorizing an invader

If a B-lymphocyte reacts with an antigen under suitable conditions, it can become active in one of two ways. It may become a short-lived plasma cell, an immunoglobulin factory which produces much more of the reactive immunoglobulin and releases it into the bloodstream. It may reproduce more B-cells like itself, with the reactive immuno-globulin on their surfaces. Thus, once exposed to a particular antigen, the body contains more B-cells with the right antibody to combine with that antigen, should it ever appear again. This is the basis for immunity against reinfection. If the challenge is not repeated, these "memory cells" gradually die and immunity slowly decreases. Some infections seem to confer little immunity, though this is often because the organism, when next met, has evolved and thus changed its antigenic determinants (as with influenza) or because the disease is caused by many different organisms (as with the common cold).

Specificity is absolute, but different materials can share antigenic determinants. In such cases, if the immune system has reacted to one of the materials, it will subsequently react to the other as if it had been exposed to it already. The sharing of antigenic determinants by the organisms which cause smallpox (◗ page 242) and the related but milder disease, cowpox, led to the scientific discovery of immunization by Edward Jenner (1749-1823). In this case, the organisms involved are closely related, so the cross-reactivity is not surprising. In some cases, the similarity of antigenic determinants is coincidental and may be harmful, as in the case of rheumatic fever (◗ page 230).

Triggering the system

The interaction between T-cells and antigens is a major contributor to the immune response, largely because of chemical substances called lymphokines which are released by an activated T-cell. Some of these signal macrophages to come to the site of invasion, while others stimulate B-cells into activity. Although a B-cell can form an antibody-antigen complex, no immune response will occur unless there is co-operation from a T-cell. Nevertheless, in the case of some foreign matter such as bacterial toxins, formation of the complex may be enough to render it harmless.

The situation is more complex and more effective because there is more than one kind of T-cell. Some "helper" T-cells provoke the immune response, while "suppressor" cells limit it. They recognize antigens through surface receptors, similar to immunoglobulins.

A T-cell will react with an antigen only when it is associated on the surface of a macrophage with a major histocompatibility complex (MHC). These genes produce molecules, present on all cells which an organism recognizes as characteristic of itself. Known as human leuk-ocyte antigens (HLAs), they are tolerated by the organism's immune system. They differ between all individuals except identical siblings, so one person's HLAs will elicit an immune response in someone else. This is why organ and tissue transplants are frequently rejected.

Helper T-cells react to the antigen, particularly if it has been ad-sorbed on the surface of a macrophage, and consequently stimulate B-cells. For this to happen, the T-cells have to recognize the HLAs on both the macrophage and the B-cells as similar to those on its own surface. Another type of T-cell, which attacks virally-infected body cells, does so only if the infected cell has HLAs in common with it. These cytotoxic T-cells are activated by helper T-cells through the lymphokine gamma-interferon.

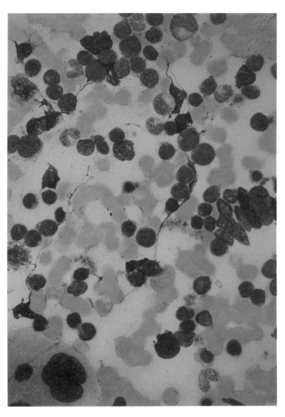

▲ *Artificially colored micrograph of human bone marrow in the spaces within spongy bone. Bone marrow is the source of stem cells, "general purpose" cells from which both B- and T-cells are produced after maturation in the thymus, spleen and other lymph organs.*

Cross-reactivity and double-cross

Cross-reactivity of antigens – the basis of modern immunization, discovered by Jenner – saved lives in Poland in an unusual way during World War II.

Vast numbers of Poles died as a result of the harsh conditions imposed upon them by the German occupation. The insanitary conditions led to outbreaks of typhus, a disease spread by lice. The disease had been kept out of Germany for a quarter of a century, which meant that the natural resistance of the population was low, so the Germans were determined that it should not find its way back. As many Poles were being sent to forced-labor camps in Germany, the Germans instituted typhus testing and refused to take any whose blood gave a positive result.

The test used, known as the Weil-Felix reaction, depends on the ability of typhus antibodies to form clumps with a bacterium called Proteus. This clumping is characteristic of antibody-antigen interaction and works because of cross-reactivity between typhus and Proteus. Two doctors working in southeastern Poland reasoned that an injection of Proteus would induce antibodies which would also give a positive Weil-Felix reaction. They tried this and it worked so successfully that, after repeating the injection on many local inhabitants and submitting blood samples to the Germans, the entire area of about a dozen villages was declared an epidemic zone and remained free of German interference for several years.

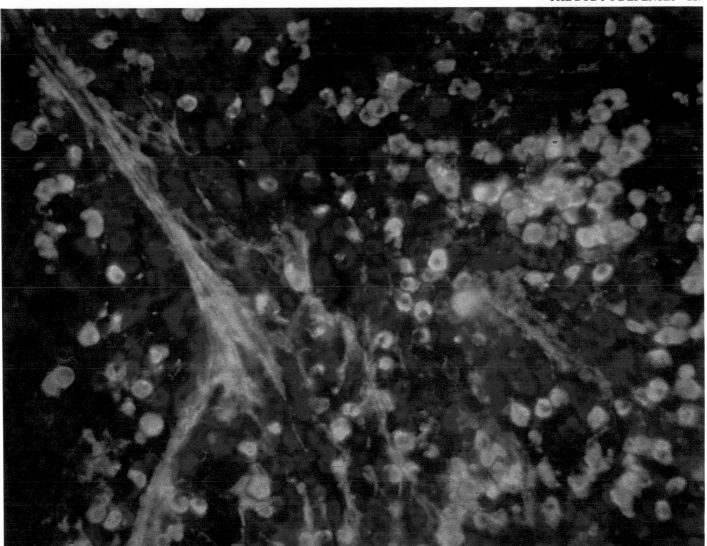

"Self" and "not self"

The Australian immunologist Sir Frank Macfarlane Burnet (1899-1985) noted that the immune system matures at a late stage of embryonic development, by which time most of the substances in the body which could be antigenic already exist. He proposed that any substance present when the immune system develops will be tolerated.

The basis for Burnet's theory was the mutual tolerance shown by some non-identical twin cattle. Identical human twins share immunological tolerance, whereas non-identical twins do not. The difference between humans and cattle in this case is that non-identical cattle twins share the same placenta and mixing of the fetal blood occurs. Consequently, according to this theory, each cow would recognize its non-identical twin as "self", because this mixing predated the development of its immune system.

Sir Peter Medawar (b. 1915), a British biologist interested in skin grafts, set out to test Burnet's theory. He had found that skin grafts between different people were unsuccessful. If one such graft was followed by another between the same donor and recipient, the second graft was rejected more quickly, indicating the development of immunological memory.

He then took two strains of highly interbred mice. Individuals of each strain would accept grafts from each other, but not from the other strain. He injected spleen cells from one into newborn mice of the other strain; these were then found to tolerate skin grafts from both strains. They had developed immunological tolerance.

Although this explains immunological tolerance on one level, it does not explain how it arises or continues. The answer seems to lie with the T-lymphocytes. T-cells can be made tolerant towards antigens, so that they no longer effect an immune response. B-cells still recognize the antigen, but do not become active because of the missing T-cell response. T-cells probably develop their tolerance towards "self" during development in the thymus. In some cases, the protective system breaks down and the immune system treats "self" as foreign, causing auto-immune diseases (◆ page 230).

▲ Micrograph of plasma cells producing antibodies IgM (colored red) and IgG (green). It has been calculated that, during an immune response, each plasma cell makes 2,000 antibody molecules a second for several days.

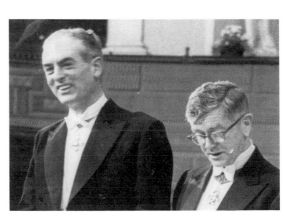

▶ Sir Peter Medawar and Sir Frank Macfarlane Burnet shared the Nobel Prize in Physiology in 1960 for their research into how an organism's immune system learns how to recognize "self" and differentiate it from "non-self".

Because the immune system's reaction is specific to a particular antigen, exposure to that antigen can be used to produce immunity artificially. This is the basis of vaccination. In the case of a microbial infection, the microbe may be killed without damaging its outer coat. Injection of the dead microbe induces an immune response to the antigenic determinants on it, so that subsequent infection with live microbes of the same species produces a rapid immune response.

The manifold nature of T-cells reflects the multiple functions of the immune system. Not only does the body need to defend itself from outside invasion; it also needs to defend itself from enemies within, such as cells which become cancerous. Characteristically, the surface of cancer cells differs from that of normal cells; in other words, they develop new antigenic determinants or may lack normal ones. The majority of potential cancer cells are destroyed by the immune system before they can gain a hold in the body (◆ page 224).

People who suffer exceptional stress, such as a bereavement, may be more prone to develop cancer than the population at large. From this and related observations, it has been postulated that psychological events can depress the level of activity of the immune system. Some lymphocytes carry receptors which can recognize peptide hormones found in the brain. Some T-cells produce lymphokines, including interferon, in response to them. Ultimately, the immune system must be modulated or influenced by the central nervous system, but how this is effected is not yet understood.

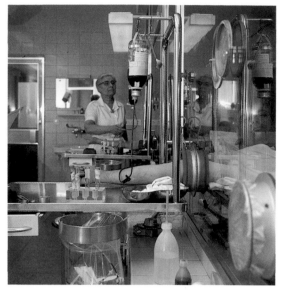

▲ *When transfusing blood, the blood groups of donor and recipient must be matched; the blood groups O, A, B and AB indicate the presence or absence of immunogenic substances, which must match.*

▼ *18th-century cartoon by James Gillray (1757-1815) satirizing the dangers of inoculation with cowpox vaccine against smallpox.*

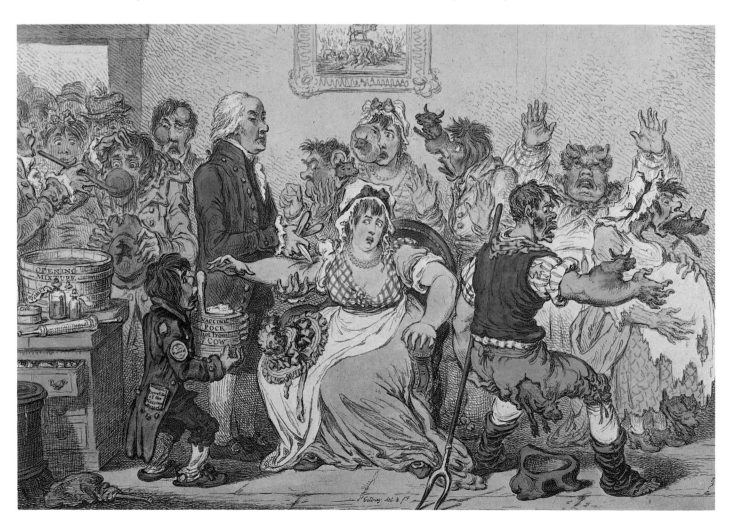

What is cancer?...The universality of cancer...Defining tumors...Viruses and malignancy...Oncogenes... The progress of cancer...Detection and monitoring... Treatment...PERSPECTIVE...Cancer incidence around the world...Smoking and lung cancer...Cancer in Africa... Can cancer be prevented?...Some unorthodox cures.

The body's cells usually regulate their growth and maintenance with exquisite delicacy. They multiply only when required – during childhood, and later to replace those lost through injury, disease and the continual shedding of cells from areas such as the skin and intestinal tract. When this self-control breaks down, the result is a malignant tumor (cancer). What may be a fatal process begins when just one healthy cell becomes cancerous and, free of normal constraints, transmits its abnormality to succeeding cell generations.

A fundamental aberration of cell behavior, cancer is found in all animals except the very simplest. There are even cancer-like growths in plants. For this reason, and because ancient skeletons interred in Egypt have shown deformations suggesting bone cancer, the condition is assumed to have affected all populations at all times.

Defining cancers

There are hundreds of different cancers, in two principal groups. Solid malignant tumors (which should be distinguished from benign, non-invasive ones) include those of the breast and womb in women; the prostate gland in men; and the stomach, lung and colon in both sexes. Systemic cancers are leukemias, affecting the blood-forming organs; and lymphomas, affecting the lymphatic system. Pathologists classify cancers further, according to the type of tissue and cell in which they arise. Carcinomas are based on tissue covering the body's external surfaces (for example, tumors of the skin and breast) or internal surfaces (such as intestinal, prostate and liver cancer). Sarcomas originate in muscle, bone, and other connective tissues. In addition to leukemias and lymphomas, the other principal category contains nerve tumors such as gliomas.

At first, malignant cells may resemble their healthy parents and even conduct some of their normal functions. But as the disease progresses they become increasingly abnormal in behavior and appearance. As well as proliferating out of control (usually rapidly) and invading adjacent tissues, cancers can spread to distant parts of the body. Breaking away from the primary growth, cells travel through the bloodstream, lymphatic vessels or body cavities, where they establish secondary tumors elsewhere. The whole process is known as metastasis.

Metastatic interference with essential organs and a draining of the body's vital resources are the reasons why cancers are sometimes fatal. But the disease can often be treated successfully – by surgery, irradiation, drugs, or any combination of these three. The chances are particularly good when cancer is detected before it has metastasized (which is the reason for regular screening using tests such at the cervical smear). Many patients are cured, and more than one in three survive five years or longer.

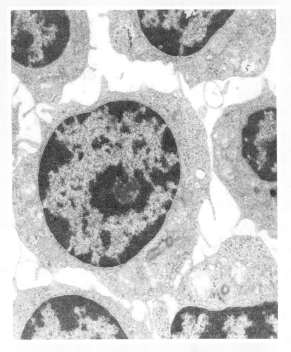

▲ The white blood cells of a patient with leukemia multiply quickly as the bone marrow and other tissues in which they are made become unusually active, and become destroyers, rather than defenders, of the body tissues.

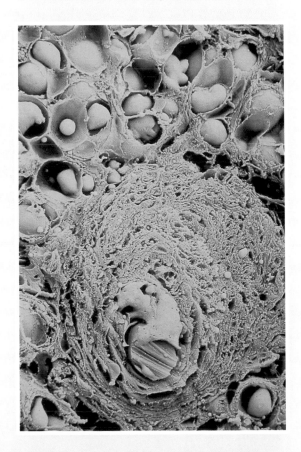

▲ A tumor in an ovary, with the normal tissues severely displaced by the growth; the Graafian follicle, consisting of a mature egg and its surrounding tissue, is visible towards the top of the picture.

Thousands of chemicals are known to be carcinogens

The incidence of cancer

Some 5·9 million people develop cancer each year. The organs most commonly affected are the stomach (with 680,000 new cases annually), lung (590,000 new cases), breast (540,000), colon and rectum (510,000), cervix (460,000), mouth and pharynx (340,000), esophagus (300,000) and liver (260,000). About half these cancers, and over half the 4·3 million deaths each year, occur in the Third World: cancer is one of the three major causes of death after the age of five in developed and developing countries alike.

Whereas the mortality rate from stomach cancer is highest in Japan, liver cancer occurs mainly in tropical Africa, Southeast Asia and the western Pacific, with 40 percent of all new cases appearing in China. The picture changes dramatically with time too. In the United States between 1950 and 1980 the number of children under 15 dying of leukemia fell by 50 percent from 1965 onwards. Kidney cancer and other tumors declined by 68 percent. Lung cancer (70 percent of which is attributable to smoking) is becoming less prevalent in many Western countries – but it has been increasing among women, who were later than men in adopting the smoking habit, and is now rising quickly in the Third World.

Carcinogens of many kinds

Such trends reflect differences in the causation of cancers and/or their detection and treatment. Just as cancer itself is a collective term, so there are different factors which initiate malignancy. Thousands of chemicals are now known to be carcinogens: blue asbestos has been incriminated as a cause of the otherwise extremely rare mesothelioma, affecting membranes lining the body cavities. Toxins from the mold "Aspergillus flavus", which promote liver cancer in fish and turkeys, are also thought responsible for some human liver tumors in sub-Saharan Africa, and in part for the high rate of stomach cancer in Japan.

There is evidence linking breast and colon cancer with a high fat uptake, and some other dietary constituents, both natural and synthetic, have been under suspicion. Cancer-causing agents sometimes have a delayed-action effect, so it may be decades before the dangers of presently-used materials come to light. In addition to over 50,000 synthetic chemicals now being marketed, nearly a thousand new ones are introduced each year, some of which may prove to be long-term human carcinogens. In the mid-1960s the high-dose contraceptive pill was shown to cause inflammation of the cervix, which may be a precursor to cervical cancer. The introduction of low-dose pills overcame this problem, although it 1983 it was claimed that long-term users suffered a slightly higher risk of breast and cervical cancer.

Cancer of the esophagus exemplifies the multiple causes which can make the charting of the disease so hard. It is related to both tobacco and alcohol, and is 44 times more common among French people who smoke or drink heavily than those who indulge in moderation. But even higher rates are found in northeastern Iran, where both habits are rare – the cause seems to be shortage of Vitamin A.

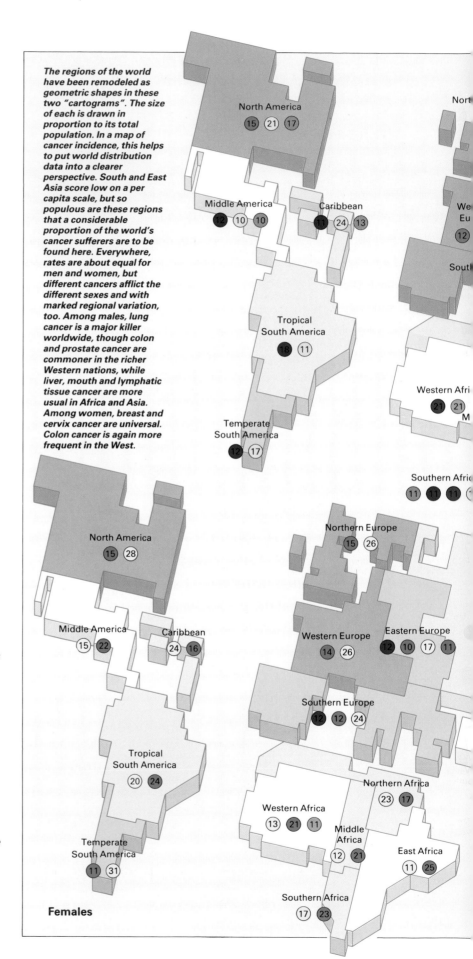

The regions of the world have been remodeled as geometric shapes in these two "cartograms". The size of each is drawn in proportion to its total population. In a map of cancer incidence, this helps to put world distribution data into a clearer perspective. South and East Asia score low on a per capita scale, but so populous are these regions that a considerable proportion of the world's cancer sufferers are to be found here. Everywhere, rates are about equal for men and women, but different cancers afflict the different sexes and with marked regional variation, too. Among males, lung cancer is a major killer worldwide, though colon and prostate cancer are commoner in the richer Western nations, while liver, mouth and lymphatic tissue cancer are more usual in Africa and Asia. Among women, breast and cervix cancer are universal. Colon cancer is again more frequent in the West.

Females

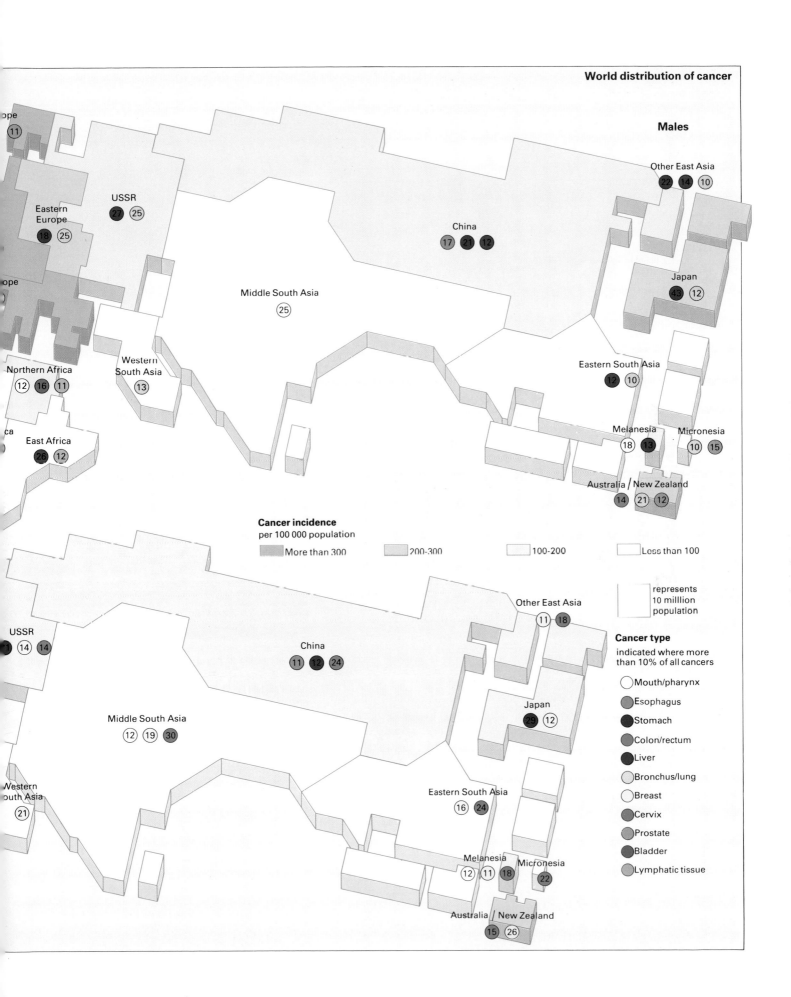

World distribution of cancer

Males

Other East Asia
㉒ ⑭ ⑩

USSR
㉗ ㉕

China
⑰ ㉑ ⑫

Japan
㊸ ⑫

Eastern
Europe
⑱ ㉕

㋋ope
⑪

㋋ope

Middle South Asia
㉕

Eastern South Asia
⑫ ⑩

Western
South Asia
⑬

Northern Africa
⑫ ⑯ ⑪

Melanesia
⑱ ⑬

Micronesia
⑩ ⑮

East Africa
㉖ ⑫

Australia / New Zealand
⑭ ㉑ ⑫

Cancer incidence
per 100 000 population

More than 300   200-300   100-200   Less than 100

□ represents
10 milllion
population

Cancer type
indicated where more
than 10% of all cancers

○ Mouth/pharynx
● Esophagus
● Stomach
● Colon/rectum
● Liver
○ Bronchus/lung
○ Breast
● Cervix
● Prostate
● Bladder
● Lymphatic tissue

Other East Asia
⑪ ⑱

USSR
● ⑭ ⑭

China
⑪ ⑫ ㉔

Japan
㉙ ⑫

Middle South Asia
⑫ ⑲ ㉚

Eastern South Asia
⑯ ㉔

Western
South Asia
㉑

Melanesia
⑫ ⑪ ⑱

Micronesia
㉒

Australia / New Zealand
⑮ ㉖

Carcinogens have to "hit" specific genes in the body's cells to cause cancer

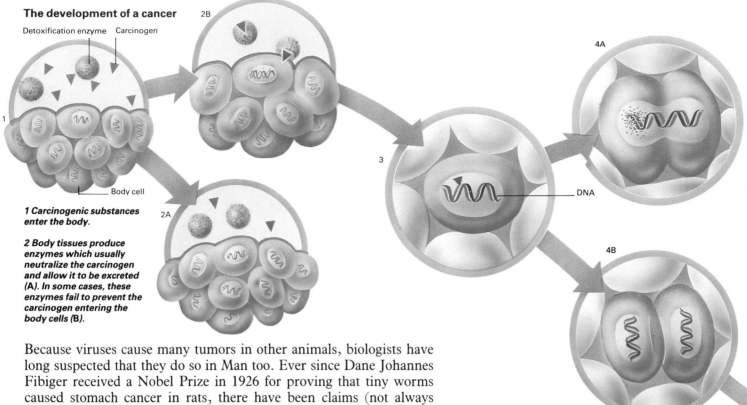

The development of a cancer

Detoxification enzyme   Carcinogen

Body cell

1 Carcinogenic substances enter the body.

2 Body tissues produce enzymes which usually neutralize the carcinogen and allow it to be excreted (A). In some cases, these enzymes fail to prevent the carcinogen entering the body cells (B).

DNA

Because viruses cause many tumors in other animals, biologists have long suspected that they do so in Man too. Ever since Dane Johannes Fibiger received a Nobel Prize in 1926 for proving that tiny worms caused stomach cancer in rats, there have been claims (not always justified) linking infectious organisms with the disease. Epstein-Barr (EB) virus, the agent of glandular fever, certainly plays a role in the development of African lymphoma, though it does so only if some ancillary factor (thought to be malaria) comes into play. Similarly, about 80 percent of liver cancer is strongly associated with the virus responsible for hepatitis B – prevalence of which partly explains the uneven global distribution of this cancer. In 1981 Dr Robert Gallo and colleagues at the US National Institutes of Health discovered what they called human T-cell leukemia virus in two patients with that disease. Unlike many similar finds in the past, further reserch has strengthened the link between this virus and cancer.

As with many other diseases whose relationship to HLA antigens has been uncovered recently (◀ page 32), heredity also plays a role in cancer. Familial susceptibility is now known to be based on genes which makes us slightly more vulnerable to particular sorts of malignancy. And in 1960 came the first of a group of discoveries linking cancer with abnormalities in patients' chromosomes. Bone-marrow cells from an individual with chronic myelogenous leukemia proved to be missing a segment from one of their small chromosomes. About ten years later, new staining techniques revealed exactly what had happened – part of the DNA from chromosome number 22 had moved to number 9. Called the "Philadelphia chromosome" after the city where it was first found, this defect has been followed by several similar discoveries, raising the prospect that people at risk might be identified before their cancers develop.

During the early and mid 1980s, came a series of even more far-reaching breakthroughs, which began to answer two riddles. Why, despite exposure to potent carcinogens or radiation did people such as heavy smokers sometimes escape cancer? And how did aberrations like the Philadelphia chromosome actually produce the disease? Scientists had long believed that known causes of malignancy were really

3 The carcinogen may bind with several sites in the cell, notably with a particular site on the cell's DNA.

4 Normally the cell repairs the DNA without further problem (A); sometimes the cell reproduces and duplicates the DNA, thus creating a mutant gene (B).

5 A promotor substance may encourage the replication of the cells with the mutant gene over normal body cells; the carcinogen enters the body for a second time and again binds with the DNA causing a second mutation. It is this second mutation that makes the cell a cancer cell.

Can cancer be prevented?

Arguments about the degree to which cancer is preventable have become polarized in recent years. Some experts argue that because migrant populations tend to lose the cancer patterns characteristic of their native lands and acquire those of their new homes, most tumors are environmental in origin and thus avoidable. Opponents say that comparatively few causes of tumors are known for certain (although the elimination of smoking would certainly reduce lung cancer dramatically). Likewise, some dietary guidelines are uncontentious (such as reductions in smoked and pickled foods, linked with increased risks of stomach and esophagal cancer); others are debatable (such as curbs in fat consumption to diminish the dangers of colon and breast cancer). Others (for example, megadoses of vitamins to combat cancer in general) are challenged by most experts. The sharp increase in cervical cancer over the past three generations, paralleling greater sexual freedom, has encouraged the notion that "lifestyle" is the key to cancer avoidance. This is repudiated by those who see involuntary exposure to environmental carcinogens as more significant.

secondary agents, which initiated cancer only after scoring a certain number of hits on target genes. This hypothesis would explain the element of chance in the process, but was founded on little real evidence. The watershed in understanding began with the uncovering of "oncogenes". These are the genes which chemicals need to hit in order to produce tumors, and they are also those disrupted by chromosome abnormalities related to cancer. Suddenly, the once-confusing mosaic of cancer research began to be unified.

The key experiment, by Geoffrey Cooper at Harvard University and Robert Weinberg at the Massachusetts Institute of Technology, was to chop up human tumor-cell DNA into gene-sized fragments and feed them to normal mouse cells, which then became cancerous. When reisolated and identified, the oncogenes responsible proved familiar, having been extracted earlier from tumor viruses in animals. It seems that they were appropriated originally by the viruses from cells they infected. The specific difference between an oncogene and its normal counterpart has since been discerned by Weinberg and Mariano Barbacid at the US National Cancer Institute. They found that an oncogene was abnormal in the coding of just one of the units in its DNA. The result is that it produces a correspondingly abnormal protein, which presumably accounts for the conversion of a healthy cell into a malignant one. Researchers have since identified the same oncogene in lung and gut tumors that Weinberg and Barbacid found in bladder tumors. From studies on the rare childhood disease retinoblastoma, which develops when a particular gene stops working, it also seems that there may be other cancer-suppressing genes.

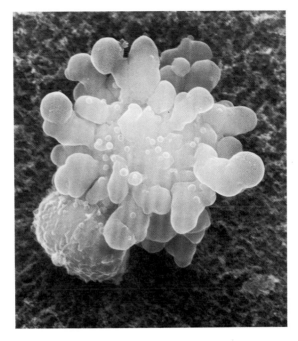

▲ A cancer cell in the process of being destroyed by a white blood cell, at one of several stages at which the body may invoke its defenses to protect itself against the onset of cancer.

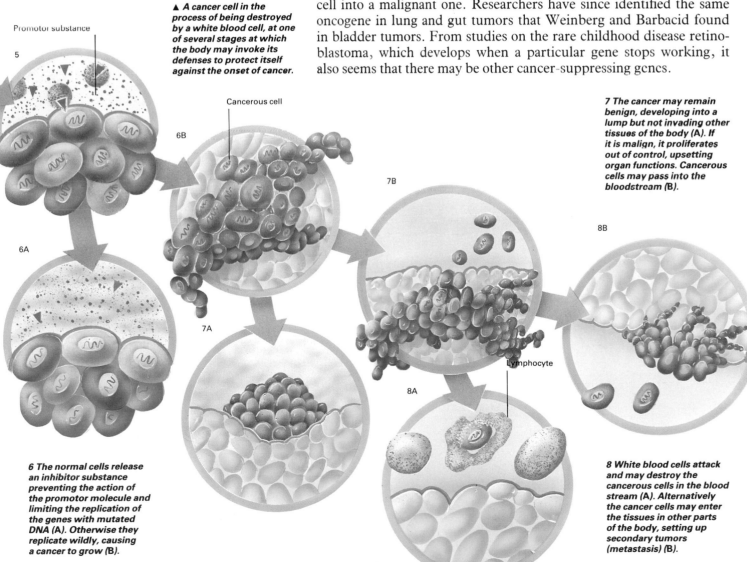

Promotor substance

5

Cancerous cell

6B

7B

6A

7A

8B

8A

Lymphocyte

6 The normal cells release an inhibitor substance preventing the action of the promotor molecule and limiting the replication of the genes with mutated DNA (A). Otherwise they replicate wildly, causing a cancer to grow (B).

7 The cancer may remain benign, developing into a lump but not invading other tissues of the body (A). If it is malign, it proliferates out of control, upsetting organ functions. Cancerous cells may pass into the bloodstream (B).

8 White blood cells attack and may destroy the cancerous cells in the blood stream (A). Alternatively the cancer cells may enter the tissues in other parts of the body, setting up secondary tumors (metastasis) (B).

People who give up smoking reduce the danger of lung cancer – until they begin again

The oncogene investigations, and related work with vaccines based on either cancer viruses or tumor "markers" which characterize malignant cells, could revolutionize cancer prevention over the next decade. The first hope is for immunization against liver cancer using hepatitis B vaccine. For the moment, the major strategies are avoidance of carcinogens and routine screening of high-risk groups for early signs of disease. Figures from Holland in 1984 confirmed a 50-70 percent reduction in mortality from breast cancer in women given regular physical examinations and mammography (an X-ray technique showing tumors not large enough to be felt). The Papanicolaou test, which identifies cancerous and pre-cancerous cells from a woman's cervix, is also effective in revealing a treatable but otherwise potentially fatal disease. Radiography has proved a disappointing tool in identifying lung cancer, which is often too advanced for effective therapy by the time it is detectable. Computer tomography (CT) and nuclear magnetic resonance (NMR) scanning, already successful in locating brain tumors, should allow smaller cancers to be picked up earlier; and further improvements may come from using radioactively-labeled monoclonal antibodies to home in on a tumor site.

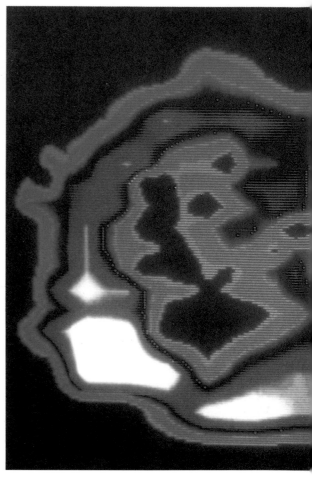

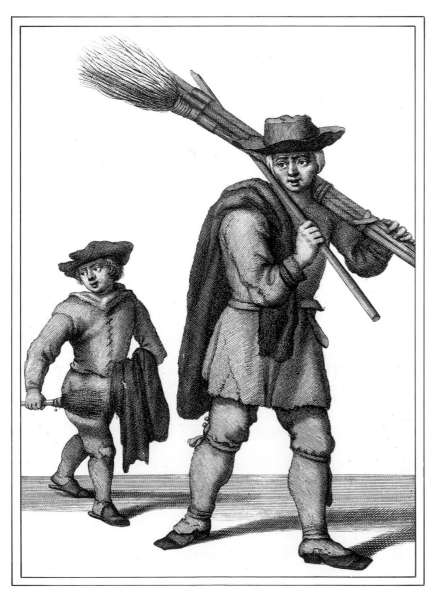

Tumor safaris in Africa
A classic of modern medical sleuthing was the paper by Denis Burkitt, an English surgeon working in Africa, which appeared in the British Journal of Surgery in 1958 and contained the first correct description of a cancer later known as African lymphoma. Burkitt's interest had been aroused by seeing characteristic jaw tumors in African children, often associated with tumors in other parts, which seemed to affect youngsters in a particular age bracket. Although clinicians had long classified these cancers according to the organ affected, Burkitt suspected that they had more in common than a typical primary tumor and its secondaries elsewhere. Intent on studying the natural history of the disease, he organized "tumor safaris" during which he examined hundreds of patients and discerned that the condition did indeed have a common cause and was confined to a warm, moist strip of Africa lying mostly between 10°N and 10°S of the Equator. This led to the idea that an insect might be transmitting a micro-organism responsible for "African lymphoma", and to the subsequent discovery of the Epstein-Barr virus which is now heavily implicated as its cause.

◄ *Percival Pott (1713-1788) produced a pioneering study of cancers in 1775, when he observed the high incidence of a cancer of the scrotal skin among chimney sweeps. He was able to relate this to the particular cause of the contamination: a chemical in the soot affecting the skin of the boys who climbed chimneys.*

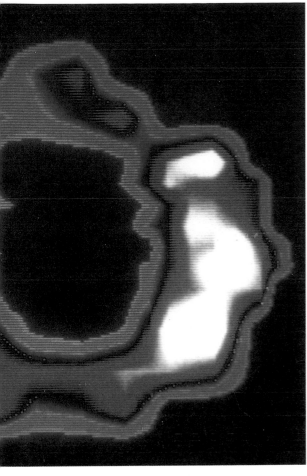

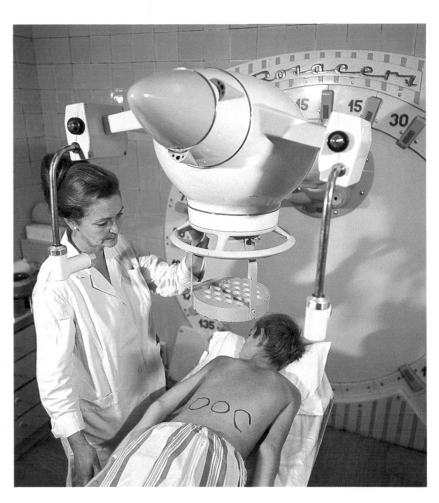

▲ *Oat cell cancer of the lung (shown here in the left lung by NMR) is one of the commonest and deadliest cancers, killing almost all victims within two years. Its name reflects differences between it and other cancer cells under the microscope. The cells secrete hormones, causing some patients to develop Cushing's syndrome (♦ page 85).*

Smoking and lung cancer

To establish cause and effect in medicine can be a harder task than it seems, as shown by disputations about the link between smoking and lung cancer. During the first half of this century, physicians noticed that people who smoked cigarettes heavily appeared more likely to develop the disease than those who smoked little or not at all. The common-sense conclusion was clear. But it could have been utterly wrong; perhaps the smoking habit and a propensity to develop lung cancer resulted from a third, inbred factor. If this were true, anti-tobacco propaganda would have been both ill-founded and ineffective. It took meticulous studies by British epidemiologists Richard Doll, Austin Bradford Hill and others during the 1950s before the "obvious" conclusion was accepted. One of their key findings was that smokers who gave up the habit thereby reduced their risk of contracting lung cancer. This evidence, virtually impossible to square with alternative explanations of the association between smoking and disease, clinched the argument, although the tobacco companies continued to argue that no direct link between smoking and lung cancer had ever been demonstrated.

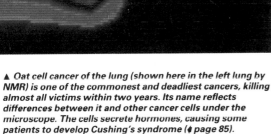

Cigarettes smoked in 1950 (number per adult)

| 0 | 500 | 1,000 | 1,500 | 2,000 | 2,500 | 3,000 | 3,500 |

USA
Eire
UK
Greece
Holland
Australia
Portugal

| 0 | 20 | 40 | 60 | 80 | 100 | 120 | 140 |

Deaths from lung cancer in 1975
(per 1 million population aged 35-44)

Deaths from lung cancer in ex-smokers
(as %age of numbers expected in continuing smokers)

Less than 5 years
5-10 years as ex-smoker
10-14 years as ex-smoker
More than 15 years as ex smoker

| 0 | 25 | 50 | 75 | 100 |

▲ *Screens of X-rays and other forms of radiation, focused onto cancer tissue, are the basis of radio-therapy. Although cells near the tumor may be harmed too, they are usually able to repair the damage. Modern machines allow millions of electron volts to be targeted deep inside the body, without causing the skin reactions associated with earlier, lower voltage treatment. Some cancers, particularly those of varied cell types, are relatively resistant to radiation.*

◄ *The link between smoking and lung cancer has been demonstrated statistically, and it is now clear that cigarette smoke contains many different carcinogens. Low-tar cigarettes can reduce the danger of contracting lung cancer, but it remains true that 25 percent of all regular smokers will die killed before their time by the habit.*

Modern methods of treating tumors

The three main weapons in the modern armory for the treatment of cancer are surgery, chemotherapy and radiotherapy. For treatment to be entirely successful it must obliterate all cancer cells if the disease is not to recur. Operations vary in scale, as with the alternatives of mastectomy (removal of the entire breast) or lumpectomy (removal only of the cancerous lump) for breast cancer, and surgery may be augmented by the other therapies. Drugs alone usually produce "remissions", particularly when used in combination. They can completely cure African lymphoma, Hodgkin's disease, choriocarcinoma and certain childhood leukemias, though some cause side-effects such as hair loss because they interfere with normal as well as malignant tissues. Interferon, now made by genetic engineering, could prove a more potent and safer weapon in future. X-ray, neutron and other beams of radiation, which at low levels *cause* cancer, also destroy malignant cells. The latest machines allow huge doses to be directed to deep-seated tumors without destroying the surrounding tissues. Warming patients up to around 42°C while under general anesthetic is another promising therapy, because cancer cells are particularly sensitive to heat.

Improving one's chances of surviving

While disagreements persist about the roles of external and internal factors in producing cancer, few specialists dispute the emerging view that a patient's state of mind can have a decisive effect on the outcome of malignant disease. Steven Greer, at King's College Hospital, London, has found that women treated for breast cancer are more likely to have a favorable outcome if they react to their illness either by showing a fighting spirit or by denying their diagnosis, than if they respond with stoic acceptance or with feelings of helplessness and hopelessness. He believes the mind may affect the body by impairing the immune system – which, as well as manufacturing antibodies to defeat infection, also helps to rid the body of tumor cells. Support for this thesis comes from research in America showing that antibody production is often reduced in efficiency after personal tragedies such as bereavement.

Tumors and chemotherapy

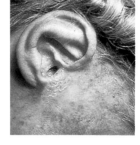

Cure
Childhood lymphoblastic leukemia
Burkitt's lymphoma
Wilm's tumor
Choriocarcinoma
Hodgkin's disease
Testicular teratoma

Palliation
Breast cancer
Many lymphomas
Chronic leukemia
Myeloma

Symptom relief
Squamous cell
    head and neck cancer
Oat-cell lung cancer
Adult leukemia
Ovarian cancer

Little benefit
Lung cancer
Renal cancer
Pancreatic cancer
Colo-rectal cancer
Gastric cancer
Melanoma

► *Chemotherapy, usually involving a combination of several drugs, can prove effective against many forms of cancer, either as the sole treatment or with other forms of therapy.*

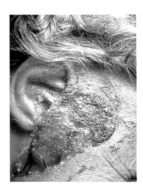

▲ *A squamous-cell carcinoma, before and after radiotherapy. The radiation is aimed to destroy the cancerous tissues.*

Other cures for cancer?

Cancer has been tenuously linked to mind-induced diseases (◀ page 72). But more than any other disease, it has been the subject of unorthodox therapeutic claims, with innumerable, plausible but eventually useless remedies on offer.

One which enjoyed considerable fame during the 1970s was laetrile, usually administered in the form of bitter almonds. A combination of folklore, a feeling that in a desperate situation anything is worth trying, and pressure from practitioners of "alternative medicine" aroused sufficient interest among American politicians to persuade over half the states to legalize laetrile therapy. Eventually in a decisive study, 178 cancer patients were given the material and their progress monitored. The results, published in 1982, showed "no substantive benefit in terms of cure, improvement, or stabilization of cancer, improvement of symptoms related to cancer, or extension of life span." But laetrile was found to be dangerous – because its active ingredient releases cyanide.

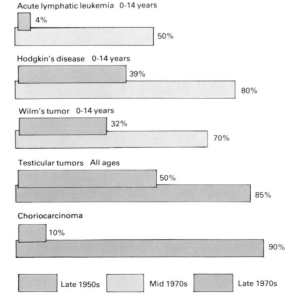

Acute lymphatic leukemia 0-14 years
4%
50%

Hodgkin's disease 0-14 years
39%
80%

Wilm's tumor 0-14 years
32%
70%

Testicular tumors All ages
50%
85%

Choriocarcinoma
10%
90%

| Late 1950s | Mid 1970s | Late 1970s |

◀ *The five-year survival rate for cancer patients has improved significantly in the past 30 years thanks to earlier diagnosis and a wider range of effective treatment. Whereas only a tiny percentage of sufferers survived some childhood leukemias in the 1950s, the chances of survival today are 50 percent or more.*

*How allergies occur...Wasp and bee stings...
Rheumatoid arthritis...Autoimmune diseases...Immune
deficiences in childhood...AIDS...PERSPECTIVE...Food
allergies..."Total" allergies?*

The origin of an allergy

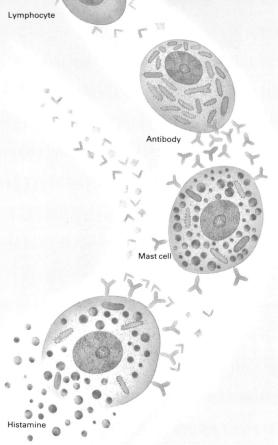

▼ *An allergic reaction
results when the immune
system has made anti-
bodies to a certain
substance or allergen.
These antibodies attach to
"mast-cells" in the body
tissues: when the allergen
returns, even in tiny
quantities, the mast cells
release histamine, causing
inflammation.*

Allergens

Lymphocyte

Antibody

Mast cell

Histamine

For about one person in every two hundred an insect sting is not a minor inconvenience, but a life-threatening event that produces ana-phylactic shock – breathing becomes difficult and irregular, rashes suddenly appear and the subject may collapse and die within minutes. Between 50 and 100 deaths from this cause are reported annually in the USA. Other people – about one in ten – suffer in a more limited way. Their hypersensitivity is localized, generally in areas which produce mucosal fluids – the eyes, nose and throat. Asthma, a disease characterized by constriction of the airways, and hay fever can both be caused by allergens such as pollen and the feces of house dust mites. Both types of response are caused by over-reaction of the specific immune system (◀ page 213).

The same type of over-reaction can also be localized on the skin, causing rashes and swellings. Because of the way in which the im-mune system works, the first exposure to allergen causes no un-pleasant reaction. But it sets in motion the production of antibodies specific to that substance.

Anaphylactic shock and allergic reactions are caused by the class of antibodies known as immunoglobulin E (◀ page 216) bound to a particular type of cell, called a mast cell. When immunoglobulin E reacts with an antigen, it activates the mast cell to release inflam-matory substances, such as histamine and leukotrienes, which produce the unpleasant effects associated with allergy. In a normal way these substances are part of the body's defenses against invasion; in the case of an allergic reaction they are released in large amounts in response to miniscule amounts of the allergen.

Allergic-type reactions can occur without involving the immune system. Wasp and bee stings contain substances that act in the same way as those released by mast cells, and so cause irritant swellings even in those whose immune system is not sensitized to antigens in the sting. Jellyfish tentacles and some foods, such as strawberries and fish which is not fresh, contain histamine or closely-related substances. These are known to cause both irritant rashes and asth-matic attacks.

Atopic individuals – those who suffer from allergies – are often allergic to many substances. They can reduce the effects of allergy by avoiding those substances to which they are most sensitive. Prick tests are used to measure susceptibility. In these, a small quantity of a suspected allergen is inserted just beneath the skin and the strength of the subsequent reaction monitored.

Some allergies can be cured by repeated doses of an allergen, in increasing amounts. The course of treatment is usually long and there is a remote danger of anaphylaxis. In other cases, allergies may disappear spontaneously. Some childhood ailments, such as infantile eczema, fall into this category.

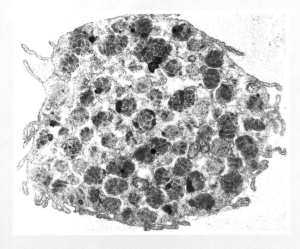

▲ *A mast cell containing granules of histamine and heparin.*

Destructive complexes

The immune system can also cause illness when circulating antibodies form insoluble complexes with antigens. The harm depends on where these complexes are deposited, as neighboring tissues can be damaged by the phagocytic response. In systemic lupus erythematosus (SLE), antibodies to nucleic acids are produced. These frequently form complexes which deposit in the central nervous system and kidneys, which are subsequently damaged.

Antibody-antigen complexes also play a part in rheumatoid arthritis, which usually affects joints but may be found in organs such as heart, lungs and nervous system (◀ page 109). Deposition of the complexes in the synovial membranes leads to inflamed joints as a result of complementary activation by the immunoglobulin G responsible. Both SLE and rheumatoid arthritis are autoimmune diseases, in which the antigens are part of the sufferer's "self" and should be tolerated by his or her immune system but are not. The precise agent of rheumatoid arthritis is still not known, but it has been suggested that a virus, as yet unidentified, is involved.

High concentrations of antigens from an external source can also trigger diseases of this type. Farmer's lung, for example, is produced by breathing in spores from moldy grain; these cause antibody-antigen complexes to deposit in the lung, where the tissue is subsequently damaged. In some other diseases, including leprosy, viral hepatitis and quartan malaria, some of the harmful effects may be caused by immune complex deposition.

Circulating antibodies can also cause tissue damage by reacting with an antigen on a cell surface. Some drugs, including penicillin, may bind to cell-surface protein to create a new antigenic determinant (small molecules that do this are called haptens) which the body does not recognize as self. The result can be destruction of tissues, such as red blood cells. A similar type of immune defect which used to occur commonly was rhesus babies (◀ page 193).

Tissue damage may also result from the activation of T-lymphocytes. Contact dermatitis can occur in various occupations, following exposure to metals (particularly platinum) and other industrial materials. It may be produced also by cosmetics and topically applied drugs. The dermatitic agent acts as a hapten. T-cells are attracted to the site and release lymphokines. These attract phagocytes which release hydrolytic (digestive) enzymes; it is these enzymes that then damage surrounding tissue.

Cases of mistaken identity

Immune disease can arise through mistakes in the immune system's recognition process. A particular type of streptococcal infection, which causes sore throats, occasionally also provokes rheumatic fever which may damage the heart. This occurs because the cell wall of the relevant micro-organism shares antigenic determinants with the surface of the heart muscle. The infection consequently produces large quantities of antibody which contravene the immune system's self-tolerance and attack the heart muscle, most frequently causing scarring of valve tissue. As rheumatic fever develops only if the streptococcal infection is left-untreated, the rise of antibiotic treatment in developed countries has led to a reduction in its incidence. Ulcerative colitis (◀ page 137) is thought to be a similar disease. Exposure to intestinal bacteria produces cross-reacting antigens which trigger autoimmune attack on the colonic mucosa.

Asthma

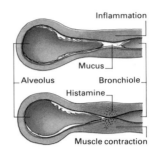
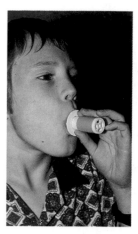

▲ ► *An inhaler reduces the inflammation of the bronchi which causes asthmatic breathlessness.*

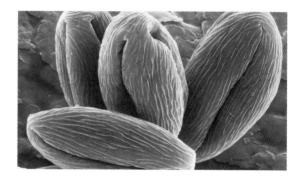

▲ ► *Two of the wide variety of pollens which are frequent causes of the common allergic reaction known as hay fever. Cornflower (above) and hollyhock (right) pollen, here magnified some 1,000 times.*

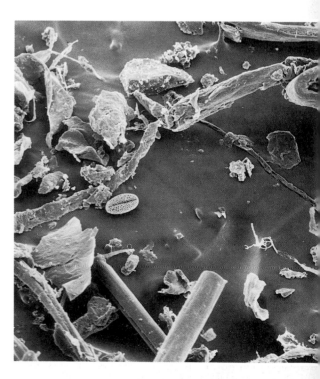

▲ *House-dust with pollen grains, fibers and soot particles; the feces of dust mites are often allergenic.*

► *The Portuguese man o' war ("Physalia utriculis"), uses histamine as a poison with which to sting its prey.*

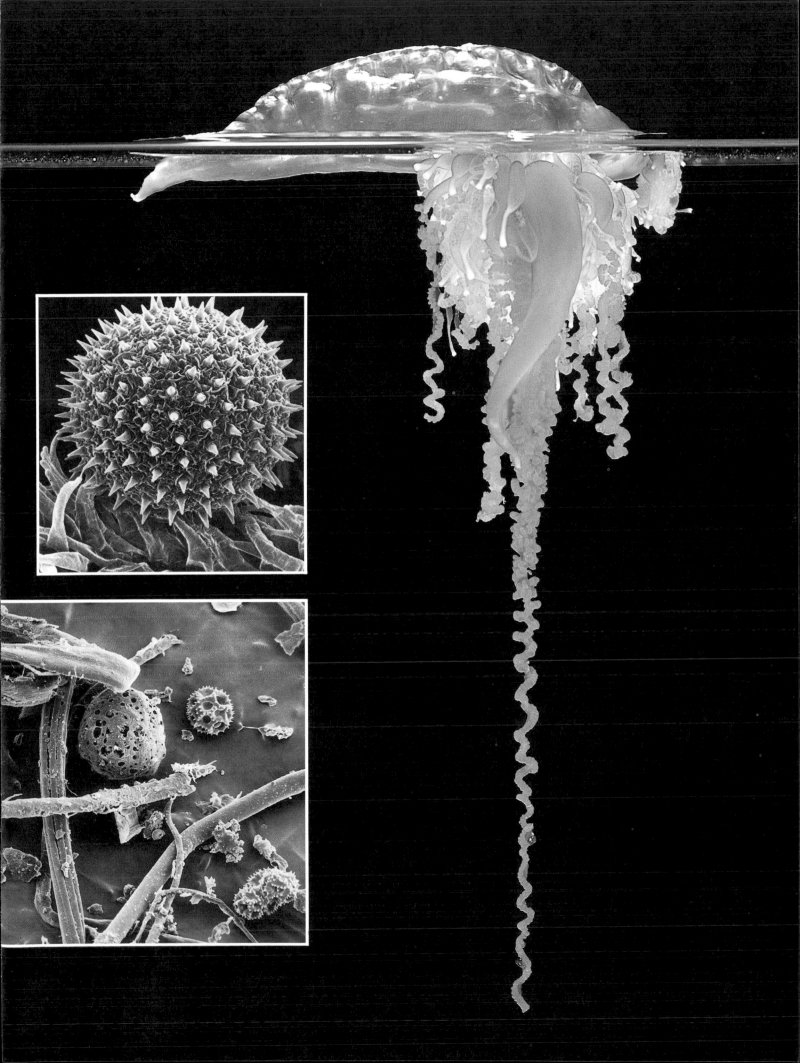

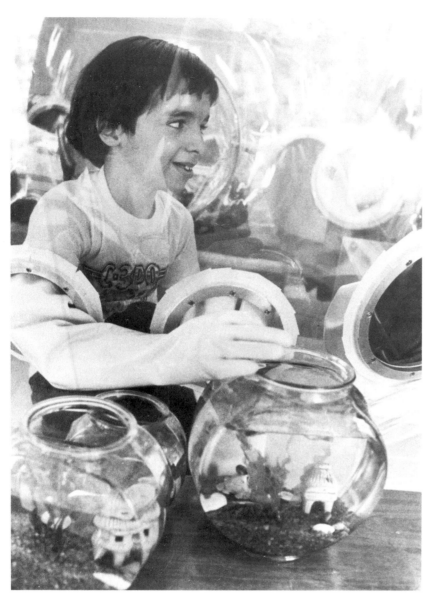

Food allergies or food intolerance?

Behavior and physical condition may be affected dramatically by "food allergy". Many studies have tried to show that hyperactivity and emotional disturbance in children are a result too.

"Allergy" strictly refers to ailments involving only an immune response. Food allergies do exist; proteins in cows' milk are probably the most frequent cause. Even in breast-fed babies, such an allergy may show up if the mother drinks milk. True allergies can also develop to carbohydrates and proteins in such foods as fish and cereals.

When tests show no immune reaction to a specific food, but the food nevertheless causes bad effects, it is known as "food intolerance". Migraine attacks can result from specific foods, chocolate for example, containing substances related to psycho-active chemicals in humans. This is a toxic rather than an allergic reaction.

It has been claimed that food intolerance is caused by food processing and artificial additives. Some synthetic colorants can produce an immune response by combining with protein to form new antigenic determinants. However, in many cases, processed foods are likely to be less allergenic than unrefined foods, because processing reduces the number of protein and carbohydrate types.

An extension of the idea that the modern treatment of food makes it harmful, is "total allergy syndrome". Sufferers are said to develop allergy or intolerance to an increasing number of modern materials, as well as to both polluted air and tapwater. Ultimately, they live in increasing isolation from the outside world. The underlying cause remains unidentified. Some immunologists are even sceptical about its reality, arguing that the symptoms are psychological in origin.

◄ *David, an American boy with severe combined immune deficiency (SCID), spent his life in a sterile "bubble" which protected him from bacteria and viruses. Untreated sufferers usually die by the age of 2. Low numbers of T-lymphocytes are produced, and immunoglobulins do not function as antibodies. SCID can be treated with bone marrow grafts.*

Immune deficiencies

In addition to over-reaction, the immune system can cause disease through deficiency. The most common form is deficiency of immunoglobulin A, found in mucosal tissue, which provides a line of defense against invasion. Sufferers are prone to repeated mild respiratory infections. Infantile eczema may also result.

Less frequent, but sometimes more serious, are diseases in which immunoglobulin G levels are low. In some babies they are slow to start, and infections, especially respiratory diseases, increase in the period between the baby using up reserves from its mother and developing its own. Far more serious is X-linked infantile agammaglobulinemia. Immunoglobulin G is very low and all other immunoglobulins are absent. A genetically-determined disease, it affects only males, who usually die from infection as children.

No treatment has yet been devised for the seemingly new immune deficiency disease, acquired immune deficiency syndrome (AIDS), which appeared in the USA in 1979/80 (◄ page 202). It is caused by a virus which attacks T-lymphocytes. Characterized by a drastic loss of natural immunity, it is usually fatal.

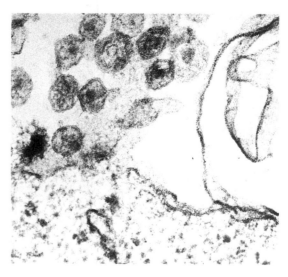

▲ *Acquired immune deficiency syndrome (AIDS) is caused by the virus HTLV-III, (human T-lymphotropic virus III), shown in this electron micrograph.*

The body's internal environment...External threats to internal balance...Poisons and their effects... Homeostasis hazards...Radiation...Natural poisons... The liver and poisons...Alcohol...PERSPECTIVE...Smog... Metal poisons

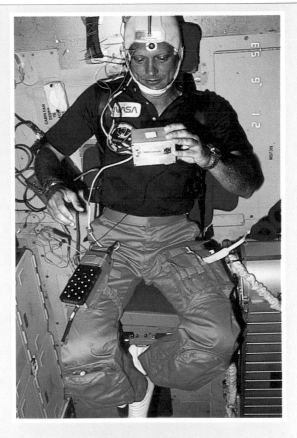

The human body's complex set of interrelated chemical reactions is viable only within a narrow range of physical conditions. Two of the basics of civilization – clothing and shelter – have developed in order to help us stay within these limits despite variations in the evironment itself. We cannot stand being too hot or too cold, too "hydrated" or too dehydrated; nor can we endure a serious change in the chemical composition of the air we breathe or in the amount of exposure to radiation and electrical charge – both natural and artificial.

Homeostasis is the mechanism that keeps the internal environment of the organism stable, but it cannot always succeed (◀ page 12). A rise in external temperature, for example, triggers heat receptors in the skin which cause vasodilation and sweating. The former cools the body provided that the skin's temperature is at least 1°C less than the internal, or core, temperature. If the external temperature is too high for this difference to be maintained, the only available means of cooling the body is sweating, in which the energy used to evaporate water has a cooling effect.

▲ *In addition to motion sickness, the harmful effects of weightlessness suffered by astronauts include loss of strength in muscles, breakdown of red blood cells, a shift of blood from legs to the head, and loss of calcium from bones.*

The effects of poisons

A poison is a substance which harms a living organism. Almost any substance, including water, is poisonous if administered in sufficient quantity, though most substances commonly classed as poisons produce a harmful effect in small doses.

If a single dose of a substance causes harm, it is an acute poison. Swallowing less than a quarter of a gram of potassium cyanide will kill most people within a few minutes. On the other hand, chronic poisoning is caused by long exposure to small concentrations of a substance. Liver damage produced by high alcohol consumption over a decade or more is an example of chronic poisoning.

Poisons work in different ways. A common effect is to interfere with the activity of one or more enzymes, which act as catalysts and promote the body's normal metabolism. Many toxic metals bind with an enzyme and alter its molecular structure, preventing it from working. Some enzymes require a particular metal atom for their activity. If this becomes linked to another substance, such as cyanide, or is replaced by a different metal atom, the enzyme can be inactivated. Alternatively, the poison may compete with the enzyme's natural substrate (the substance which it changes), and thus disrupt a metabolic process. Carbon monoxide (CO), on the other hand, competes with oxygen for binding sites on the hemoglobin molecule (◀ page 158), thus preventing the oxygen reaching the body tissues. Other poisons attack and interfere with particular cells – digitalis (◀ page 164) makes the heart muscle work faster, neurotoxins interfere with nerve impulse transmission and cytotoxins (◀ page 228) kill cells which are dividing by interfering with nucleic acid synthesis.

Skin temperature

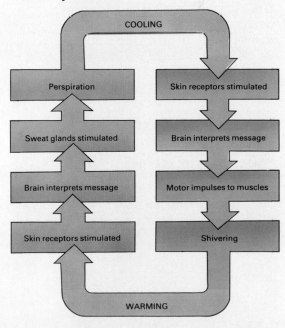

COOLING

Perspiration	Skin receptors stimulated
Sweat glands stimulated	Brain interprets message
Brain interprets message	Motor impulses to muscles
Skin receptors stimulated	Shivering

WARMING

▲ *The body maintains its temperature by protective action whenever the skin temperature rises or falls beyond acceptable limits. If the environment is too extreme for these mechanisms to cope, internal distress results.*

The body is finely tuned to respond to external threats to its internal balance

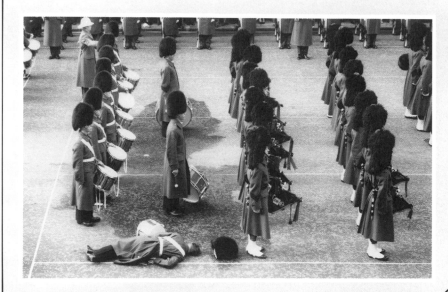

◀ Usually, it takes many hours exposure to heat before the core temperature rises to a dangerous level. This induces heat stroke. Characterized by mental confusion, heat stroke can also be brought on by exercise in temperatures near normal body heat. Heat may also cause salt loss and dehydration.

The body tends to be more tolerant of cold than of heat, depending on how fat a person is. A drop in skin temperature of more than 4°C below normal induces vasoconstriction and shivering. These prevent further heat loss, and the muscle activity of shivering generates more heat. Fat people can tolerate a skin temperature as low as 12°C. If the core temperature drops by only 2°C, however, the body can no longer warm itself by internal activity and hypothermia results.

As the core temperature drops, hemoglobin becomes less efficient at releasing oxygen (◀ page 158). This can cause cardiac arrhythmias (◀ page 164) and cerebral disturbances. Hypothermia can occur as a result of living in cold surroundings, coupled with some other factor such as alcohol or barbiturate consumption, or malnutrition.

A combination of cold and pressure (from tight clothing, for instance) can cause minor damage in the form of chilblains. Extended cooling of parts of the body below 12°C can lead to more permanent damage even if no freezing occurs. Frostbite only develops if the cell fluid freezes, though it is only a portion of the fluid that usually freezes.

Temperature control is essential in the maintenance of homeostasis. The body is heated by vasoconstriction, adrenal and thyroid hormones which boost the metabolic activity of the cells, and activity of the skeletal muscles, and cooled by vasodilation and sweating. Core temperatures above or below normal may disrupt cell proteins, and affect the body's fluid electrolyte balance. As well as heat stroke, a condition in which brain cells may be quickly destroyed, overheating may lead to heat exhaustion, in which there is heavy perspiration but the heart beat is weakened.

The metabolic balance of the body comprises the chemical reactions of both breaking down food (catabolism) and reconstituting the elements into the proteins required by the body (anabolism). The body requires a balance of protein, glucose and lipids in the bloodstream, and these are affected by the food intake and hormones, such as insulin, which affect the deposition of fat and activity of the liver. Metabolic activity affects the temperature balance of the body, burning excess glucose as fuel, and allowing the body to create layers of fat to protect against cold.

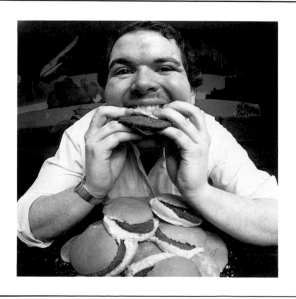

◀ The body may be poisoned by tiny quantities of some materials, or by gross overconsumption of a single food that, in normal quantities, might be nutritious. In extreme circumstances, the stomach rejects the food by vomiting; otherwise absorbed nutrients are oxidized, stored or converted, assuming vitamins and enzymes are available. The rise of obesity, diabetes and other dietary "diseases of civilization" are the result of the longterm failure of the body to maintain metabolic homeostasis. Other metabolic imbalances include phenylketonuria (◀ page 196), cystic fibrosis (in which vitamin absorption is inadequate), coeliac disease and protein-energy malnutrition (◀ page 130).

▶ *Divers surfacing too quickly may suffer from decompression sickness or bends – nitrogen bubbles form in the bloodstream, cutting the oxygen supply to the body tissues. Similarly, climbers at very high altitudes without extra oxygen deprive their body tissues of the gas and raise acid levels.*

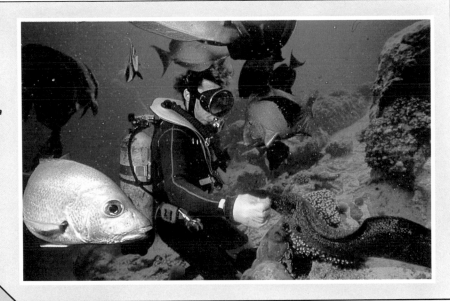

The acid-base balance of the body is related to the level of hydrogen ions in the extracellular fluid. This in turn is related to the level of carbon dioxide in the blood, since an increase in CO_2 levels raises the acidity of the blood. Detectors in the carotid artery are linked to the inspiratory center of the brain, thus ensuring the body breathes in fresh oxygen when it is underventilated; hyperventilation makes the body more alkaline. The kidney is responsible for the maintenance of the acid-base balance, by excreting uric acid from the blood. The stomach's acid level may also affect blood acid level.

The fluid-electrolyte balance between the intracellular and extracellular fluids is crucial to ensuring that the cells do not become waterlogged or dried up. Two-thirds of the body's fluid is in the cells, and this moves through the membranes by osmosis. The concentration of salts and other solutes – mostly in the form of electrolytes – is therefore critical. The balance is affected by the level of excretion of fluids in urine or sweat, and by the freezing of the intracellular fluid; this may cause frostbite by raising the salt concentration in the remaining fluid, and thus damaging cell proteins.

Death by drowning occurs less quickly in cold rather than warm water; cooling slows body chemistry, so survival times increase. Children have been resuscitated as long as 30 minutes after drowning in cold water and ceasing to breathe, without suffering brain damage. Cell liquids cannot freeze, if immersed in very cold fresh water, as the salts in the cell make its freezing point lower than that of pure water. The concentration of salt in the sea, however, is greater than in the body, so seawater remains liquid at a lower temperature than the cell liquids.

Cardiac arrest is a major cause of death by electrocution. Many bodily processes depend on ionic impulses, and these can be disrupted by electric shock. The extent of disruption depends on many factors, including the voltage and amperage of the shock, the site of contact and the resistance of the skin. The effects are not always immediate. In some people who have survived electric shocks to the head or neck, cataracts of the eye have developed up to three years afterwards. Because the skin has a higher electrical resistance than soft tissues, a shock may cause damage even when the skin appears to be intact.

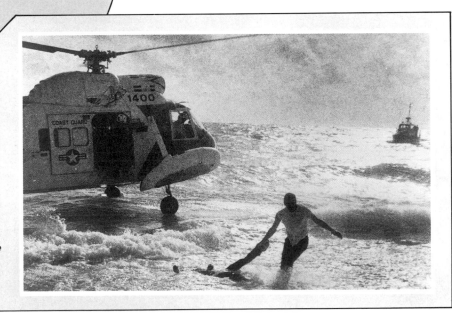

▶ *Inhalation of seawater leads to uptake of calcium and magnesium ions by the bloodstream; these then cause cardiac arrest. Fresh-water inhalation causes hemolysis; it also upsets the fluid-electrolyte balance and affects the potassium ion balance in the bloodstream. This can induce fibrillation and death.*

We are continually exposed to radiation from naturally-occurring radioactive substances in the environment

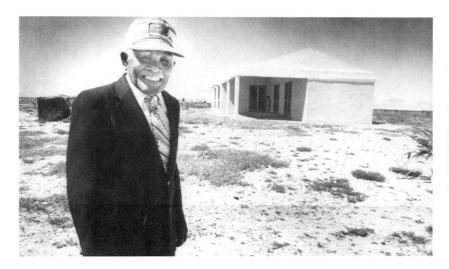

▲ *After 10 years, a resident returns to the Marshall Islands – site of US atomic tests.*

Radiation from Sun, Earth and nuclear technology

Non-ionizing radiation includes ultraviolet rays, a component of sunlight which can release energy on the skin and cause sunburn (◀ page 118). The effects of this are well documented. Other forms of non-ionizing radiation, such as high frequency radiowaves, may also be harmful, but the evidence is unclear and not widely accepted.

Ionizing radiation includes the X-rays, gamma-rays, and the alpha- and beta-particles emitted by radioactive substances. This dissipates its energy by knocking electrons out of molecules, thus converting them to ions. In the case of complex biological molecules, this can destroy their function.

There has been much debate in recent years about the safe level of ionizing radiation; this debate has mostly been conducted in connection with the development of nuclear power. Even without nuclear power, we are continually exposed to radiation from space and from naturally-occurring radioactive substances in the environment. In some places, such as parts of Scotland, the major exposure comes from living or working in buildings of granite.

The biological effectiveness of absorbed ionizing radiation is measured in Sieverts (Sv), of which ten at once constitute a lethal dose. The International Committee on Radiological Protection has set some 50mSv (milliSieverts) per year as the maximum safe level for radiation workers. Annual average radiation exposure in Britain and the United States is less than 2mSv, of which more than 50 percent is natural background radiation. Medical sources such as X-rays and radio-isotopes account for most of the rest.

The only likelihood of critical exposure to ionizing radiation comes from nuclear accident or war. An acute dose of 1Sv causes some signs of radiation sickness, including nausea and a drop in lymphocyte numbers (◀ page 213). It may also increase the risk of leukemia and solid tumors in the long term. A 10Sv dose of radiation causes vomiting and diarrhea; death is almost inevitable within a month of exposure. A major effect of this size of dose is to damage the lining of the small intestine and the stem cells from which it is normally replaced. As a result, the intestinal wall becomes smooth. Its surface area and, consequently, its ability to absorb nutrients are much reduced. Lesions occur and intestinal contents mix with the bloodstream, leading to infection and loss of body fluids.

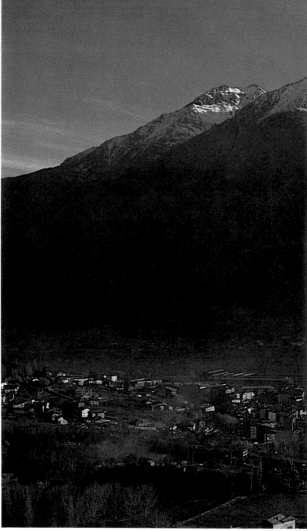

▲ *A factory chimney in the Alps: as well as smog, such chimney emissions of sulfur oxides may cause sulfuric acid to form in the clouds, devastating crops when it falls as "acid" rain, often many hundreds of kilometers away.*

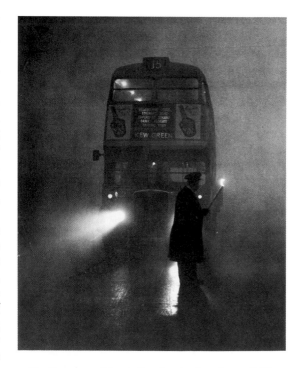

▲ *The "peasouper" fogs of London, such as those of 1952 and 1956, became a thing of the past when a Clean Air Act was passed in 1956 and restrictions were placed on the smoke output of domestic fires and factories.*

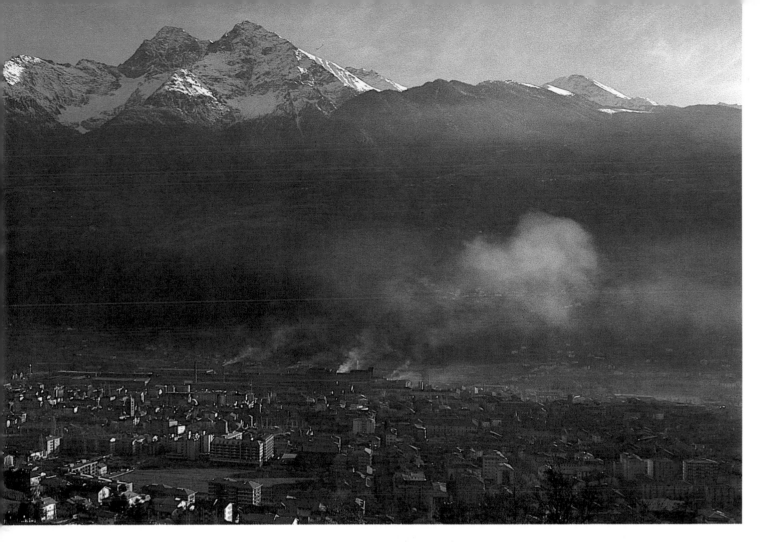

Smog now and then

In December 1952, London was enveloped in thick fog. In the week ending 13 December, 2,851 excess deaths were reported. Subsequently a further 1,224 deaths were attributed to this unusual combination of air pollution and weather conditions.

At the time, much domestic heating in Britain was by coal fire and the atmosphere was laden with particulate material and gaseous pollutants, including carbon and sulfur oxides. Cold air moving in from continental Europe trapped the pollution, which condensed in the atmospheric moisture to form a mixture of smoke and fog called smog. The deaths caused by it were mainly in elderly people who succumbed to respiratory complaints such as bronchitis.

More recently, a different type of smog has caused problems in Los Angeles and other US cities. In this case, the pollution arises from automobiles and the smog is created by the action of sunlight on reactive components in their exhaust gases. A characteristic component of this type of smog is peroxyacyl nitrate, which causes eye irritation as well as respiratory problems.

Air pollution may cause or aggravate disease. It can occur naturally, but is mostly associated with industrial activity. In addition to large quantities of particulate matter, volcanic eruptions throw out poisonous materials, such as sulfur dioxide, cyanides and fluorides.

▶ *Several tons of methyl isocyanate escaped into the air from Union Carbide's pesticide plant in Bhopal, India, on 2 December 1984, killing over 2,200 people and affecting the lives of 50,000 others, many with serious eye injuries.*

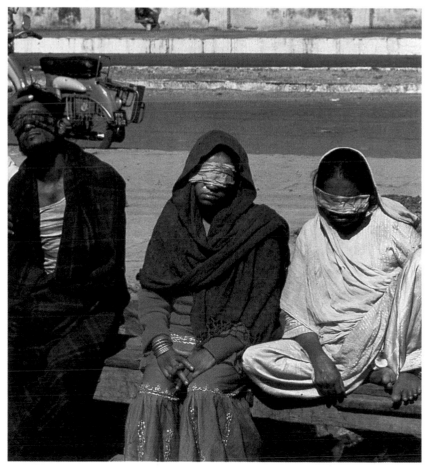

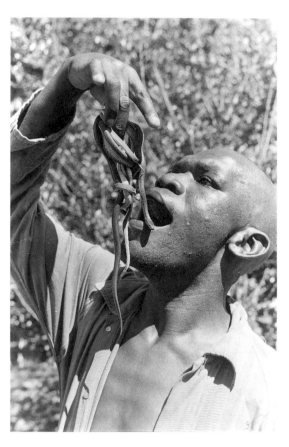

▲ *Poisonous snakes have enlarged, hollow front teeth which puncture the skin and through which venom is injected from a venom sac in the snake's head. It may be possible to ingest snake venom safely, provided the skin is not punctured. This street performer in South Africa puts poisonous snakes in his mouth and completes his act by eating a live puff adder.*

▼ *It is with the larger fungi that we most commonly associate natural poisoning. Many fatalities are caused by mistaking Amanita phalloides, shown here, for the edible field mushroom. This fungus contains very toxic peptides which inhibit an enzyme involved in RNA production, thus destroying the normal functioning of the body cells.*

Natural poisons

Many plants and animals defend themselves against predators by the use of poisons. Thousands of deaths are caused each year by snakebites, with cobras, rattlesnakes, puff adders, carpet vipers and Russell's vipers being among the most freqent attackers.

Snakes attack only if provoked, although in some cases the provocation need only be slight disturbance. The venoms are complex mixtures, but the major active components are usually toxic peptides, non-toxic proteins and enzymes. All three may cause damage by stimulating an immune response (◀ page 213). The toxic peptides often interfere with nerve cell transmission, while the enzymes can damage cells near the site of the bite as well as breaking down some blood components.

Illness can be caused by ingesting toxins from fish. The puffer fish, considered a delicacy in Japan, where it is called fugu, can contain a potent neurotoxin, tetrodotoxin. Paralytic shellfish poisoning is caused by eating shellfish which themselves have eaten toxin-containing micro-organisms.

Neurotoxins are found in some other foods as a result of microbial activity. Botulism is a form of paralysis caused by botulinus toxin, a poison produced by the anaerobic micro-organism, *Clostridium botulinum*. This substance, a protein, is inactivated by heating. Cases of botulinus poisoning usually result from eating smoked, canned or fermented foods which are not heated before consumption. The micro-organism spores are heat-resistant and survive processing, thus allowing growth and toxin formation in the product during storage.

A more commmon and less severe form of food poisoning is caused by staphylococci, notably *S. aureus*. This grows particularly well in protein-rich foods held at room temperature and produces a toxin that causes severe vomiting. It is found where hygiene conditions in food preparation are unsatisfactory. Recovery is usual within two or three days, although the poison can cause death through shock.

Molds growing on plants can also cause food poisoning. Aflatoxin, produced by a mold which grows on ground nuts, may be responsible for the relatively high incidence of liver cancer in parts of Africa where these nuts form a significant part of the diet.

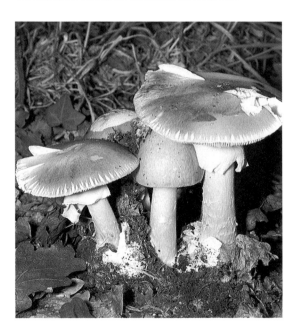

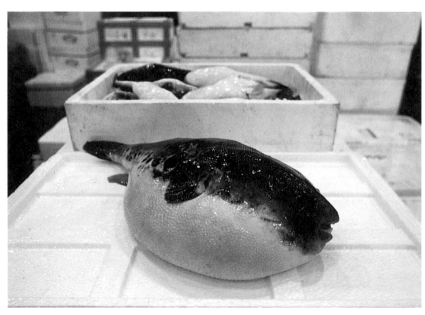

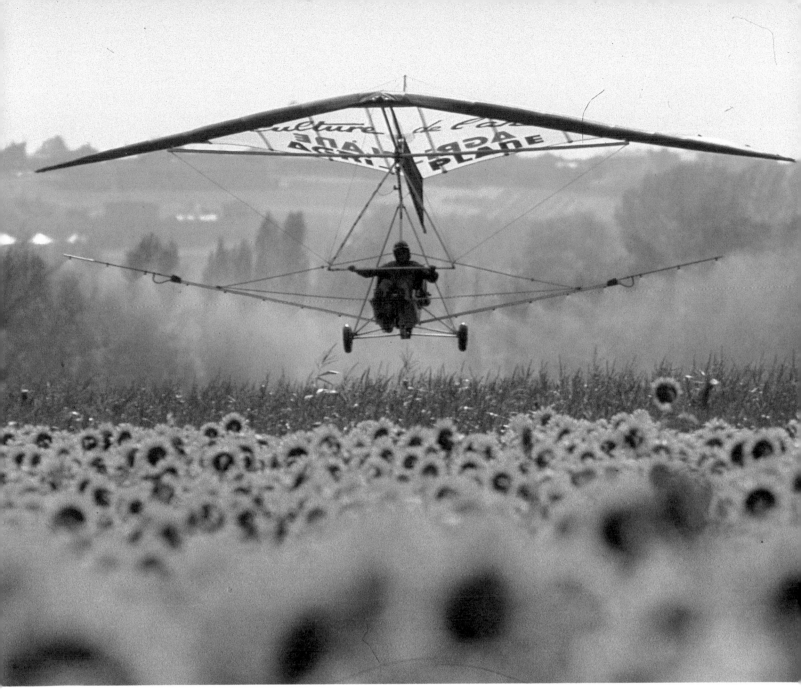

▲ Crop spraying with pesticides or weedkillers may leave traces of poisons in the crop which remain in the food. The insecticide DDT was banned in many countries when it was found to accumulate in the food chain; but many chemicals, even in minute traces, are suspected of acting as carcinogens; others are feared to cause cumulative nervous system damage, particularly in agricultural workers.

◄ One variety of puffer fish is called fugu by the Japanese. Although it is considered a fine food, fugu can seriously damage the nervous system.

Metal poisoning

Many metals can be poisonous, although their effect frequently depends on the way in which they are taken into the body. Some metals bind strongly to foodstuffs which hinder their absorption and reduce their effective toxicity. Similarly, different salts of a metal can have widely varying solubilities which affect their absorption.

Lead is probably the best-studied metal from a toxicological viewpoint. It has been suggested that the decline of the Roman Empire was caused by chronic poisoning from lead water pipes and storage tanks. Recently, concern has centered on the effect of airborne lead from automobile exhausts. In many countries, tetraethyl lead is added to gasoline to improve its performance. In the engine this is converted to an inorganic lead salt which may be inhaled. One toxic effect of lead is to attack the central nervous system. Children may be particularly prone to such attack and suggestions that chronic exposure to low levels of lead cause mental retardation have encouraged governments to restrict the use of lead in gasoline.

The striking difference in toxicity between some metals and their compounds is shown by mercury. This liquid metal is widely used in industry, and some escapes into the environment where micro-organisms can convert it to methylmercury. Like tetraethyl lead, it is an organo-metallic compound, and as such is more readily taken up by biological systems. If ingested, nearly all of it is absorbed by the gastro-intestinal tract, while less than 0·01 percent of metallic mercury is absorbed in this way.

Cadmium is also widely used in industry and has led to occupational poisoning, through inhalation of cadmium fumes. The metal is found in ores which also contain lead and zinc and the three metals are usually purified in a single refinery. Itai-itai ("ouch ouch") disease, characterized by severe arthritic pain, was first diagnosed in Japan in the late 1940s among elderly people who had eaten rice grown in water containing effluent from a smelter. It has since been suggested that people who eat vegetables from cadmium-rich soils for many years may suffer chronic effects, including high blood pressure.

The main organ for detoxification is the liver. If a poison is absorbed via the stomach or intestine, then it passes through the liver. If absorbed via the mouth or injected directly into the bloodstream, it can avoid the liver and may have a greater effect. The liver contains a large number of enzymes that react with foreign substances and make them less toxic. Often this is done by converting them into substances which are more water-soluble and thus more readily excreted.

Equal doses of a poison may affect two people quite differently. This depends in part on the means and rate of absorption of the poison. It can also depend on other substances to which a person is exposed. Carbon tetrachloride, once used as a dry-cleaning fluid, is mildly poisonous. If inhaled it sensitizes heart muscle, making it more reactive towards adrenaline. This effect is increased dramatically if carbon tetrachloride is inhaled after drinking alcohol, when collapse and death may result from small doses. Doctors are increasingly aware of the possibility of such harmful drug interactions and may warn patients to avoid certain combinations. This can often necessitate abstaining from alcohol while undergoing treatment.

Poisoning by alcohol

Ethanol, the active ingredient in alcoholic beverages, is probably responsible for more chronic poisoning than any other chemical substance. Among US white adult males, liver disease is the fourth most common cause of death. More than two-thirds of the cases are alcohol-related.

Alcohol interferes with the normal metabolic processes, mainly through its metabolic product, acetaldehyde. This can cause acute poisoning, the lethal dose being between 300 and 500ml consumed within an hour (equivalent to about 1 liter of gin or whisky). Related chemical substances are more toxic, and alcohol is sometimes used to prevent death from acute overdoses of both methanol and ethylene glycol. A major ingredient of automobile antifreeze, the latter is not poisonous itself – its metabolic products, though, cause harm. These are produced by the same enzyme that normally metabolizes alcohol. If large doses of alcohol are given to a person who has taken a lethal dose of ethylene glycol, the two substances compete for the limited amount of enzyme available. This slows down metabolism of the glycol and prevents the metabolic products from reaching a lethal concentration.

Ethanol dissolves easily in both water and lipids, so that it can be taken up readily by body tissues. In pregnant women, it can cross the placental barrier and poison the developing embryo. Substances with a toxic effect on embryos are called teratogens (◀ page 199).

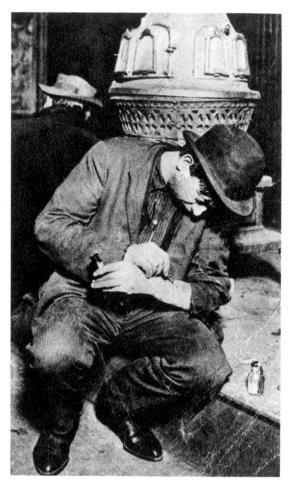

▲ *Morphine, the principal alkaloid in opium, is a uniquely powerful pain-killer. But its euphoria-inducing qualities have also made it and the related diacetyl morphine (heroin) an increasingly widely-used and dangerous drug of addiction.*

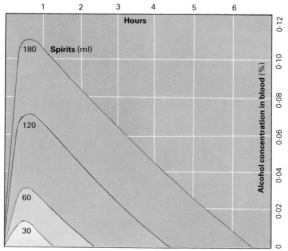

▲ *Alcohol remains in the bloodstream for many hours after drinking. There is some evidence that regular, moderate consumption may help protect against the build-up of fats causing heart disease; in other respects it acts as a poison.*

◀ *Chronic alcohol poisoning leads to the depositing of fat in and enlargement of the liver. In cirrhosis, the liver becomes fibrous and nodular, with a "hobnail" appearance. In 20 percent of cirrhoses, cancer of the liver also develops.*

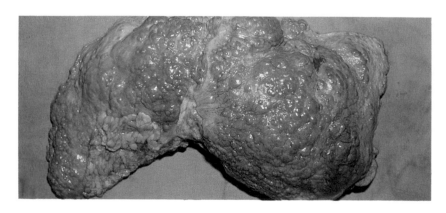

The sites of infections...Kidney diseases...The eradication of smallpox...Measles and polio...Skin infections...Infections caught from animals...Malaria and yellow fever...Rabies and plague...PERSPECTIVE... Scarlet fever, fading away?...The threat of meningitis... Hepatitis...Blood poisoning and toxic shock syndrome... Opportunistic pathogens

All the body's tissues are vulnerable to invasion by microbes. Among well-nourished people with good hygiene, some tissues are attacked comparatively rarely. Conjunctivitis, for example, is uncommon in the West – partly because tears, which bathe the conjunctiva (the eye's transparent layer of skin) and cornea, contain the potent antibacterial agent lysozyme. Yet one agent of conjunctivitis, trachoma virus, is the world's commonest cause of blindness. Transmitted by touch and flies, trachoma is particularly prevalent among the poor of Africa and the Middle East. There is no satisfactory vaccine, and antibiotics act only against bacteria as they attack tissue which has already been infected by the virus.

Infections and sanitation

Two exceptions prove the rule about cleanliness and infection. The first, poliomyelitis, is much less serious when mediocre living conditions expose children to the virus in their earliest years. Entering the body by mouth, it multiplies in the throat and intestine, often causing no ill effects whatever. Occasionally, though, the virus travels to the spinal cord, where it destroys nerve cells, producing potentially fatal paralysis. But the chances of this happening became far greater when improved sanitation in the West began to postpone infection until later years. This led to the first-ever epidemic (in Sweden in 1887), then to outbreaks in the USA, and then to identification of the virus and the development of vaccines. Two vaccines are now used – a live, weakened poliovirus taken by mouth, developed by Albert Sabin (b. 1906), and a killed virus given by injection, developed by Jonas Salk (b. 1914). Polio has declined dramatically since their introduction.

Glandular fever caused by Epstein-Barr (EB) virus also passes unnoticed among children under ten – most of whom, in developing countries, become infected and develop antibodies against it without being aware of the fact. The better-known and often lengthy illness of fever, sore throat and swollen glands is much more likely when infection is delayed until adolescence or adulthood. Often known as the kissing disease, after one mode of transmission, it can be passed on by any form of close contact. Time is the only healer. Neither EB nor the other viruses which cause a minority of cases respond to drugs.

The importance of access

Certain infections are rare the world over simply because the target tissue is so inaccessible. One is osteomyelitis, caused when a bacterium (usually *Staphylococcus aureus*) travels from an abscess or wound infection and invades the long bones in a growing child. Effective treatment requires that large doses of antibiotics are given promptly and for a long period of time. Permanent deformity can result if the infection spreads to a joint.

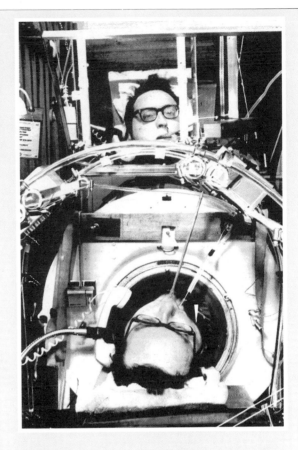

▲ *The iron lung was developed in the 1930s to help patients whose respiratory muscles had been paralyzed by polio. The decline of polio since the advent of mass immunization made it obsolete, but a new use has been found for the machines in helping patients suffering from nervous disorders that impede breathing. The lung automatically expands and contracts the patient's chest.*

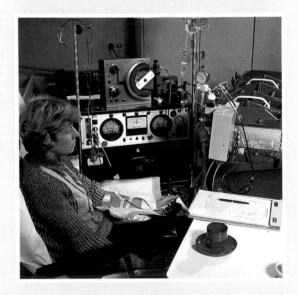

▲ *Invented by Willem Kolff in wartime Holland, the artificial kidney rids the blood of waste products such as urea which normally filter out through the body's own kidneys to produce urine. Blood flows between the machine and the patient's circulation via a permanent "shunt" in the arm or leg. It passes to a membrane with a vast surface area, across which the impurities leak away into liquid on the other side.*

The urinary tract is a highly inviting site for colonization by bacteria. Bladder infection (cystitis), with its characteristic burning pain on urination, is commoner in females because of anatomical differences and usually responds to antibiotic therapy. Kidney infection, which is potentially much more serious, can be caused by bacteria migrating from the bladder or other parts of the body (virulent streptococci from a throat infection are particularly dangerous). The resulting damage prevents the kidney from purifying the blood (◀ page 135). When untreated or unresponsive to treatment, such infections are one of the major cases of kidney failure. Two solutions are then possible – transplantation of a carefully matched healthy organ (◀ page 16), or dialysis in which impurities are removed from the patient's blood as it passes through an artificial kidney (◀ page 241). Some specialists believe that people should be screened regularly for urinary infection – which, though it can be so mild as to be unnoticeable, may lead to irreversible kidney failure.

A killer wiped from the face of the Earth

Smallpox (*variola*) begins with a rash similar to that of chickenpox, but the spots soon become ugly pustules, which may bleed. One of the most severe infections ever known, smallpox killed 60 million people during the 18th century. But an immunization campaign, started by the World Health Organization (WHO) in 1967, ended in Somalia a decade later with the last known natural case. Smallpox is now extinct – the first infection ever to be completely eradicated worldwide. This achievement was possible by using a modern version of the vaccine developed by the English physician Edward Jenner (1749-1823) in the late 18th century. Smallpox itself used to appear in both its devastating, Asiatic form and also as the much milder alastrim. Working in a Gloucestershire village, Jenner decided to investigate the local tradition that farm workers became immune to smallpox if they acquired a similarly mild condition, cowpox, from cattle. Although controversial for decades afterwards, Jenner's inoculation of material from cowpox vesicles into peoples' skin to prevent smallpox was taken up in Britain and abroad, leading to a massive decline in smallpox deaths. WHO field teams were able to eradicate smallpox because immunization is long-lasting, because there is no animal "reservoir" for the virus, and because they could vaccinate large populations very quickly, propelling vaccinia virus directly through the skin with a jet injector.

If another disease is ever to be made extinct, the two most realistic possibilities are polio and measles. Like smallpox, the viruses do not occur in other animals, and similarly effective vaccines are available. Even in developed countries, the rash, fever and respiratory tract infection of measles can be followed by serious, life-threatening complications such as encephalitis or secondary bacterial invasion. But while measles has been virtually eradicated in some North American states, and several other countries are progressing in that direction, the disease remains a killer elsewhere. Its ferocity worsened by malnutrition and accompanying diarrheal illness, measles virus is responsible for 900,000 deaths annually in Africa and other parts of the Third World. Some authorities believe the WHO should embark on a global eradication program. Others feel this is impracticable because the vaccine has to be given in the brief period between infants losing antibodies received from the mothers and becoming vulnerable to infection (unlike vaccinia, which can be administered at birth).

Measles epidemics

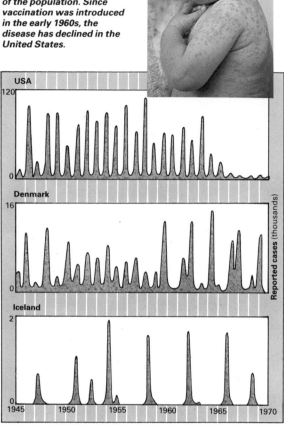

► ▼ *Measles is one of the most contagious childhood infections, involving fever, running nose and a rash. Measles occurs in epidemics, the frequency of which apparently corresponds to the density of the population. Since vaccination was introduced in the early 1960s, the disease has declined in the United States.*

USA
120
0

Denmark
16
0

Iceland
2
0
1945   1950   1955   1960   1965   1970

Reported cases (thousands)

Staphylococci and blood poisoning
One bacterium whose impact on humanity has altered over the decades is Staphylcoccus aureus, an organism well adapted to cause disease by producing toxins and chemicals which allow it to spread by breaking down tissues. Before the antibiotic era, it was feared as a microbe which, having invaded the bloodstream from its primary site such as a carbuncle, boil or infected wound, produced shock, heart damage, and other life-threatening conditions. Some 80 percent of those with such "blood poisoning" died. The advent of sulfa drugs and then penicillin changed this situation dramatically, staphylococci being particularly sensitive to these drugs. But heavy use of antibiotics has led to a worrying increase in the proportion of resistant strains. And during the early 1980s Staph. aureus was incriminated as the agent of a condition among menstruating women: toxic shock syndrome. Characterized by rapid onset of high fever, nausea, vomiting and watery diarrhea, possibly leading to severe illness, this is thought to have been caused by staphylococci proliferating in tampons and producing a toxin absorbed through the membranes of the vagina.

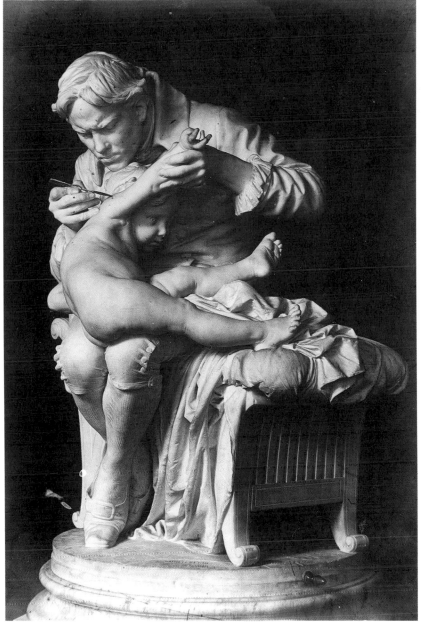

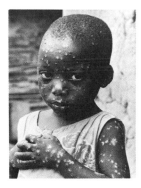

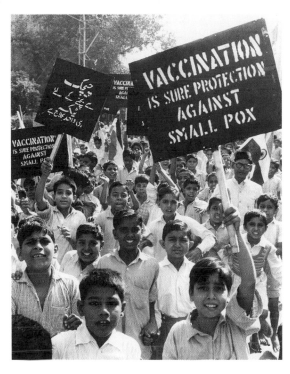

◄ ▼ *Smallpox affected 10 million and killed over 1 million people annually before the eradication campaign which began in 1967. To wipe out the disease it was necessary to inoculate large numbers of people in affected areas after a thorough publicity campaign. Jet injector guns with high-pressure sprays rather than needles meant that it was possible to inoculate up to 1,000 people an hour.*

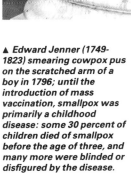

▲ *Edward Jenner (1749-1823) smearing cowpox pus on the scratched arm of a boy in 1796; until the introduction of mass vaccination, smallpox was primarily a childhood disease: some 30 percent of children died of smallpox before the age of three, and many more were blinded or disfigured by the disease.*

Chickenpox, shingles and mumps

Chickenpox (varicella) is an infection related both to herpes simplex (♦ page 244) and to smallpox. It is clearly identifiable from the crops of spots it causes, first on the trunk and then the face and limbs, when a young child is infected. Usually mild, the disease is highly infectious as these skin eruptions release more virus particles. Far less common is shingles (zoster). This occurs in adults when the same virus, persisting in nerve cells after recovery from chickenpox, becomes reactivated. The skin rash is similar, but the disease is extremely painful because nerves are affected. Although there is no treatment for chickenpox, idoxuridine helps shingles lesions to heal. A chickenpox vaccine has recently been developed, but its use remains controversial because the disease is so mild. But the same vaccine might help prevent the much more disabling condition of shingles too. A similar argument applies to infection of the salivary glands by mumps virus, which also tends to be mainly a childhood infection. Though a vaccine exists, and could forestall the testicular inflammation that follows mumps in 20 percent of men, the disease is rarely dangerous in children.

The dangers of rubella

Rubella (German measles) is not in itself a major health problem. In childhood the rash often goes unnoticed. Even adult victims, who may develop joint pains, usually have only a brief, mild illness. But rubella during pregnancy can cause deafness, heart and other defects in the child. First identified during the Second World War by Australian eye specialist Dr Norman Gregg, who noticed that congenital cataract was common among children of mothers who contracted rubella while pregnant, such teratogenic (fetus-poisoning) effects are the principal reason for immunization. Whereas the 1960s saw an estimated 12·5 million cases of rubella and about 20,000 malformed infants in the USA, the licensing of a vaccine in 1969 prefaced a massive reduction in the disease. Once, young girls were encouraged to attend "rubella parties" at which they allowed themselves to become infected (by droplet transmission from those with the disease), but most countries now have programs to ensure immunization of all girls at 12-14 or all children at an earlier age (thus reducing the possibility of pregnant women being exposed to the virus).

Leprosy still affects over 11 million people, mainly in Africa and Asia

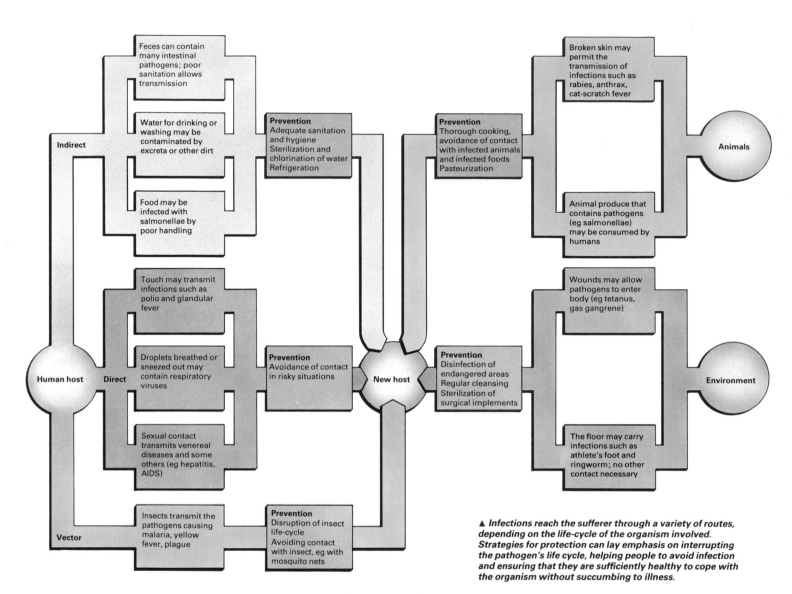

▲ *Infections reach the sufferer through a variety of routes, depending on the life-cycle of the organism involved. Strategies for protection can lay emphasis on interrupting the pathogen's life cycle, helping people to avoid infection and ensuring that they are sufficiently healthy to cope with the organism without succumbing to illness.*

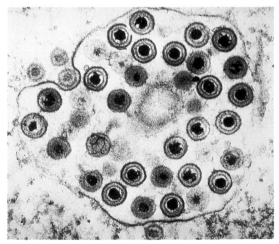

▲ *Herpes simplex, the virus responsible for persistent cold sores on the lips, and closely related to the genital herpes virus. It is thought that the virus is usually acquired during childhood, becomes dormant for many years, and becomes evident after stimulation by sunlight, infection etc. The cold sores may last for two weeks.*

The most disfiguring skin infections

Apart from orifices offered by respiratory, intestinal, reproductive and urinary tracts, the skin is an obvious target for invasion. Like the eyes, it too has defense mechanisms, but these can be breached. One of the commonest occurrences is when a normally harmless skin inhabitant, *Propionibacterium acnes*, proliferates inside sebaceous glands (◀ page 116). The inflammation accompanying this invasion, known as acne, affects about 80 percent of adolescent girls and over 90 percent of boys. Related to excess sebum production resulting from hormonal changes during puberty, acne is usually fairly short-lived.

This is not the case with herpes simplex, probably our commonest virus parasite. Acquired in childhood and often without causing any obvious symptoms, the virus takes up residence as a latent infection – sometimes on the genitals but usually on the lips, where it produces intermittent cold sores.

Although its mode of transmission is still uncertain, leprosy is recognized principally for "granulomas" which appear on the skin. Related to the tubercle bacillus (◀ page 176), the leprosy bacillus produces similar nodules on internal organs but can also cause an anesthetic form of the disease, in which loss of sensitivity heightens the risk of

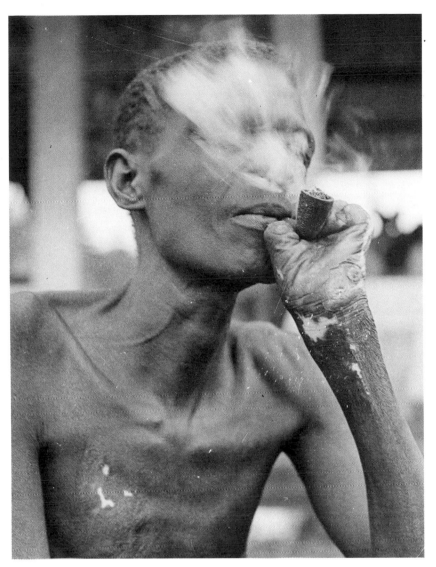

The decline of the scarlet fever bacterium
Most of us have suffered an occasional sore throat caused by streptococci. Yet scarlet fever, which at one time was a common sequel to such infections, is now very rare. Many of today's doctors are unfamiliar with the vivid red rash – feared because it in turn might be a prelude to the much more alarming rheumatic fever, which damages tissues of the heart. Treatment of serious streptococcal throat infections with antibiotics must be part of the explanation. Improved nutrition and hygiene may have helped. But another reason seems to be that the hemolytic streptococcus itself has become less virulent. Why the bacterium should change in this way is not known. Streptococci which continue to flourish in Asia, Africa and South America retain their virulence.

The new threat of meningitis
While some bacteria have faded in importance, microbiologists have become concerned about two others. Agents of meningitis (inflammation of membranes covering the brain and spinal cord), both are acquired through the respiratory tract. They produce sudden fever, headache and vomiting; are potentially fatal, and attack children in particular. Earlier this century, epidemics of "cerebrospinal, spotted fever" caused by one, Neisseria meningitidis, excited dread, notably in the USA. Today, after epidemics in countries ranging from Latin America to Europe, there is anxiety that the disease may be resurgent. And Haemophilus influenzae – a bacterium once wrongly thought to be the agent of influenza – has become the leading cause of bacterial meningitis.

◄ *The nodular "granulomas" produced in the skin and elsewhere by leprosy bacilli are sometimes accompanied by an anesthetic form of the disease in which victims lose sensation in their hands and feet, leading to injury and mutilation. The incubation period of leprosy can be several years, and drugs take several months to take effect.*

injury to the hands and feet. The disease progresses slowly over many years and is far less infectious than was thought in the days when lepers were synonymous with social outcasts. It still affects 11 million people, mainly in Africa and Asia, but is susceptible to a few drugs. Following the first, long-sought-after successes in growing the bacillus outside the human body – in armadillos – a vaccine was developed in the early 1980s and tests are now underway.

Some of the most disfiguring infections occur when fungi attack the skin, nails or hair. Although producing conditions which are often chronic and resistant to treatment, these fungi rarely affect the victim's general health. The commonest disease is Tinea pedis (athlete's foot), causing blisters between the toes. It is acquired from fragments of skin left behind by other sufferers, and is often contracted in showers and dressing rooms. Tinea corporis (ringworm) produces annular lesions on the non-hairy skin and is picked up by contact with infected children or, very occasionally, cats or dogs. Chemicals such as griseofulvin are effective, but only if used after scrupulous removal of dead and infected tissues. Fungi are also responsible for deeper infections. Many are restricted to certain geographical regions, where most people become infected though few succumb to the full-blown disease.

Opportunistic pathogens
Whereas older textbooks divided micro-organisms into those causing disease (pathogens) and those not doing so, the distinction now appears much less decisive. An individual's constitution and wellbeing may influence the chances of becoming infected with a well-recognized "pathogen", and some microbes are being identified as harmful only when given unusual opportunities. The bacterium Pseudomonas aeruginosa, for example, lives unnoticed in human intestines. But it can produce serious infections if it colonizes burned skin (where its resistance to many antibiotics poses an additional problem). Pseudomonads are also capable of proliferating in preparations such as eye drops and ointments, which can be extremely hazardous if the contamination is overlooked. Such "opportunistic pathogens" have been given further scope in recent decades with the development of substances intended to combat the rejection of transplanted organs by the body's immune system (◊ page 213). These drugs impair the immune response, making patients vulnerable to organisms that are normally harmless, so precautions are necessary to minimize the risk of infection.

Malaria affects over 400 million people worldwide

Fighting with diseases

During the Crusades, each side tried to spread disease by dumping plague-ridden bodies into enemy camps. More recently, during the Second World War, British scientists tested a possible biological weapon and Japan also tested biological agents on prisoners of war. The 1972 Biological and Toxin Weapons Convention bans offensive work on biological weapons by the superpowers, but it still permits research into defensive measures. The development of vaccines inevitably involves the manufacture of correspondingly virulent bacteria and viruses, however, and there are fears that the spirit of the convention may be being flouted. While allegations of biological attacks by the Soviet Union in Laos and Kampuchea have not been substantiated, Western observers are convinced that the USSR is stockpiling infectious organisms for use in war. The US Department of Defense is also spending heavily on research into genetically-engineered micro-organisms. These could be much more dangerous than those that have evolved naturally.

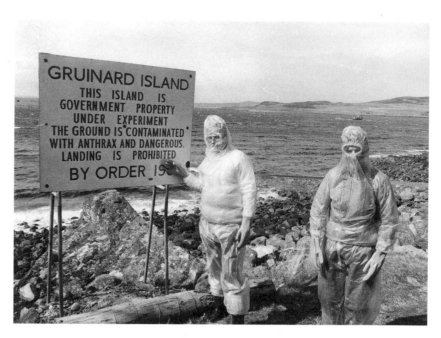

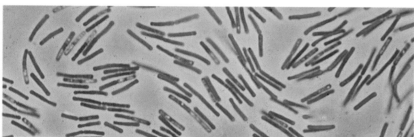

◀ *Bacillus anthracis is the agent of anthrax, a disease that is usually fatal in animals and may be so to humans if the spores are inhaled. The bacillus was first isolated and identified by Robert Koch in 1876; Pasteur then developed an anthrax vaccine which caused the disease to decline in many countries.*

▲ *In World War II the British Government experimented with the anthrax bacillus as a biological weapon. They tested its release on the uninhabited Gruinard Island in Scotland. Many sheep were killed, and it is intended that the island should remain isolated for at least one hundred years.*

Some micro-organisms attack the body only if allowed access through a wound. Best known is *Clostridium tetani*, the tetanus (lockjaw) bacterium. One of several bacteria capable of turning into hardy spores, this tolerates higher temperatures, and survives longer without food, than organisms unable to form spores. Although tetanus spores occur in soil throughout the world, the disease is rare in the West because most people are immunized in infancy (with triple vaccine, against diphtheria and whooping cough as well). Farm workers and others at risk also receive regular booster doses of anti-tetanus vaccine to keep their immunity high. *C. tetani* does not spread through the body. It triggers a potentially fatal illness by producing toxins which attack nerves, inducing convulsive muscular spasms. Penicillin has some effect on the organism, but the main tactic when a non-immune person becomes infected is to inject anti-tetanus antibodies. This confers "passive immunity", in contrast to the active immunity conferred by vaccination. In Third World countries, lack of hygiene during childbirth means that many babies are infected via the umbilical cord and killed by this most easily avoidable of infections.

Other species of clostridia include those responsible for botulism (not strictly an infection but a form of poisoning ◀ page 238) and gas gangrene. So-called because they liberate gases (and foul-smelling substances), the clostridia of gas gangrene gain entry to the body's tissues either through a dirty wound or, in the case of surgical wounds, from the patient's own intestines. Gas gangrene has been a potent threat during warfare – from the trench campaigns of the First World War to the more recent Falklands conflict.

Jaundice and the hepatitis virus

Hepatitis (inflammation of the liver) has emerged as a major public health problem in recent years. Symptoms are nausea, fever, weakness, loss of appetite, sudden distaste for tobacco smoking and (except in the mildest form) jaundice. Although in the earliest days of medicine Hippocrates recognized "epidemic jaundice", knowledge of the viruses responsible dates back only to the late 1960s.

Most serious is hepatitis B. This may persist after its acute and often severe phase to produce cirrhosis (◀ page 240). There is also strong evidence of an association between the disease and primary liver cancer. An estimated 200 million carriers worldwide includes 0·1 percent of the population in Europe and North America, compared with 20 percent in parts of Asia and Africa. Formerly called serum hepatitis because the virus is transmissible via blood and serum, it is now known to be spread by mouth and by sexual contact too; promiscuous male homosexuals are at particularly high risk.

Hepatitis A, acquired through water or food contaminated by feces carrying the virus, is incapacitating but unlike hepatitis B does not cause chronic liver damage. Vaccines against both forms of the disease are now under way – priority being given to those which can be given to groups (which range from dentists and laboratory staff to young male homosexuals) who are in particular danger of contracting hepatitis B.

Malaria

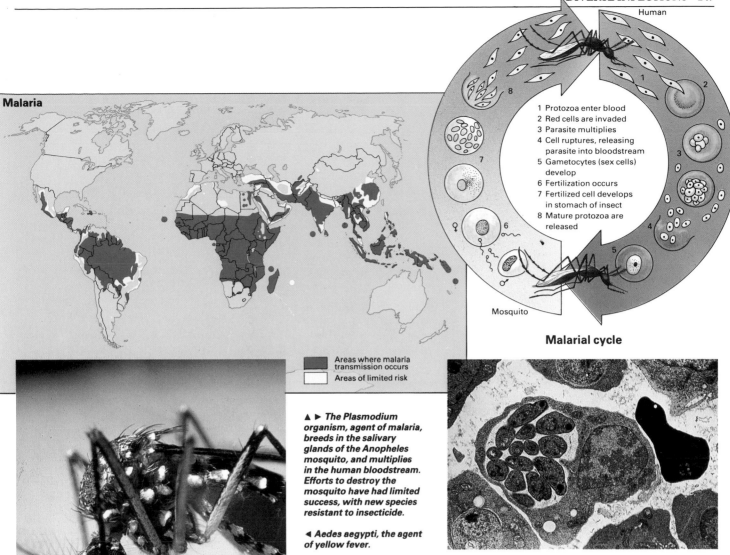

Areas where malaria transmission occurs

Areas of limited risk

Malarial cycle

1 Protozoa enter blood
2 Red cells are invaded
3 Parasite multiplies
4 Cell ruptures, releasing parasite into bloodstream
5 Gametocytes (sex cells) develop
6 Fertilization occurs
7 Fertilized cell develops in stomach of insect
8 Mature protozoa are released

Human

Mosquito

▲ ▶ *The Plasmodium organism, agent of malaria, breeds in the salivary glands of the Anopheles mosquito, and multiplies in the human bloodstream. Efforts to destroy the mosquito have had limited success, with new species resistant to insecticide.*

◀ *Aedes aegypti, the agent of yellow fever.*

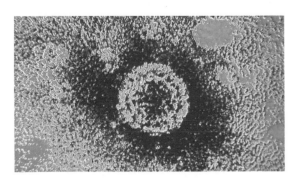

▲ *The virus of hepatitis B, which can remain in the bloodstream of healthy people for prolonged periods, perhaps indefinitely. For this reason people with the virus are never accepted as blood donors.*

Bacillus anthracis, the agent of anthrax, is related to clostridia but requires oxygen for growth whereas clostridia thrive without oxygen. Primarily a disease of sheep, cattle and horses, anthrax is occasionally acquired by humans, either through skin abrasions or by inhalation of the spores. "Hide porter's disease" and "wool sorter's disease" – names given to anthrax in the past – reflect its occupational significance. As a skin infection, it causes blisters which may become purulent; if untreated, blood poisoning may follow. When inhaled, the bacilli trigger a lung infection leading to hemorrages and blood poisoning. An effective vaccine is available, as are several antibiotics.

Anthrax is one of the zoonoses – diseases acquired from animals but which are not usually passed thereafter from person to person. Most are tropical conditions whose parasites spend part of their life cycle in intermediate "vectors". Malaria, caused by protozoa known as plasmodia which have a complex lifestyle in the human bloodstream and liver, and in the stomach and salivary glands of *Anopheles* mosquitoes, is the most widespread disease of this sort, with 400 million cases worldwide. Next come filariasis, whose thread-like worms, carried by various species of mosquitoes, affect 250 million people; schistosomiasis (bilharzia), with 200 million cases, caused by flat worms transmitted by water snails; and onchocerciasis (river blindness), another threadworm infestation, purveyed by a blood-sucking black fly and affecting 40 million people in Africa, central America and the Yemen. Others include sleeping sickness (African trypanosomiasis), caused by protozoa carried by the tsetse fly; Chaga's disease; and yellow fever, spread by *Aedes* mosquitoes.

See also
The Human Body 9-20
Medicine, Doctors and Health 33-40
Intestinal Infections 141-8
Respiratory Infections 167-76
Sexual Infections 201-4

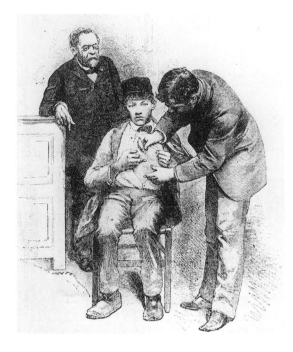

▲ *In July 1885 Joseph Meister became the first person to receive the rabies vaccine developed by Louis Pasteur; Pasteur himself was unsure that the vaccine would work but Meister lived to become caretaker of the Pasteur Institute.*

Some mysterious infections

Although the conquest of infectious disease is one of the great achievements of medical science, puzzles remain. One is that of multiple sclerosis – MS (◊ page 62) – which produces unpredictable defects in the nervous system. MS is probably attributable to a "slow virus" – one causing symptoms which take months or years to appear. The search for the MS agent continues. Another mystery is the cause of a type of encephalitis (inflammation of the brain) which first appeared in China between 1917 and 1927, affecting 65,000 people before spreading to North America and Europe and then disappearing. Several other encephalitides are known – some produced by viruses transmitted by ticks or mosquitoes, some arising as complications of conditions like measles. But the brief history of encephalitis lethargica has never been explained. Virtually unknown since the 1930s, it caused highly variable symptoms – including stupor, coma, fits and visual defects, which suggested that a virus was responsible. As the disease often led to the involuntary movements, paralysis and compulsive behavior of parkinsonism, microbiologists suspect that a slow virus was to blame. Paranoia and psychoses were common among victims, and historians have even speculated that the rise of National Socialism in Germany, with the violent, aggressive behavior and gesticulation of Hitler, may have been due at least in part to this extraordinary historical malady.

▶ *The rat flea, Xenopsylla cheopis, which carried the bacillus of bubonic plague and was responsible for spreading the Black Death and many recurring epidemics throughout the Middle Ages and 17th century. These epidemics spread across the whole of Europe in a few years, carried in ships and bags of wool.*

Offensive tactics are possible against several vector-borne diseases (vaccination to prevent yellow fever, drugs to treat, or better still prevent, malaria). For some recently recognized and highly lethal zoonoses such as Lassa fever (carried by rats), the only measure is to inject antibodies from blood serum donated by victims fortunate enough to recover. The main means of control is to attack the intermediate host though this, in turn, is bedevilled by the increasing resistance of mosquitoes and other vectors to chemical pesitcides.

Rabies, a zoonosis contracted when rabies virus passes into a person's bloodstream following a bite by a rabid dog or other animal, is an acute infection of the central nervous system. Also known as hydrophobia, because victims develop a dread of water, rabies causes vomiting, high fever and seizures, and is invariably fatal if untreated. But because rabies has a long incubation period in man (up to 16 weeks), patients can be helped by both active and passive immunization with pre-formed antibodies. Found in wildlife in many parts of the world (including jackals in India, skunks in the USA and foxes in Europe), rabies has been kept out of countries such as Britain by strictly imposed quarantine on imported animals.

Bubonic plague, the cause of three appalling historic pandemics (worldwide epidemics), begins as a zoonosis, when rat fleas leave their natural host and bite humans. This transfers *Yersinia pestis*, the plague bacillus, which spreads to lymph nodes and proliferates there, producing grotesque nodules called buboes, before colonizing many other organs and killing the victim. Pneumonic plague develops if the lungs are affected, so that bacilli are coughed up, spreading the infection from person to person. Both forms of the disease occured during the second pandemic – the Black Death, which began during the 14th century and killed 25 million people (a quarter of the population) in Europe alone. Now curable by antibiotics, plague remains a public health hazard in many parts of the world.

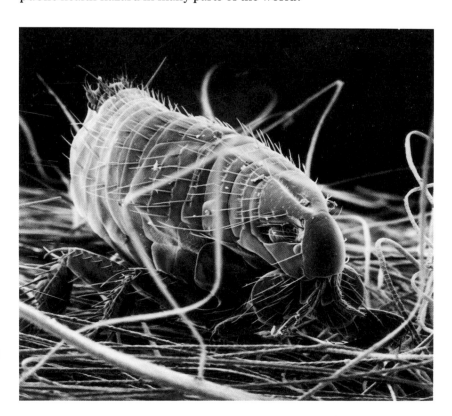

Credits

1 SPL 2-3 John Watney 4-5 SPL/Michael Abbey 7 SPL/Frieder Michler 8 Susan Griggs Agency, London 10-11tl Robert Harding Associates/Walter Rawlings 10-11tr, cl, cr, Camerapix Hutchison 10-11bl Natural History Picture Agency/Peter Johnson 10-11br Robert Harding Associates 16 SPL 18bl SPL 18tr SPL/Eric Grave 18bc, br SPL/Michael Abbey 23l John Reader 23r Cleveland Museum of Natural History 25bl, br Mansell Collection, London 26bl SPL/Jan Hinsch 26c SPL/ Dr G. Schatten 26br SPL/Omikron 27tr SPL/National Institute of Health 29tr Gregor Mendel Memorial Museum, Brno 31 Jan Massys: Lot and his daughters / Musée de Cognac SPL 32bl Tecknik photo, Cognac 33 BBC Hulton Picture Library, London 34tl Zentralbibliothek, Zürich 34bl BBC Hulton Picture Library br Mansell Collection 35tl Royal Library, Windsor Castle, RL 19003v. Copyright reserved. Reproduced by gracious permission of Her Majesty the Queen 34bl Rembrandt: The Anatomy Lesson / The Bridgeman Art Library, London 34br BBC Hulton Picture Library 36t John Watney, London 36c Mansell Collection 36b Popperfoto, London 37tl Ann Ronan Picture Library 37tr BBC Hulton Picture Library 37br *Illustrite Zeitung*, Leipzig 38t SPL/Guy Gillette 38b SPL/R. Clark, M. Goff 39tl SPL 39tr SPL/Ohio Nuclear Corporation 39bl Frank Spooner Pictures, London 39br SPL/Dr R. Damadian 40 Camerapix Hutchison 41 Rob Judges, Oxford/R.N.I.B. 8942 SPL 43 SPL/Dr Ralph Eagle 44-45 SPL/Dr G. Bredberg 45 Frank Spooner Pictures 46tr SPL/M.I. Walker 46b SPL/Omikron 47 John Watney 48 Zefa/F. Walther 49 Equinox Archive 50t SPL/Argentum 50b Rob Judges, Oxford 51t SPL/Argentum 51b Biophoto Associates, Leeds 52 John Watney 55 SPL/Manfred Kage 56t Biophoto Associates 56b Warren Anatomical Museum, Harvard University 59t SPL/Cosmos/Eric Gravé 59b SPL/Manfred Kage 61b SPL/Bill Longcore 62-63 Camera Press, London 63b Ken Moreman 64 Network/Barry Lewis, London 65 Fotomas Index 66 Tom Nelson/Gerardo Campos/Betty Edwards/J.P. Tarcher Inc. 67t SPL/Phelps/Mazziotta 67bc SPL 67br SPL/Jerry Mason 69tr John Topham Picture Library, Markbeech 69b Rob Judges, Oxford 70 Richard and Sally Greenhill, London 71tl, c, tr Rob Judges, Oxford 72 Mary Evans Picture Library, London 73 Frank Spooner Pictures 74-75 Rex Features, London 76t Rex Features 76b Zefa/G. Sirena 77t BBC Hulton Picture Library/Bettman Archive 77b Mary Evans Picture Library 78 Ann Ronan Picture Library 79l Chim/Magnum Archive, Paris 79r Richard and Sally Greenhill 80l Ann Ronan Picture Library 80r Rob Judges, Oxford 81l Mike Abrahams/ Network,

London 81r Laurie Sparham/Network 82 Frank Spooner Pictures 83l Laurie Sparham/Network 83r Mike Abrahams/ Network 84t SPL 84b Hogarth: Rake's Progress/Fotomas Index 86 SPL/David Parker 86b SPL/Prof. T. Blundell, Birkbeck 90t SPL/David Parker 90b SPL/Manfred Kage 91t SPL/David Parker 91b Biophotos Associates, Leeds 93 SPL/Science Source 94-95 SPL/Manfred Kage 95c Camera Press 95b John Watney 96bl WHO Photo/Best Institute 96c Dr J.J. Bending/Guy's Hospital, London 100 Bodleian Library, Oxford 102 Equinox Archive 103l SPL/Science Source 2,3 SPL/Eric Gravé 106 Janet Hughes/Northwick Park Hospital 107 SPL 108 SPL 109l SPL 109r John Watney 110-111 Gower Medical Publishing, London 110t Dr J.C. MacLarnon/Nuffield Orthopaedic Hospital, Oxford 110b Zefa Picture Library, London 111t SPL/James Stevenson 111t John Watney 111br Biophoto Associates 111bl Gower Medical Publishing 112t Gibbs Dental Division, London 112b Lawrence Clarke, Witney 113t Camerapix Hutchison 113b Gower Medical Publishing 114 SPL/Nancy Hamilton 115l SPL/Michael Abbey 115r SPL/Manfred Kage 891 1687 SPL/Manfred Kage 117l SPL/Martin Dohrn 117r Mansell Collection 118tl Zefa/J. Röhrich 118tr, cr SPL/John Radcliffe 118cl SPL/Russ Kinne 118 SPL/Hank Morgan 119 Camera Press/Colin Davey 120tl John Watney 120bl SPL/R. Stepney/M. Aumer 120br SPL/Dr Tony Brain 121l Equinox Archives 121r Bodleian Library, Oxford 124 SPL 126 British Library, London 127 John Watney 128 Rex Features 129 Frank Spooner Pictures 130 Camerapix Hutchison 131tl Zefa/Teasy 131tr Bryan and Cherry Alexander 131c, b Camerapix Hutchison 132 BBC Hulton Picture Library 134 SPL 135 SPL/Michael Abbey 136t Mansell Collection 136b SPL 137 C. James Webb, Mitcham 138tr, c SPL/ Manfred Kage 138br Gower Medical Publishing 139t John Watney 139b Ken Moreman 140 BBC Hulton Picture Library 142 WHO/Dr Henrioud 143tl from *Illustrirtes Lexicon der Verfalschungen*, H. Klenske, Leipzig, 1879 143b Mansell Collection 146 SPL/John Durham 147 Biophoto Associates 148t SPL 148b SPL/Gene Cox 149 from *Movement of the Heart and Blood in Animals*, by William Harvey, 1628 150 SPL 151 SPL/Manfred Kage 152 SPL/K.R. Porter 153 SPL/Manfred Kage 155 SPL 156 Allsport/Tony Duffy 158tr John Watney 158c John Watney 159 John Watney 160tr SPL 160b Martin v. Wagner Museum der Universität Wurzburg 161 Biophoto Associates 162 SPL 163 SPL/Jim Stevenson 164-165 BBC Hulton Picture Library 164b John Watney 165bl John Watney 165 Ken Moreman 166 Rob Judges 167 Natural History Picture Agency 170 BBC Hulton Picture Library 171 SPL/Division of Computer Research and Technology, National Institute of Health 171b SPL/Dr S. Patterson 172 WHO Photo/P.Larsen 173t Gower Medical Publishing 173b SPL/Dr E.H. Cook 174-175l,2 Biophoto Associates, 3a SPL/John

Durham, 3b John Watney, 4a SPL/Dr E.H. Cook 4b SPL/Lee Simon/Sinclair Stammers 175t Michael Salas/Image Bank, London 176t SPL 176b Popperfoto 177 September Press, Wellingborough / Copyright reserved. 178c Biophoto Associates 178b, 179 SPL 181t SPL/Manfred Kage 181b Frank Spooner Pictures 184t, b, Petit Format/Nestle/Susan Griggs Agency 186 Anthea Sieveking/Vision International 187t, b, Sally and Richard Greenhill 187c Pictorial Press 188 Zefa/W. Imaehl 189 Ken Moreman, inset: Gower Medical Publishing 190l Topham Picture Library 190r Rex Features 191 SPL/Dr J. McFarland, inset: Gower Medical Publishing 192 Richard and Sally Greenhill 194t Gower Medical Publishing 194c, b John Watney 195 Frank Spooner Pictures 196l Frank Spooner Pictures 196r BBC Hulton Picture Library 197t Sally and Richard Greenhill 197c SPL 198 Chemical Design Ltd., Oxford 199t, b SPL 201t, b WHO Photo, Geneva 202-203 Frank Spooner Pictures 203b SPL/Eric Gravé 204 WHO Photo 208t Age Concern/Photo Co-op 208b Age Concern/ Ian Cook 209 Frank Spooner Pictures 210 From DREAMSTAGE Scientific Catalogue (c) J. Allan Hobson, M.D., and Hoffman La-Roche Inc. 211 SPL 213 SPL 214b SPL/Biology Media 214-215 SPL/Dr D. J. McLaren 216t SPL/ Division of Computer Research and Technology, National Institute of Health 218 SPL/Manfred Kage 219t SPL/Dr A. R. Lawton 219b Associated Press 220t Zefa/Reichelt 220b Fotomas Index 221t SPL/Dr Brian Eyden 221b SPL/Manfred Kage 225 SPL/Andrejs Leipins 226 Mansell Collection 226-227 SPL/Dr R. Damadian 227 Zefa/V.W.S. 228 SPL/Dr Karol Sikor 229 SPL/Dr Rosalind King 230t John Watney 230-231cl, cr, b Biophoto Associates 231 Natural History Picture Agency 232t, b Frank Spooner Pictures 233 Frank Spooner Pictures 234t Topham Picture Library 234 Rex Features 235t, b Frank Spooner Pictures 236tl Topham Picture Library 236br BBC Hulton Picture Library 236-237 Salim Patel 237br Frank Spooner Pictures 238tl, br, Frank Spooner Pictures 238bl Natural History Picture Agency 239 Frank Spooner Pictures 240t BBC Hulton Picture Library 240bl Biophoto Associates 241t Popperfoto 241b Zefa/W. H. Mueller 242 SPL/Lowell Georgia 243tl BBC Hulton Picture Library 243tr Popperfoto 243cr WHO Photo/T. S. Satyan 244bl SPL/Science Source 245 Popperfoto 246tr Popperfoto 246cl SPL/Dr R King 247cl SPL/Martin Dohrn 247cr SPL/Omikron 247b SPL/E.H. Cook 248t BBC Hulton Picture Library 248b SPL/Dr Tony Brain.

Artists Principal anatomical artwork by Dave Mazierski; other artwork by Lynne Brackley, Kai Choi, Chris Forsey, Alan Hollingbery, Kevin Maddison, Julia Osorno, Mick Saunders, Linda Stevens. **Indexer** Susan Harris. **Typesetting** Peter Furtado / Peter MacDonald, Hampton.

Further Reading

General

Anthony, C.P. and Thibodeau G.A. *Textbook of Anatomy & Physiology* (C.V. Mosby Company)
Cunningham, D.J. *Textbook of Anatomy* (11th edition – Romanes)
Hole, J.W. *Human Anatomy and Physiology* (2nd edition – Wm C. Brown)
Mason, W.H. and Marshall, N.L. *The Human Side of Biology* (Harper & Row)
Purves, W.K. and Orians, G.H. *Life: the Science of Biology* (Blackwell Scientific)
Singer, C. and Underwood, E.A. *A Short History of Medicine* (Oxford University Press)
Soper, R. and Smith, S.T. *Modern Human and Social Biology* (Macmillan)
Tortora, G.J. and Anagnastakos, N.P. *Principles of Anatomy and Physiology* (2nd edition – Harper and Row)

The Human Body

Andrews, M. *The Life that Lives on Man* (Taplinger)
Eden, J. *The Eye Book* (Viking Press)

Ekholm, E.P. *The Picture of Health* (Norton)
Emery, A.E.H. *Elements of Medical Genetics* (Churchill Livingstone)
Frisbee, J. *Seeing, Illusion, Mind and Brain* (Oxford University Press)
Gilling, D. and Brightwell, R. *The Human Brain* (Orbis)
Glasser, R.J. *The Body is the Hero* (Collins)
Julian, D.G. *Cardiology* (Ballière Tindall)
Leakey, R.E. *The Making of Mankind* (Michael Joseph)
Lewontin, R, *Human Diversity* (Edward Arnold)
Mottram, R.F. *Human Nutrition* (Edward Arnold)
Nossal, G.J.V. *Reshaping Life* (Cambridge University Press)
Rowland, A.J. and Cooper, P. *Environment and Health* (Edward Arnold)
Schiffman, H.R. *Sensation and Perception* (J. Wiley)
Selye, H. *The Stress of Life* (McGraw Hill)
Singer, P. and Wells, D. *The Reproductive Revolution* (Hutchinson)
Smith, A. *The Body* (2nd edition – Penguin Books)
Smith, A. *The Mind* (Hodder & Stoughton)

Medicine and Disease

Abbott, D. *New Life for Old* (Muller)
Baldry, P. *The Battle against Bacteria* (Cambridge University Press)
Berkow R. *The Merck Manual of Diagnosis and Therapy* (14th edition – Merck and Co. Inc.)
Boyd, W. and Sheldon, H. *Introduction to the Study of Diseases* (Lea and Febinger)
Dixon, B. *Beyond the Magic Bullet* (Allen & Unwin)
Doll, R. and Peto, R. *The Causes of Cancer*
Dowling, H.F. *Fighting Infection* (Harvard)
Goodwin, P. *Can you Avoid Cancer?* (BBC)
Illich, Ivan *Limits to Medicine* (Penguin Books)
Kedzi, P. *You and Your Heart* (Penguin Books)
Muir Gray, J.A. *Man against Disease* (Oxford University Press)
Parish, P. *Medicine: a Guide for Everybody* (Penguin Books)
Pascoe, D. *Toxicology* (Edward Arnold)
Trowell, H.C. and Burkitt, D. *Western Diseases, their Emergence and Prevention* (Edward Arnold)
Tudge, C. *The Famine Business* (Penguin Books)

Glossary

Abdomen
The lower part of the trunk, between the diaphragm and the pelvis.

Abortion
The ending of pregnancy and expulsion of the FETUS before it is viable. Abortion may be natural or induced.

Absorption
The process whereby substances cross through MUCOUS MEMBRANES or skin, as when the products of digestion are absorbed through the lining of the intestine.

Abscess
A local collection of pus.

Acute
Describes a sudden, short episode of illness, usually severe.

Addiction
A craving for a potentially harmful drug with increased bodily tolerance for it.

Adipose
Of a fatty nature.

Alimentary canal
The digestive tract, from mouth to anus.

Allergy
Abnormally sensitive reaction of the body's immune system to a foreign substance.

Amino-acid
Basic chemical unit from which PROTEINS are synthesized by the body.

Anabolism
The process whereby more complex chemicals are built up from less complex ones.

Anemia
Disease in which the number of red blood cells circulating in the body, or their ability to carry oxygen, is lowered.

Anesthesia
The absence of bodily sensation, usually defined with respect to loss of pain sensations. Anesthetics may be local or general (causing a total loss of consciousness).

Analgesia
The absence of normal sense of pain.

Anatomy
The study of the basic structure of the body, and the relationship of the parts to each other.

Aneurysm
The swelling or bulging of a blood vessel.

Antibiotic
Chemical produced by a MICRO-ORGANISM and used as a drug to kill or inhibit the growth of other micro-organisms.

Antibody
Defensive substance produced by the immune system to neutralize or help destroy a specific foreign substance (ANTIGEN).

Antigen
A foreign substance that provokes the body to produce ANTIBODIES.

Antiseptic
Any chemical used to destroy harmful MICRO-ORGANISMS.

Articulation
A joint.

ATP
Adenosine triphosphate, the energy-carrying molecule manufactured in all cells as a way of storing energy.

Atrophy
Wasting away or shrinkage of a part or ORGAN.

Auto-immune disease
A disease in which the body rejects some of its normal tissues and mobilizes the immune system against them.

Autonomic nervous system
The system of nerves controlling many of the body's organs outside normal conscious control. It comprises the sympathetic and the parasympathetic systems.

Bacillus
A rod-shaped BACTERIUM.

Bacteria (singular bacterium)
A large and varied group of MICRO-ORGANISM, classified by their shape and staining ability. They live in many environments; only a few are harmful to the human body.

Basal metabolism
The rate of METABOLISM when the body is resting.

Benign
Not malignant (of cancers).

Biopsy
The removal of living TISSUES for examination.

Bolus
A soft, rounded mass of food after swallowing.

Calorie
The amount of heat required to raise 1g of water through 1°C. The calorie value of food is calculated as the number of calories it would yield as energy if completely used. Nutritionally the kilocalorie (Calorie) is used.

Cancer
A malignant TUMOR.

Capillaries
The smallest blood vessels forming a fine network in all tissues.

Cardiac
Relating to the heart.

CAT scan (also **CT scan**).
Computerized axial tomography, a technique of building up an X-ray image of a slice through the body.

Catabolism
The breakdown of complex substances into simpler ones.

Chromosome
A thread of genetic material contained in the cell nucleus and duplicated when the cell divides.

Chronic
Describes an illness of slow onset and long duration.

Cilia
Small hairlike structures on the outer surface of some cells.

CNS
Central nervous system; brain and spinal cord.

Collagen
A PROTEIN that is the main organic constituent of CONNECTIVE TISSUE.

Conception
The moment of fertilization.

Connective tissue
One of the main tissue types in the body, including bone, cartilage and fat, that acts to bind and support other tissues.

Coronary
Relating to the arteries which supply the heart's own muscle.

Cortex
The outer surface of an organ, such as the brain or the adrenal glands.

CSF
Cerebro-spinal fluid.

Cyst
Abnormal swelling containing a fluid.

DNA
Deoxyribonucleic acid; its structure contains the blueprint that contains genetic information.

Diastole
The phase of relaxation or dilation of the heart muscle in the cardiac cycle.

Dilation
Expansion, widening or swelling.

ECG
Electrocardiogram, the recording of the electrical changes accompanying the cardiac cycle.

ECT
Electroconvulsive therapy, a treatment for psychosis.

Edema
The abnormal accumulation of fluid in body tissues.

EEG
Electroencephalogram, the recording of the electrical impulses of the brain.

Embolus
A blood clot, air bubble, fat, mass of bacteria or other foreign material carried in the blood.

Embryo
The developing baby in the womb from conception to the end of the tenth week.

Endemic
A disease always present within a population or region.

Enzyme
An organic catalyst, usually a PROTEIN, that affects the speed of a metabolic reaction.

Epidemic
An outbreak of an infectious disease affecting a significant proportion of a population.

Etiology
The study of the causes of disease.

Fascia
A sheet of thin fibrous tissue, covering, supporting or separating muscles.

Fetus
The developing baby, from the tenth week after conception to birth.

Fever
The elevation of the body temperature above normal.

Follicle
A small cavity, sac or gland in the body.

Gene
The unit of heredity, made up of DNA and located on a CHROMOSOME in a cell nucleus.

Genetics
The study of heredity.

Gland
Group of specialized epithelial cells that secrete substances for specific effect.

Gonad
A male or female sex gland.

Graft
The transplant of a healthy tissue or organ to replace a damaged or diseased one.

Hepatic
Relating to the liver.

Heredity
The passing of genetic characteristics from parents to children.

Histology
The microscopic study of the structure of TISSUES.

Homeostasis
The maintenance of a stable internal environment despite changes in external conditions.

Hormone
Chemical secreted by an endocrine gland which has a specific effect on a target cell in another part of the body.

Hypertension
High blood pressure.

Hypertrophy
The increase in size of a tissue through enlargement of its cells.

Immunity
State of resistance to an INFECTION, through the existence of ANTIBODIES specific to that PATHOGEN.

Infant
A baby up to one year old.

Infarct
The death of body tissues caused by blockage in their blood supply.

Infection
The invasion of and multiplication within the body by harmful living organisms.

Inflammation
A localized response to INFECTION, characterized by swelling, redness and pain.

In vitro
In glass; outside the living body and within an artificial environment such as a testtube.

In vivo
In the living body.

Ischemia
The reduction in blood circulation in a tissue through blockage of its blood vessels.

IUD
Intra-uterine device; a coil or loop inserted into the uterus to prevent conception.

IVF
IN VITRO fertilization.

Lipid
Fat or fatlike substance such as cholesterol.

Macrophage
White blood cell specialized to circulate through the body tissues and consume foreign bodies and cell debris.

Malignant
Relating to a disease that tends to worsen and cause death, notably some TUMORS.

Meiosis
The process of cell division within the reproductive organs which results in the manufacture of sex cells.

Meninges
The three layers of membrane covering the brain and spinal cord.

Metabolism
The sum of all biochemical reactions in the body, including ANABOLISM and CATABOLISM.

Microbe
See MICRO-ORGANISM.

Micro-organism
A living organism too small to be seen without a microscope.

Mitosis
The normal process of cell division, in which the cell's chromosomes are fully reproduced.

Mucous membrane
A membrane lining a body cavity that opens onto the exterior.

Mucus
The thick fluid secreted by the mucous glands and MUCOUS MEMBRANES.

Necrosis
The death of a cell or group of cells as a result of disease or injury.

Neoplasm
A mass of new and abnormal cells; a TUMOR.

NMR
Nuclear magnetic resonance; a technique of imaging the interior of the body using the magnetic resonance of the atoms comprising the elements of the body tissues.

Organ
A structure of definite form and made up of two or more kinds of TISSUE.

Orthopedics
The study of bone disease.

Pandemic
A universal outbreak of a disease.

Pathogen
An organism that produces disease.

Peristalsis
Wavelike muscular contractions along the wall of a hollow muscular vessel, moving the contents along that vessel.

Physiology
The study of the functions of an organism and its parts.

Plaque
A cholesterol-containing mass in the lining of arteries; also a mass of bacterial cells and other debris that accumulates on the surface of teeth.

Prosthesis
An artificial device implanted to replace a defective natural part of the body.

Protein
An organic compound made up of AMINO-ACIDS.

Protozoon
Simple, single-celled organism.

RNA
Ribonucleic acid; a single-stranded nucleic acid that cooperates with DNA for protein synthesis.

Sarcoma
A CANCER arising from CONNECTIVE TISSUE, muscle or bone.

Sepsis
The presence of harmful BACTERIA or TOXINS in the bloodstream or tissues.

Septum
A wall dividing two cavities.

Serum
Blood plasma minus the clotting proteins.

Sphincter
A circular muscle constricting an orifice.

Spirochete
Spiral-shaped BACTERIUM.

Stenosis
An abnormal narrowing of a duct or opening.

Stroke
The sudden disturbance of the activity of a part of the brain through the disruption of its blood supply.

Synovial
The space between the articulating bones of a joint, filled with synovial fluid.

System
An association of ORGANS that have a common function within the organism.

Synapse
The junction between the processes of adjacent neurons, across which nerve impulses are carried by TRANSMITTER SUBSTANCES.

Systole
The phase of contraction of the heart muscle in the cardiac cycle.

Teratogen
An agent that deforms or causes physical defects in an embryo.

Threshold
The minimum stimulus required to trigger an action potential in a nerve.

Thrombosis
The formation of a clot in an unbroken blood vessel.

Tissue
A group of similar cells and their intercellular substance performing a specific function within an organ of the body.

Transmitter substance
One of a variety of chemicals that carry nerve impulses from one neuron to another across the synaptic cleft.

Trauma
An injury, either a physical wound or a psychological disorder, caused by a physical blow or shock.

Tumor
A growth of excess tissue due to abnormal cell division.

Ulcer
An open lesion of skin or MUCOUS MEMBRANE, with loss of substance or NECROSIS of the tissue.

Vibrio
A comma-shaped BACTERIUM.

Villus
Microscopic projections of MUCOUS MEMBRANES.

Virus
The smallest form of living organism, dependent on living cells for replication.

Vitamin
An organic molecule necessary to act as catalyst for specific metabolic activities.

Word Stems

Many medical words are composites of frequently occurring word stems; these describe parts of the body, activities or relationships. With a knowledge of these stems, technical terms can be more easily understood.

Acou-, acu- hearing (acoustic, relating to hearing)
Aden-, adeno- gland (adenitis, inflammation of the glands)
Alg-, -algia pain (neuralgia, a nervous pain)
Angi- vessel (angiocardiography, recording the activity of the heart's blood vessels)
Ante- before (antenatal, before birth)
Artero- artery (arteriosclerosis, hardening of the arteries)
Arthr- joint (arthritis, inflammation of the joints)
Audio- sound (audiometry, measuring the sensitivity of hearing)
Aut- self (autolysis, destruction of cells of the body by their own enzymes)
Bili- bile (bilirubin, a pigment found in bile)
Bio- living (biopsy, study of tissue from a living body)
-blast bud (osteoblast, cell that creates bone)
Brachi- arm (brachialis, a muscle of the arm)
Bronch- windpipe (bronchitis, inflammation of the bronchi)
Carcin- cancer (carcinogen, a substance that induces cancer)
Cardi- heart (cardiography, measurement of heart activity)
-cele enlarged cavity (meningocele, enlargement of the meninges)
Cerebro- brain (cerebrospinal, relating to the brain and spinal cord)
Chemo- drug (chemotherapy, the treatment of cancer with drugs)
Chol- bile (cholangitis, inflammation of the tubes leading to the gall bladder)
Chondr- cartilage (chondrocyte, cartilage cell)
Cortico- outer part (corticoid, hormone of the adrenal cortex)
Crani- skull (craniotomy, surgical opening of the skull)
Crypt- hidden (cryptorchism, the failure of testicle to descend into the scrotum)
-cyst- sac (cholecyst, gall bladder)
Cyto-, -cyte cell (cytoplasm, the fluid contained in a cell)
Derma-, -derm skin (dermatology, skin of skin diseases)
Dys- difficult (dysentery, intestinal disorder)

-ectomy removal (mastectomy, removal of the breast)
-emia blood condition (anemia, shortage of red blood cells)
Entero- intestine (gastroenteritis, disorder of the stomach and intestines)
Eu- well (eupnea, normal breathing)
Gastr- stomach (gastrectomy, removal of the stomach)
-gen agent that produces (pathogen, organism that causes disease)
-gloss- tongue (hypoglossal, under the tongue)
-gram record (electrocardiogram, record of the electrical activity of the heart)
Gyne- woman (gynecology, study of disorders of the female anatomy)
Heme-, hemato- blood (hematuria, blood in the urine)
Hepat- liver (hepatitis, inflammation of the liver)
Hydro- water (hydrocele, accumulation of fluid in a saclike cavity)
Hyper- excessive (hyperthyroidism, excess activity of the thyroid gland)
Hypo- below, deficient (hypodermic, beneath the skin)
Hyster- womb (hysterectomy, removal of the uterus)
-iatrics medicine (pediatrics, medicine for children)
-itis inflammation (neuritis, inflammation of the nerves)
Lacrim- tear (lacrimal gland, tear gland)
Laparo- abdomen (laparoscopy, insertion of a fiber-optic tube into the abdomen)
Leuko- white (leukocyte, white blood cell)
-lysis dissolve (hemolysis, dissolution of red blood cells)
Mammo- breast (mammography, X-rays of the breast)
Mega-, megalo- large (megakaryocyte, large marrow cell)
Morpho- shape (morphology, study of the shapes of organs)
Myelo- marrow, spinal cord (poliomyelitis, inflammation of the grey matter of the spinal cord)
Myo- muscle (myocardium, heart muscle)
Naso- nose (nasopharynx, nose and throat)
Necro- death (necrosis, death of cells)
Nephro- kidney (nephritis, inflammation of the kidneys)
Neuro- nerve (neurotransmitter, substance transmitting nerve impulses)
-odont- tooth (orthodontics, straightening of teeth)
-oculo- eye (binocular, with two eyes)
Oligo- little (oligospermia, shortage of sperm)
-oma cancer (fibroma, tumor of mainly fibrous material)
Onco- cancer (oncogene, a gene that promotes cancer)

Oo- egg (oophoritis, inflammation of the ovary)
Ophthalm- eye (ophthalmology, study of the eye)
Orch- testicle (orchitis, swelling of the testicle)
Ortho- correct (orthoptics, straightening of the eyes)
-osis condition (sclerosis, condition of hardening)
Osteo- bone (osteomalacia, softening of the bones)
Oto- ear (otitis, inflammation of the ear)
Patho-, -path disease (pathology, study of diseases)
-penia shortage (thrombocytopenia, shortage of clotting cells)
Phag- consume (esophagus, the gullet)
Pharm- drug (pharmacology, study of drugs)
-phobia fear (hydrophobia, fear of water)
-plasm, -plasty development (neoplasm, new growth or tumor)
-plegia paralysis (quadriplegia, paralysis of all the four limbs)
-pnea breath (apnea, inability to catch the breath)
Pneumo- lung (pneumonia, disease of the lung)
Poly- many (polyarthritis, inflammation of many joints)
Psycho- mind (psychiatry, medicine for the mind)
Pyo- pus (pyogenic, pus-forming)
-rrhage, -rrhea flow (hemorrhage, flow of blood)
-sclero- hard (arteriosclerosis, hardening of the arteries)
-scope view (endoscope, device for viewing within the digestive tract)
-stasis condition (homeostasis, even condition)
-stomy hole (colostomy, creating a new opening in the colon)
Tachy- fast (tachycardia, fast heart beat)
Thrombo- clot (thrombosis, inflammation caused by a clot)
-tomy cut (lobotomy, excision of the frontal lobes of the brain)
Tox- poison (toxemia, the presence of poisonous organisms in the blood)
-trophy relating to growth (hypertrophy, growing excessively)
-tropic influencing (gonadotropic, influencing the activity of the reproductive organs)
Uro-, -uria urine (polyuria, excessive passing of urine)
Vaso- tube (vasoconstriction, narrowing of the blood vessels)
Xero- dry (xerophthalmia, abnormal dryness of the eyes)

Index

S

Sabin, Albert 241
sacrum 108
sadism *81*
salivary glands *57*, 121, *123, 243*
Salk, Jonas 241
Salmonellae 143, 146, *147, 204*
salpingitis *191*
salt loss *234*
sarcomas *108, 221*
scarlet fever *245*
scarring 117, 119, 165, 212
Schally, Andrew *89*
schistomiasis 247
schizophrenia *28*, 60, *80, 82, 82, 83*
Schwann cells 60, 212
sciatica 64, 108
SCID *see* severe combined immune
   deficiency
scoliosis 109
screening techniques 194, 226
scrotum *177, 178, 226*
scurvy *127*, 132
sebaceous glands *113*, 116, 244
Selye, Dr Hans 73, 88
semen 178, 180, *189*
semicircular canals *45, 52*
seminal vesicles 178
sensitization 70, 72
sensory focusing 71
"sensory homunculus" *57*
sensory impulses *54*
septum *150*, 168, *187*
severe combined immune deficiency
   (SCID) 16, *232*
sex cells *see* gametes
sex hormones 88, 90, *90, 91*, 209
sexual deviations *81*
sexual intercourse *95, 177*, 179, 180, 201
sexually transmitted diseases 201-4
Sherrington, Sir Charles 56
Shigella 147
shingles *see* herpes zoster
Shumway, Norman *163*
Siamese twins *188, 196*
sickle-cell anemia 30-1, *32, 32, 108*,
   198
sight 42-3, *43, 53*, 114
   defects 49-51; loss of 62, 63
silicosis *172*
skeleton *13*, 97-9
skin *14, 41*, 53, 92, 113-6, 117-20, 135,
   144-5, 208, 213, 235, 247
   color 10, 114, *114*; diseases 117-20;
   grafts *16*, 117, 118-9, *118, 219*;
   infections 244; regeneration 212, *212*
skull 97, *98*
sleep *20*, 63, 210-11, *210, 211*
sleeping pills *210*
sleeping sickness *see* African
   trypanosomiasis
slipped disk *see* prolapsed disk
small intestine 121, 122, *124*, 132
   infections *147*, 148
smallpox 218, 242, *243*
smell 25, 46-7, 53, *57*
Smith, John Maynard *209*
smoking
   and cancer *221, 227;* and
   cardiovascular disease *161*, 164, *166,
   167*, 168; and respiratory infection
   172, *173*
sneezes *160*
spare parts surgery *16, 17*
spastic paralysis *108*
specific etiology *37*, 40
speech 53, *62*, 66, 68, 69, *69*, 154
   loss of 62, 63
sperm 25, *26*, 90, *91*, 177, 178, *178*,
   180, *181, 189*, 189, 190, *190*
spermatic cord *178*, 190
spermicide *181*

sphincter muscles 209
spina bifida 194, 200
spinal cord 53, *56*, 60, *64*, 108, 205
spine 108, 109 *see also* scoliosis
spleen 133, *153, 154*, 213
spots *see* acne
sputum 172
squints *51*
Staphylococcus aureus 174, 241, *242*,
   238
starch 121, 122, *124*
steatorrhea 132
stem cells *218*
stenosis *109*, 165
sterility 191
sterilization *182*
stethoscope 152, 165
Still's disease *see* rheumatoid arthritis
stings 229
stomach 122, *123, 138*, 160, *235*
   cancer *221*
stomach ulcer *see* gastric ulcer
stones *see* gall bladder stones, kidney
   stones, urinary stone disease
strabismus *51*
streptococci *245*
Streptococcus mutans 112
streptomycin 176
stress 52, *58*, 64, 73-4, *75*, 77, *79, 86*
   antidotes 76; and cancer 220; control
   88
stretch receptors 160, *160*
stroke 63, *162*, 168
subclavian veins 154
sublingual gland 121
subluxations 106
submandibular gland 121
substantia nigra *54*, 62, *62*, 64
sucrose 122
sugars 99, 121, 122, *124 see also*
   glucose, sucrose
sulfa drugs 40, 172, *242*
sunburn *118*, 236
suppressants *144-5*
surgery *37, 110, 111*, 221, 228
surrogate mothers *190, 191*
Swammerdam, John *102*
sweating 114, 116, *116*, 233, *234*
synapses 59, *59*, 60
synovial joints 100
synovial membranes 230
syphilis 201, *201*, 202, *204*
syringomelia 41
systemic lupus erythematosus 230
Szasz, Thomas *82*

T

tachycardia 137, 165
Taenia saginata 148
Taenia solium 148, *148*
tapeworms 148
taste 46-7, 53
taste buds 46, *46, 57*
tattoos *120*
Tay-Sachs disease 197
TB *see* tuberculosis
tectum *54*
teeth 104, *104*, 112, *112*, 121, *123*, 209
telepathy *72*
temperature control 113, 233, *233*, 234,
   234 see also body temperature
tendons *97*
tennis elbow *105*
teratogens *199*, 240, *243*
Terrace, Herbert *69*
testicles *16, 26*, 85, 90, 177, *177, 178*,
   189
testicular varicose veins *see* varicoceles
testosterone 90, *91*, 177
test-tube babies *190*
tetanus 246

tetracycline *144-5*, 202
tetraplegia *64*
thalamus *54, 57*
thalassemia 198
thalidomide *199*
thermography *38, 109*
thiamine (vitamin B1) 126, *127*
thorax 154
threadworms 148
thrombin *153*
thrombophelitis 168
thrombosis *see* coronary thrombosis
thrush *see* vaginal thrush
thymosins 92
thymus gland 92, *153*, 213
thyroid gland 85, 91, 92, 93, 126
thyrotoxicosis *see* hyperthyroidism
thyrotropin 92
tics 64
Tinea corporis 245
Tinea pedis 174, 245
tissues 18, *97*
Tizard, Barbara *70*
toes 97, 109
tongue 46, *46*, *98*, 121, *123*, 160
tonsillectomy 215
tonsillitis 169, *215*
tonsils 46, 154, 213, *215*
tooth decay *see* caries
torticollis 64
"total allergy syndrome" *232*
touch 41, 53, 113, *115*
toxemia 166
toxic shock syndrome *242*
trachea *16, 68*, 154, *173*
trachoma 50, 202, 241
tranquillizers *81, 82*, 84, *144-5*
transferrin 213
transplants *16*
transvestism *81*
trapezium *98, 101*
trauma 105, *105*
Treponoma pallidum 201, 204
triceps *101*
trichomoniasis 204
tricuspid valve 149
triglycerides 122, *124*
trypanosomes *174*
trypsin 122
tuberculosis 105, 109, *172, 173*, 176,
   176
tumor necrosis factor 215
tumors *108*, 221, *221*, 236
Turner's syndrome 196, *197*
twins *28, 65, 188*, 196, 218, 219
typhoid bacillus 146, *146*
typhoid fever 146, *146*
typhus 218
tyrosine 114

U

ulcerative colitis 138, 230
ulcers 138, *138*
   drugs for *144-5 see also* duodenal
   ulcers, gastric ulcers, mouth ulcers,
   peptic ulcers
ultrasound scans *38, 39, 61, 139*, 194
umbilical cord 184, *187*, 246
urea 116, 135
ureter *135*, 136
urethra 140, *160*, 178, 179, 191, 204
urethritis 201
uric acid 96, 116, *235*
urinary stone disease 138, *139*, 140
urinary system *14*, 135-6
urinary tracts 137, 138, 209
   infections 140, 242
urination *see* micturition
urine 136, 138, *160, 174*
uterine contractions 86, *185*, 186, *186*
uterus 90, *90, 179*, 180, 184, 188, *191*

V

vaccination *see* immunization
vaccines *36*, 112, 142, *144-5*, 169, 171,
   172, 173, 174, 220, *220*, 242, *243*,
   248
vaccinia 242
vagina *177*, 179, *179*, 180, *181*, 186,
   204
vaginal thrush 204
valvular disease 165
varicella *243*
varicoceles 168, 190
varicose veins 168
vas deferens *60*, 178, *178*, 182
vasectomy *182*
vasoconstriction 234, *234*
vasodilation 164, 233, *234*
vasomotor center *55*
veins 149, *149*, 150, *150, 151*, 152, 168
vellus 114
vena cava 150, 152
"venereal diseases" *see* sexually
   transmitted diseases
venous blood 158
ventricles
   of the brain 53; of the heart 149, *149*
ventricular septal defect 168
venules 150, 212
vertebrae 97, *99, 101*, 109
Vesalius, Andreas *34, 102*, 150
vestibular complex 55
Vibrio cholerae 141, 142
Vinci, Leonardo da *35*, 150
viruses 142, 169, 170, *174-5, 200*, 230,
   247, 248, *248 see also* names of
   individual viruses
visual cortex 67
vital capacity 154
vitamins 40, 64, 92, 93, *108*, 113, 122,
   124, 126, *127*, 132, *144-5*
   deficiencies *127*, 132, 222
vitiligo 94, *95*
vocal cords 68, *68*, 160
Volkmann's canals *97*
vomiting 63, 141, *160*

W

Waksman, Selman 40
warts *120*
Weil-Felix reaction *218*
Weismann, August *28*
Wernicke, Carl 68
"wet dreams" 178
whipworms 148
white blood cells *see* leukocytes
white polymorph cells 212
whooping cough *see* pertussis
Wilson's disease *94*
windpipe *see* trachea
wisdom teeth 104
wrist 97, *101*

X

X-rays 29, *37, 38, 39, 61*, 105, *107*,
   110, 112, *159*, 194, 227, 228, 236
xenon arcs 50
Xenopsylla cheopsis 248
XXY syndrome 196

Y

yawning *160*
yellow fever 247
Yersinia pestis 248